T0199926

Regenerating Japan

CEU Press Studies in the History of Medicine
Volume X

Series Editor: Marius Turda

Regenerating Japan

*Organicism, Modernism and National Destiny
in Oka Asajirō's* Evolution and Human Life

Gregory Sullivan

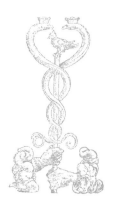

Central European University Press
Budapest—New York

Published in 2018 by

Central European University Press

Nádor utca 9, H-1051 Budapest, Hungary

Tel: +36-1-327-3138 or 327-3000 · *Fax*: +36-1-327-3183

E-mail: ceupress@press.ceu.edu

Website: www.ceupress.com

224 West 57th Street, New York NY 10019, USA

ISBN 978-963-386-210-0

ISSN 2079-1119

Library of Congress Cataloging-in-Publication Data

Names: Sullivan, Gregory (Gregory F.), author.
Title: Regenerating Japan : organicism, modernism and national destiny in Oka Asajiro's evolution and human life / Gregory Sullivan.
Description: Budapest ; New York : Central European University Press, 2018. |
Series: CEU Press studies in the history of medicine ; volume 10 |
Includes bibliographical references and index.
Identifiers: LCCN 2018005824 (print) | LCCN 2018032439 (ebook) | ISBN 9789633862117 | ISBN 9789633862100
Subjects: LCSH: Biology--Social aspects--Japan. | Biology--Study and teaching--Japan. | Evolution (Biology) and the social sciences--Japan. | Oka, Asajirō, 1868-1944.
Classification: LCC QH333 (ebook) | LCC QH333 .S85 2018 (print) | DDC 570.76--dc23
LC record available at https://lccn.loc.gov/2018005824

Printed by Prime Rate Kft., Hungary

For Kumiko

TABLE OF CONTENTS

LIST OF FIGURES

A time that tries to suppress and bypass science with ideological beliefs will be retarded in the progress of the world. We have no choice but to be enveloped by things like the theory of evolution.

EMPEROR HIROHITO, 1935

PREFACE AND ACKNOWLEDGEMENTS

As the first step toward a comprehensive reinterpretation of the role of evolutionary science and biomedicine in pre-1945 Japan, this book tackles the early writings of that era's most influential exponent of *shinkaron* (evolutionism)—the German-educated research zoologist and popularizer of biomedicine, Oka Asajirō (1868–1944). Concentrating on a series of highly prominent essays that Oka published in major journals and magazines in the years during and after the Russo-Japanese War (1904–5)—writings which were later anthologized as *Evolution and Human Life* (*Shinka to Jinsei*) in 1906 (with expanded versions in 1911 and 1921)—*Regenerating Japan* describes the process by which Oka came to articulate a programmatic modernist vision of national regeneration that would prove integral to the ideological climate in Japan during the first half of the twentieth century. In contrast to other scholars, who insist that Oka was merely a rationalist enlightener bent on undermining state Shinto orthodoxy, the book explains how Oka enlisted notions of organic individuality—especially that of the nation as a superorganism—from evolutionary biology to underwrite the social and geopolitical aims of the Meiji state. Though during the Russo-Japanese War Oka believed he had articulated a metapolitical formula for the national cohesion desired by this state, the book shows that a postwar crisis of unity and, most especially, the state Shintoist reaction to this crisis spurred him to expand his *shinkaron* into something Japan had never seen before: a modernist program that would rejuvenate the collective body of the nation, overcome disaggregating decadence, and supplant the emerging theistic orthodoxy with a scientistic faith. [1]

---

[1] In Japan, the first name follows the family name. In this book Oka Asajirō is usually referred to in the Japanese name order. The same is applied to other Japanese persons discussed in the text.

In the epilogue to the book I suggest that this generative scientism, as I call it, gained wide currency among early-twentieth-century political and intellectual elites, including Emperor Hirohito himself—who had personal connections to Oka—and that wartime ideology may represent an unfinished attempt to synthesize Shinto fundamentalism and the eugenically oriented scientistic programmatic modernism that Oka was the first to articulate.

The audience for this book will be scholars and students in Japanese history, Asian studies, the history of science (especially biology, evolutionary theory, or eugenics), and, secondarily, the philosophy of science, history of education, fascist studies, religious studies, history of medicine, military history, and world history. *Regenerating Japan* should be of particular interest to anyone interested in how evolutionary ideas spread internationally, how they helped establish the foundations for eugenics, and how they fared within non-Western educational systems, sociopolitical orders, and ideological contexts.

A longer list of colleagues, friends, advisors and institutions than this preface can accommodate are deserving of thanks for the moral and intellectual support they have lent over the years.

To start off, I would like to express my gratitude to the philosophy department at the University of California, Berkeley, where I received my bachelor degree. This project would not have been possible without the intellectual rigor and sense of problem I was exposed to as an undergraduate.

Regenerating Japan expands upon my Yale dissertation and during my years as a graduate student I received generous assistance in the form of a University Dissertation Fellowship, a Council on East Asian Studies Dissertation Research Supplementary Grant, a Council on East Asian Studies Summer Research and Travel Grant, and a Sumitomo Fellowship. I also benefited tremendously from a year of study the Inter-University Center for Japanese in Yokohama. Appreciation is also owed to the staff of the East Asian Reading Room at the Sterling Memorial Library for assistance in locating materials. In a similar capacity, the Schuyler-Otis Bland Memorial Library at the US Merchant Marine Academy in Kings Point, NY, has been of tremendous help in obtaining books and articles through its interlibrary loan service. I am particularly grateful to George Billy for his patient hard work on my behalf.

Other individuals to whom gratitude should be extended include Georgia Durant, Adam Mayes, Christopher Trogan and Laury Magnus in New York, and Stanly Weinstein, the Nomoto Family, Edward Kamens, Simon Kim, Michael Auslin, Paul Groner, Edwin McClellan, Frances Rosenbluth, and Jonathan Spence in New Haven. A very special expression of thanks is in order for Conrad Totman, who invited me into his home for long afternoons to discuss this project during its fledgling stages.

Finally, no words of appreciation can capture the degree to which I have relied on the love and wisdom of my wife, Kumiko. Her strength of character and innate optimism were what enabled me to persevere through the many obstacles placed in my path.

INTRODUCTION

MOSS ANIMAL NATION

In the summer of 1907 the popular journal *Jiji Shinpō* ran an article that purported to identify a species whose ideal lifestyle qualified it as worthy of human emulation. Though generally dwelling in "old ponds, large lakes" and "near where haze hovers over the inlets of muddy creeks," this variety of invertebrates, which the author referred to as *kokemushi* or moss animals, could also be found in ponds around Tokyo in such places as the Sho-Ishikawa Botanical Gardens, the Tokyo Higher Normal School, and, before recently going extinct there, the grounds of the Tokyo Imperial University (Todai). Entitled "Ideal Group Life," the article in question began by describing the exemplary existence of these moss animals:

> Taken one by one these creatures are really very small. Each is formed into a cylindrical shape which is barely three millimeters in length. One end of this cylinder sticks to the surface of water, grass, leaves, and other such things. At the center of the opposite end of the body there is a mouth around which are arrayed several dozen thin, threadlike fingers. These fingers are employed to catch and eat the minute bits of food which are washed toward the moss animal through the water. Individually these moss animals take on such a form, but that is not the whole story. From a place which we should call, as it were, the flank of both sides of this cylindrical creature, it reproduces by sprouting buds. Such buds grow up very rapidly and each one becomes an individual in its own right. Furthermore, because these buds, which emerge from the sides of the creature, go on to reproduce, after a short time the original individual moss animal multiplies until finally there is a cluster of several hundred or several thousand of them. Since parents, children and siblings are all connected to one another, the same blood circulates through the entire group

even when there are such great numbers of sprouts. In addition, because a nervous system, which each moss animal possesses in nervelike form, links them all together with thin threads, sensations are transmitted from the individual to the entire group and feelings of joy and anger can be shared.[1]

The author of this article was Meiji Japan's foremost popularizer of the theory of evolution (*shinkaron*), Oka Asajirō (1868–1944), a German-trained, internationally respected zoologist and research scientist. By the time "Ideal Group Life" appeared, Oka, a professor of zoology at the Tokyo Higher Normal School, had published cutting-edge research on moss animals and other varieties of freshwater invertebrates, written a slew of textbooks on zoology and evolution, overseen the first full translation of Darwin's *Origin of Species* into Japanese, put out a best-selling overview of evolutionary theory, and, with the outbreak of the Russo-Japanese War, established himself as a popular essayist on all questions pertaining to the intersection of human affairs and evolutionary science. A household name and, in the coming years, a major inspiration to the biological avocation of Prince Hirohito,[2] Oka had a transformative impact on the Japanese milieu until his death in 1944.[3] Circa 1907 Oka's writings were inspiring a Darwin boom which would make him the definitive voice of evolutionism in Japan during the first half of the twentieth century. What Oka's *shinkaron* offered his Japanese readership was apparently straightforward: insights into political and societal trends that were authoritatively informed by evolutionary science and its iron laws of necessity.

Oka placed moss animals at the crux of his evolutionism. The blood-bound, psychically integrated colonial life of bryozoans—which is the phylum into which moss animals fit[4]—became his scientistic paragon for biopolitical survival. Called "overindividuals" or "corms" by his contemporaries, and referred to as superorganisms in current scientific literature, the "ideal group" of the moss animal collective was presented as a *kuni* or nation in

1   Asajirō Oka, "Risōteki Dantai Seikatsu" [Ideal group life], in Asajirō Oka, *Shinka to Jinsei* [Evolution and Human Life] (Tokyo: Yūseidō Shuppan, 1968), 66–67.
2   Bix, *Hirohito and the Making of Modern Japan*, 60. See also Migita, *Tennosei to Shinkaron*.
3   Matsunaga Toshio claims Oka's writing had an impact on "many famous writers." See Matsunaga, "Evolutionism in Early Twentieth Century Japan," 221. Tsukuba Hisaharu mentions that returnees from Manchuria after the Second World War regretted not being able to bring their copies of Oka's writings with them. See Tsukuba, "Kaisetsu" [Commentary], 430–55.
4   Ryland, *Bryozoans*, 23.

Oka's article of 1907. "Ideal Group Life," in fact, features a vivid portrayal of the qualities that make moss animal superorganisms exemplary nation-states, especially in an era of geopolitical contestation. Not only do the individual zooids—the technical term for individual bryozoans—that comprise the "higher self" of the nation share the same blood and the same experiences, but, more fundamentally, they are united by social instincts. Such instincts ensure perfect altruism within moss animal nations, conditions that Oka likens to a physical embodiment of the Golden Rule of the world's major religions. That is, moss animals, as Oka explains, "do to others what they would have others do to them—and they chose not to do to others what they would not have done to themselves."[5] With egoism eliminated, labor equitably divided, and individuals in a state of spontaneous mutual harmony, subordinating and even sacrificing their lives for the commonweal, the need for various phenomena associated with life in human nation-states is also obviated: private property, class divisions, unemployment, political dissent, crime, laws, police, government agencies, and even organized religion—all of these simply do not exist. The nation instinctively acts "as one man,"[6] its individual members reflexively serving as the willing cells of the superorganism.

This seamless organic unity enables moss animal "clusters" to answer their primary existential challenge: competition with other nations. Even though Oka observed individual moss animals instinctively sharing nutrients that float within reach of the "threadlike fingers," this altruism does not extend beyond political borders. Like their human counterparts, moss animal nations unify internally in order to aggressively project their concentrated power in an "entirely outward direction."[7] In other words, "the absolute peace within a nation of this species of moss animals represents just a single step up in the unit of competition, a place where competition between individuals gives way to the competition between nations."[8] Having attained a higher individuality through perfect internal harmony, the collective egoism of the nation instinctively advances on to perpetrate wars of expansion against its neighbors:

---

5   Oka, "Risōteki Dantai Seikatsu" [Ideal group life], 69.

6   Ibid., 73.

7   Ibid.

8   Ibid.

[I]f a case arises where there is something which disturbs the forward progress of the particular nation, the nation musters up all its strength, and fights violently to try to conquer whomever or whatever is in its way. When we see many moss animal nations arrayed side by side in a narrow space, each nation fiercely pushes up against the others along their mutual borders. This situation, in which the small and weak are immediately crushed to pieces, gives one the same feeling as when one looks at a geopolitical map.[9]

The seeming paradox of "cohesion within, chaos without" is resolved in Oka's unforgettable account of how fighters on the embattled frontiers and civilians on the halcyon home front achieve a macabre intimacy through the ultimate sacrifices they make for the moss animal nation:

When it comes to fighting, it is not the case that only those standing on the front lines are participating—with true national unity all are serving equally. As this variety of moss animal breeds through sprouting buds and is thus always growing out into the surrounding space, only those who are robust and in the prime of life, are standing at the front, while among the elderly staying in the interior of the nation there are those who of course gradually weaken and die. When we inquire what happens to the bodies of these dead, it turns out that they are gradually converted into fat and other such things and carried into the blood which circulates through the inside of the nation, eventually reaching the front lines at the nation's borders to become military provisions for those in the prime of life. In other words, in times of war, parents, for the sake of supplying provisions for the children at the front, pack their own flesh into cans and send it off.[10]

Pursued to such grisly extremes and evident across generations, this instinctual selflessness within the moss animal nation—a circumstance where "everyone is absolutely loyal, courageous and obedient"—translates for Oka into a kind of creed that can be read directly from nature and used to inculcate a collectivist ethos in human populations. Referred to as the "moss animal way," this creed should become, Oka suggests, the basis of moral education in schools: "Instead of listening to old-fashioned lectures

---

9   Ibid.
10   Ibid., 73–74. It should be noted that this is a reversal of Confucian filial piety, which at times cited examples of children sacrificing their own flesh for cannibalization by parents. See Jordan, "Filial Piety in Taiwanese Popular Thought," 271.

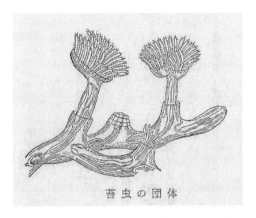

苔虫の団体

Figure 1. "Group of Kokemushi [Moss animals]."
Source: Oka, "Risōteki Dantai Seikatsu" [Ideal group life], 67.

on ethics and morals for one or two hours each week, it seems that it would be far more useful to show the students moss animal nations under a microscope and have them hear detailed explanations on the circumstances of their group life."[11] However, as these lessons of the classroom are apt to be easily forgotten, Oka believes more extreme and intrusive measures must be taken to ensure the example of moss animals insinuates itself into daily life and comes to serve as an ever-present moral compass. To this end, he makes the radical suggestion that science adopt the methods of religious inculcation: just as "Buddhism erects various images of the Buddha, arranging things so that the people will not be allowed to forget the Buddha night and day," the authorities should construct idols of the bryozoan superorganisms for public display. Embodiments of the biopolitical creed of evolutionism, these idols would inevitably come to unseat religion in every respect, for, according to Oka, "moss animals actually exhibit" a state which the sects of Buddhism and other faiths aspire to but "cannot, in the end, attain."[12] Thus, with perhaps the most beguiling image of what he hoped his evolutionism could achieve, Oka concludes that "it would be more reasonable to construct enormous images of moss animals than to build statues of sect founders and the Buddha. Especially compared to the worthless bronze statues of humans which have been erected here and there as of late, I do not

11 Ibid., 71.
12 Ibid.

5

know how many times better it is for the benefit of public morals to put up bronze images of moss animals and always have set forth before all eyes admonitions such as 'Like these moss animals, do unto others as you would have others do unto you' and 'Like these moss animals, escape the confines of the ego, proceed on to the level of the higher self.'"[13]

This book will portray Oka's startling suggestion that moss animal superorganisms supplant objects of religious devotion as a seminal moment in the application of evolutionary science to human affairs in twentieth-century Japan. Our context will be the Russo-Japanese War, its aftermath, and the final years of the Meiji era. It was during these years that Oka, in the wake of his publishing success with a primer on the biological aspects of evolutionary theory, began to give lectures and write articles that spoke to its sociopolitical application. First in 1906 and again in later editions that appeared in 1911 and 1921, these essays were gathered together in a best-selling anthology entitled *Evolution and Human Life* that will be the focus of this study. "Ideal Group Life" was the first article produced after the initial edition of the anthology came out and it represents not only a summation of the contents of the first edition but the pivotal moment at which Oka begins to consider how the example of moss animals and other "ideal groups" might invasively shape "public morals" in a fashion equivalent to that of devotional bronze statues.

Initially, Oka submitted his superorganismic vision of the Japanese ethnic nation not only as a formula for national strength but as the solution to the central problem of early-twentieth-century Japan—promoting social cohesion. His *shinkaron* was an offshoot of what we will call reformist statism and we will argue that his intention was to educate members of the nation to embrace their proper place within the national superorganism as a matter of evolutionary necessity. With such reform the normative practices and sociopolitical arrangements of the nation would be, by means of a gradual scientistic method, brought into sync with the underlying biological reality.

From about the time of "Ideal Group Life" (1907), however, Oka came to recognize the inadequacy of this "metapolitical" approach: anomic conditions within Japan in the wake of the victory over Russia were not only making it impossible to establish evolutionary science as the basis of social

---

13   Ibid., 71–72.

cohesion but they had provoked a fundamentalist movement from within the government that was threatening to permanently thwart the dissemination of evolutionary biology. Though he never abandons his moderate reformism, Oka's response to this nomic crisis would be radical, and it introduced something novel to the Japan milieu: a dynamic programmatic vision of national rejuvenation that generates a new table of ultimate values which imagines the biological transformation of humanity itself. What began as an ethos of cohesion develops into a precedent-setting scientistic formula to overcome postwar decadence, supplant religious indoctrination, and realize national destiny, all through the regeneration of social instincts. In the end, an alternate mode of modern existence came into view for the first time with Oka's evolutionism—one that identified the integrative process of organic development with the maximization of national health and power.

ANOMY IN THE MIDDLE TO LATE MEIJI

The fear of losing cohesion that prompted Oka to develop his "generative scientism"—which is the term we will use to describe the evolutionism that sought to actualize this alternative mode of modern life[14]—was not unique to him but, as Carol Gluck explains in her *Japan's Modern Myths*, a shared late Meiji concern that became especially acute around the time of the war with Russia. What she calls the "complicated society"[15] was, along with other unintended consequences of the Meiji developmental state, experienced as a series of "social fevers" or "civilization sicknesses" [*bunmei byō*],[16] all of which were connected to newly disembedded individuals who

---

14 My coinage plays off of Maistre's "Essay on the Generative Principle of Political Constitutions and Other Human Institutions" which asserts that "it is essential that the origin of sovereignty should show itself to be beyond the sphere of human power, so that even those men who appear to influence it directly are only circumstances. As for legitimacy, if its origin seems obscure, it is explained by God's prime minister in the province of this world—Time." Part of my argument in this book will be that Oka's scientism invoked the temporal process of organic development as a generative principle in order to counter a form of reactionary absolutism much like that envisioned by Maistre. As Popper argues at the conclusion of his *Poverty of Historicism*, such attempts to prognosticate and thereby harness rapid and potentially wayward change—especially where it threatened sociomoral foundations—"betray an unconscious conservatism." Though I am hesitant to label European-educated reformists such as Oka "conservatives," many share with Shinto reactionaries a concern for the perceived "loss of an unchanging world"—a loss which they seek to compensate for by "clinging to the faith that change can be foreseen because it is ruled by unchanging law." See Maistre, *On God and Society*, 40; Popper, *The Poverty of Historicism*, 149.

15 Gluck, *Japan's Modern Myths*, 26.

16 Ibid., 157–64.

were abandoning the customary concrete relations of the countryside for the pluralistic setting of industrializing urban centers. Though pundits who bewailed these rapid changes and the abstract relations of the new mass society counted "social Darwinism" as chief among such social fevers, Oka's evolutionism shared their anxieties about a creeping anomy and sought not only to match but underwrite their attempts to preserve the concrete "socio-moral bonds"[17] that ensured national unity. A central feature of the "organicist Darwinism"[18] Oka had learned in Germany as a graduate student in the early 1890s, superorganisms—as exemplified in the "ideal life" of *kokemushi*—became, during the Russo-Japanese War, his model for how to reform the polity and build a strong, modern, and enduring nomic order that would enfold individuals back into the ethnic nation.

Part II of this study, "Metapolitics," describes how Oka initially hoped to offer the consummately interdependent life inside superorganisms as an evolutionary precondition for national survival. The celebrated unity of wartime mobilization represented for him not merely a temporary expedience during a time of national emergency but the "human-way"—the definitive normative response to the permanent human condition which *Evolution and Human Life* portrayed as a perpetual global war between racially incommensurable ethnic nations (*minzoku*). The human-way prescribed both internal and external requirements for the ethnic nation to survive this never-ending struggle. In its external relations it would have to behave as a selfish individual, rejecting humanitarian illusions of a common humanity and remaining technologically and strategically primed for the reality of everlasting total war in search of autarkic living space. Internally, the human-way dictated that the individuals within the ethnic nation, like pack members of the other gregarious animals, practice altruism toward their compatriots and thereby engender, via Lamarckism, the social instincts that would facilitate the perfect organic integration needed to project national power against external enemies. While Oka's evolutionary realpolitik, as we will call it, tended toward a totalitarian identification of individuals with the whole, his orientation remained one of scientistic reform: the metapolitical requirements did not imagine a radical overthrow of the existing system of

---

17 Ibid., 110.
18 Weindling, *Health, Race and German Politics*, 48.

norms, conventions, and laws—that is, the current nomos, a term we will resort to throughout this study[19]—but their eventual approximation to the collectivist imperatives of evolutionary necessity.

By 1907—the year of "Ideal Group Life"—the inadequacy of such meta-politics was increasingly evident and, as a result, generative features that went further than mere reform began to emerge from his organicist scientism. As we will relate in Part III, "Regeneration," the social fevers of individualism had, by this time, advanced into a perilous nomic crisis in which the social foundations of the nation seemed to be rapidly disintegrating. In Walter Skya's estimation, the masses had awakened to their own subjective freedom and, as a consequence, the goals of the Meiji era, which had provided meaning and purpose in the late nineteenth century, began to lose their purchase over individuals.[20] In their place there erupted a contentious upsurge of contradictory ideological formulations that were designed to appeal to the egoistic longings of the newly self-aware masses. Though Oka's evolutionism increased in popularity over the course of the decade, eventuating in a "Darwin boom" during the final years of the Meiji era, it was quickly misappropriated by ideologues across the political spectrum. While bureaucratic elites that came out of the imperial university sought to take up evolutionism as an esoteric truth—insider knowledge used to both distinguish themselves from and establish control over the unwashed masses— anarchists, socialists, and other radical thinkers fit evolutionary theory into their campaign to attack the imperial house and overthrow the state.[21]

Most alarming of all to Oka was the reaction to the growing sense of anomy of those who shared his visceral disdain for postwar individualism: the fundamentalist promoters of state Shintoism. Like Oka, these ideologues regarded Japan's national life in this time of mass politics, precipitous socio-economic change, and nomic contestation as rudderless. Yet, in contrast to Oka's quintessentially modern solution of reconstituting social foundations through the social instincts of the "human-way," their response to the nomic crisis was purely reactionary: they called for a return to absolutism by constructing national unity around the imperial house and its historical myths.

---

19 My frequent use of this term derives mainly from Roger Griffin and Peter L. Berger. I also associate this term with the "groundless grounds" explored by Wittgenstein and Heidegger. See Griffin, *Modernism and Fascism*, 74–75; Berger, *The Sacred Canopy*, 19ff.; Braver, *Groundless Grounds*.

20 Skya, *Japan's Holy War*, 153–57.

21 Migita, *Tennosei to Shinkaron*.

As construed by the chief ideologue of such "reactionary Shinto ultranationalism," Tokyo University law professor Hozumi Yatsuka, Japan's *kokutai*, its unique national essence or body, constituted a family-state—that is, an unchanging blood community of worshipers founded by the Sun Goddess and bound together by ritual observance.[22] By the time the conflicted reality of post-1905 society was becoming undeniable, this family-state idea had begun to invade the everyday life of imperial subjects through a consolidation of the nation's Shinto shrines and the introduction of ritual practices and moral indoctrination into the school system. The backwardness and absurdity of this orthodoxy, which had been invented during his own adulthood, not only appalled Oka—it deliberately impeded what Migita Hiroki calls his primary quest: establishing evolutionism as the foundation of sociopolitical conventions for the Japanese ethnic nation (*minzoku*).[23]

Oka personally experienced this obstructionism as a member of the Ministry of Education's committee on school textbook approval between 1904 and 1918. Recruited to the committee as part of his position as a professor at the Tokyo First Normal School, Oka, already the author of several school textbooks on biology, hygiene, and zoology, hoped to use his bureaucratic role to establish a permanent place for evolutionary science in the elementary school curriculum.[24] His extensive efforts over the course of a decade and a half were utterly thwarted: no mention of evolution was included in any of the textbooks on which he worked. The year 1907, in which "Ideal Group Life" appeared, marks, among other important events, the lead up to the first of these textbooks being published in 1911. Though his best-selling primer, *Lectures on Evolutionary Theory*, was briefly threatened with censorship in 1904 and though he suffered harassment by the Special Higher Police at the behest of the Imperial Household Agency later in the decade, it was his frustrations on the textbook committee that alerted Oka to the challenge posed by the family-state orthodoxy.[25] Similarly goaded on by the anomic atmosphere of the late Meiji era, the rise of state Shinto would push Oka to offer *shinkaron* as more than just a practical, metapolitical model for scientific reform. Occupying the place traditionally reserved for religion

---

22 Skya, *Japan's Holy War*, 53–81.
23 Migita, *Tennosei to Shinkaron*, 37–44, 106–7.
24 For Oka's output before 1904 see Chapter 2.
25 Migita, *Tennosei to Shinkaron*, 108–11.

and identifying in organic processes of growth an ultimate value of health, Oka's evolutionism eventually became a scientistic program to generate an alternative mode of modern life.

An Insect's Way of Thinking:
From Modernization to Generative Scientism

In "Ideal Group Life" this longing for such an alternative registers in Oka's bemused ambivalence toward his own proposals for modernizing the nation on the model of the superorganism. This tone is perhaps most obvious in the admonitions which accompany his bronze images of moss animals, one of which pokes fun at the Christian version of the Golden Rule—"Like these moss animals, do unto others as you would have others do unto you"—and the other Buddhist enlightenment—"Like these moss animals, escape the confines of the ego, proceed on to the level of the higher self." A similarly conflicted attitude is betrayed by the Japanese term Oka employs for moss animal individuals or zooids: *mushi*, a word which is best translated as insect. At one point in "Ideal Group Life," after explaining how, upon investigating their colonies over a long period, one comes to observe and criticize human events "from the point of view of moss animals," Oka, recalling that moss animals need neither laws nor government, drolly comments:

[S]eeing how humanity proudly looks upon the loftily standing, large and imposing judicial and legislative buildings at the heart of the capital, taking photographs of them and making picture postcards, I sometimes unconsciously talk to myself wondering whether we should be proud or ashamed that we need such fabulous buildings for judicial enterprises to prosper and, when passing in their vicinity, I say such things to myself as "Even to an insect's [*mushi's*] way of thinking this is embarrassing."[26]

What Oka's self-mockery points to is a conflict between two appraisals of contemporary humanity that runs through this article and, by extension, his evolutionism. On the one hand, he at times maintains that "a perfect group life, such as we see in this species of moss animals, is not even

---

26   Oka, "Risōteki Dantai Seikatsu" [Ideal group life], 72.

a remote possibility for human beings."[27] In Oka's view, "humans are naturally self-interested, doing to others what they would not have done to themselves" and, consequently, "laws and police forces are necessary, and religion and morality cannot be abandoned." On the other hand, Oka repeatedly asserts that the moral-political perfection exhibited by moss animal nations qualify them as "valuable enough to be made the aim of our human advancement." Throughout "Ideal Group Life" he describes moss animals as "valiant" and "noble" creatures whose lifestyle humans should envy, and, even as he reiterates that attaining their cohesion is not possible, Oka states that "before trying to actualize these ideal conditions it is first necessary to recast human nature and eliminate our selfishness in order to become like moss animals."[28]

It is the aspiration to reconcile these contradictory appraisals by "recasting human nature" that would inspire Oka not only to supplant religion but, at the same time, fundamentally rethink the evolutionary ramifications of the modern social order. In particular, the anomic milieu of the period after the Russo-Japanese War raised the question whether modernization actually facilitated and should be equated with the healthy growth of the nation-state—growth, that is, which achieved the hygienic unity-in-difference that we saw in the example of moss animals sprouting buds from their sides to create an integrated superindividuality. The earlier metapolitical essays from *Evolution and Human Life* assumed this identification of modernization and healthy cohesion: the spontaneous outpouring of apparent patriotism that accompanied wartime mobilization seemed to confirm that the differentiation of society into specialized individualities during the Meiji era had not undermined the unity of the nation. According to the reformist outlook of Oka's early scientism, all that was needed was to use the educational apparatus of the developmental state to convince these individual persons that their interdependent place in the national division of labor reflected an underlying biological reality.

After, "Ideal Group Life" this faith in modernization no longer seemed warranted: its consequences, as was becoming increasingly clear, were exaggerating individualism and thereby causing members of the nation to pur-

---

27 Ibid., 75.
28 Ibid., 74.

sue self-interest apart from the common good. Without normative bonds, the nation appeared on the verge of disintegrating and the conditions of modern life came more and more to be identified with an illness that was accelerating the degeneration of the collective body toward extinction. In this decadent environment evolutionary science took on an entirely new role: instead of confirming the progress of the modern order its job became to remedy it, treating it as a process of development that had entered a corrupt and dissolute phase. Science would need to intervene in the temporal unfolding of evolution, using its knowledge of hereditary mechanisms to ensure the organic differentiation needed for national power culminated in a higher unity, not degeneration and death.

Thus, both before and after "Ideal Group Life" Oka's goal remains fixed: to "eliminate our selfishness in order to become like moss animals." Yet in his earlier scientism this selfishness is attributed to the incomplete modernization, a deficit that the internal reforms informed by modernizing evolutionary science can erase—while later on, it is the wayward mode of modern existence which evolutionism can help diagnose and return to health. Expressed as self-deprecating humor in the pages of "Ideal Group Life" Oka's ambivalence of 1907 represented his realization that the collectivist imperatives of evolutionism would be much harder to inculcate and implement than he ever imagined. Simply erecting exemplary images of altruistic moss animals in the public square would not suffice. *Shinkaron* itself would have to itself evolve, becoming a doctrine that could truly compete with religion in "recasting human nature" and ushering in a new, healthier incarnation of modern life.

Oka's regenerative vision of national destiny would come to serve this cosmological end by relying on a scientism that did more than use the "ideal group life" of superorganisms as paragons of interdependence. His pre-1907 metapolitics sought to harness the organicist logic on display in nature in just this straightforward way, as a form of scientism that would, it was hoped, gradually rectify the existing nomic structure of the nation to this exemplary cohesion as part of the process of modernization. Yet by the time Oka was ambiguously jesting about insect perspectives on modern institutions, it was obvious that modernization was not advancing nomic cohesion but its opposite—anomy. In order to counter this vital threat Oka radicalized his organicism in a manner that would propose not just reforming nomos, but generating it. In addition to an atemporal model of organic cohesion, the higher individuality of the superorganism came to offer a cosmological vision of natural development. The progress of the "consummate group," through anticipated stages of growth, came to serve as a measure of health such that health was treated as an ultimate good and the life-cycle process as an ontological substrate. Conversely, interference with such hygienic development, manifesting itself as a failure of the differentiated parts of the organism to reintegrate and support the whole—something which could be taken as a sign of impending senescence—counted as evidence of decay and decadence.

In effect, the epigenetic process described by cell biology and embryology—which were the basis of the paradigm of evolutionary morphology according to which Oka was trained and worked—delineated a value-generating ontology from which the vitality and cohesion of the nation-state derived. While Oka chided his own proposal that moss animals be set on pedestals in the public square, his apotheosis of organic development as the ultimate source of meaning and future viability achieved the equivalent. Never abandoning his reformist stance, Oka, nevertheless, put forth an organicist cosmology whose persuasive formula for national strength and cohesion even the Shinto orthodoxy would be, in the end, forced to take into account.

An example of what we will call "generative scientism,"[29] this developmental or temporal organicism enabled Oka not only to reject modern conditions as degenerate but also to articulate a eugenic program that overcomes anomy by rejuvenating lost cohesion. The organicist logic that this scientism made available agreed, in other words, with Shinto fundamentalism that the present is decadent—yet its response to this dissolution was not a return to a static nomic order from the past but a future-oriented affirmation of organicism's developmental cosmology. Once the laws of nature rendered the process of inheritance utterly transparent, the differentiation-*without*-unity on display in the degenerate present could be overcome: new humans could be engineered whose nomic disposition would bind them instinctively to the greater totality of the nation. An alternative mode of modern existence would be, in effect, brought into being, one that regained primordial unity without sacrificing the benefits of individual specialization

---

29 See note 13.

that occurred during organic growth. With individual persons eugenically reintegrated back into the superorganism, anomic egoism would be neutralized and the long-term health of the nation secured.

METAPOLITICS AND PROGRAMMATIC MODERNISM

In diagnosing modern life as decadent and prescribing a collectivist eugenic regimen for national revitalization, Oka's *shinkaron* constituted, we will argue, a form of programmatic modernism. The term comes from Roger Griffin's *Modernism and Fascism*, which portrays modernism as a response within Europeanized societies to the perception that modernization had led not to inevitable and limitless progress, but the "loss of a homogeneous value system and overarching cosmology (nomos)."[30] By the late nineteenth century modern existence came to be seen by vast numbers of intellectuals and creative elites as characterized by decadence, disenchantment, and alienation—an age of anomy had been inaugurated. In order to counteract this degenerate order, modernism evoked visions of a restored nomos—that is, norms, conventions, and laws stably grounded in an inexorable cosmological order—that could serve as the basis of an alternative, healthy mode of modern life. While "epiphanic modernism"—which is Griffin's expression for modernism in the aesthetic mode according to which it is usually understood—employed innovative artistic experimentation to offer "glimpses of a higher reality that throw into relief the anomy and spiritual bankruptcy of contemporary history,"[31] the programmatic modernism that concerns us here is more sociopolitically ambitious. It strives to overcome the decadent present and revive community cohesion and inner purpose by ushering in a new healthy incarnation of reality, a new hygienic nomos. Though it was future-oriented and employed modern techniques to realize itself, the totalizing visions of programmatic modernism entailed rejuvenating and synthesizing together healthy elements from the past nomic order which modernization had eroded. In other words, the new beginning it sought to initiate was not constructed from scratch but palingenetic: it involved the regeneration of collective life.[32]

---

30 Griffin, *Modernism and Fascism*, 116.
31 Ibid.
32 Ibid., 116–17.

The definition of fascism that Griffin advances in his book depicts it as a political variant of this programmatic modernism that aims to bring about an alternative version of modern life based on the palingenesis of the nation. According to Griffin,

> fascists conceive the nation as an organism shaped by historic, cultural, and in some cases, ethnic and hereditary factors, a mythic construct incompatible with liberal, conservative, and communist theories of society. The health of this organism they see undermined as much by the principles of institutional and cultural pluralism, individualism, and globalized consumerism promoted by liberalism as by the global regime of social justice and human equality identified with socialism in theory as the ultimate goal of history, or by the conservative defence of "tradition."[33]

Through the revolutionary seizure of power and the instantiation of a "totalizing vision of national or ethnic rebirth,"[34] fascism restores the sense of communal belonging and transcendent purpose that keeps the national organism vibrant. With the forces of decadence politically defeated, "a new era of cultural homogeneity and health"[35] will begin.

As may already be evident, the programmatic modernism imparted by Oka's *Evolution and Human Life* bears a striking resemblance to critical aspects of this revolutionary palingenetic nationalism. It is, in fact, largely on this basis that we will suggest Oka's evolutionism influenced Japanese fascism, helping to prompt "radical Shinto ultranationalism" to forgo the reactionary family-state concept for a developmental organicism that rebelled against decadence. The point, however, cannot be made strongly enough: Oka promotes neither the capturing of political power nor the radical destruction of existing ideologies and orders. His vision is neither fascist nor even protofascist. Instead, his programmatic modernism emerges out of reformist statism—a rational, moderate, and pro-modern form of universal developmentalism that is metapolitical in its intent. Although it looks to regenerate society through "collective social action or behavior that is supposed to pioneer a new source of health, spiritual or physical,"[36] this social

---

33   Ibid., 181.
34   Ibid., 182.
35   Ibid.
36   Ibid., 132.

modernism, as Griffin dubs this variant of programmatic modernism, performs its transformations within the confines of existing political orders. It was especially indicative of health professionals and natural scientists in the decades around the fin-de-siècle who found in the reformist state possibilities for rejuvenating the body of the nation and even remaking human nature to create new men.

As it happened, Oka entered the ranks of these European scientist-professionals just as their modernist confrontation with decadence was taking shape. Attending the new imperial university in Tokyo between 1886 and 1890, Oka's undergraduate thesis dealt with the very moss animals from one of its campus ponds whose "ideal group life" inspired the essay above. It was the theoretical question concerning the nature of organic individuality that led Oka, with the help of a loan from a relative, to Germany. There, after an unsatisfying stint under August Weismann, he soon became a student of the renowned zoologist Rudolf Leuckart (1892–98) whose Leipzig University laboratory was perhaps the premiere facility for investigating the nature of organic individuals.[37] We will argue that it was not only the close relationship with Leuckart but Oka's training in the research program of his field, evolutionary morphology, that set a precedent for his generative scientism and its confrontation with decadence. Though Oka's mentor Leuckart was a restrained figure, the zoologist who had synthesized evolutionary morphology, Ernst Haeckel (1834–1919), developed a speculative philosophical system around his organicist version of Darwinism that, among Oka's generation, would become the basis of a revitalization movement. Oka's years in Germany, in fact, coincide with both some of Haeckel's fiercest battles against religious reaction and the espousal of racial hygiene and eugenics among a younger cohort who were transforming Haeckel's corporatist evolutionism into a modernist program to overcome decadence. While the essays that comprise *Evolution and Human Life* depend heavily on Haeckel's evolutionary morphology with its account of organic individuality and its openness to non-Darwinian theories, it is to the regenerative visions of his contemporaries that Oka will turn to when Japan's nomic crisis appears unsurmountable after the Russo-Japanese War. For all of Haeckel's effort to convert evolutionism into a monist religion that can undergird ethics, it will

---

37   Nyhart, *Biology Takes Form*, 310.

be the replacement of the present decadent social order with the prospect of a future healthy one that will seem to offer the most promise in stabilizing a disintegrating nomos with cosmic legitimation.

EVOLUTION AND THE "EMPEROR SYSTEM"

Our argument here—namely, that the problems Oka encountered in offering *shinkaron* as a solution to the crisis of social cohesion led him to transform it into a persuasive programmatic modernist vision of national regeneration—runs directly counter to the account of Oka's career in Migita Hiroki's recent *Tennosei to Shinkaron* (The emperor system and evolutionary theory). For Migita, Oka's troubles, especially those he encountered on the textbook committee, stemmed from the heretical premises of his evolutionism. As Migita's book explains, the family-state orthodoxy of state Shinto was based on a creationist myth that enshrined an "emperor-centered historical view" by which the Sun Goddess was the divine ancestor of the imperial house and the ethnic nation (*minzoku*). In his portrayal, this narrative was utterly irreconcilable with the account in *Lectures on Evolutionary Theory*, Oka's best seller of 1904 that described the common ancestry of humankind and the rest of living nature. Such indirect yet quite deliberate calling into question of the imperial myth not only provoked government attempts to marginalize and even suppress evolutionism, but made Oka the champion of all rationalist resisters to the family-state orthodoxy to the center and left of the political spectrum.[38]

Though his struggles with orthodoxy would apparently leave Oka embittered and disillusioned, evolutionism itself could not be held down because it was widely recognized within the government from the First World War onward that science was indispensable to industrialism and modernization. As a result, in the 1920s, evolution came to occupy a position alongside the family-state orthodoxy. Migita depicts these as two completely incompatible doctrines occupying separate spheres during these years and members of the government as adopting a profoundly confused doublethink when it came to the relationship between them. Migita's supreme example of not only this paradox but the inevitable triumph of evolutionism over ortho-

---

38 Migita, *Tennosei to Shinkaron*, 14–19, 32–43, 63–65, 71–72.

doxy in twentieth century is Oka's most famous admirer, Emperor Hirohito, whose avocation in marine biology was celebrated by the government in the 1920s and early 1930s, hidden from public view after the Marco Polo Bridge Incident (1937), and used to help rehabilitate the now former living god after the Second World War.[39]

In contrast to Migita and other scholars, we will see that evolutionism in Japan was far from being merely a modernizing doctrine that remained aloof from the family-state and other ideological currents. Instead, it became entangled, nearly from the very beginning, in forging social cohesion and national unity, attempting to underwrite all ideologies, and even adapting itself to extant political orders. The immense readership of *Evolution and Human Life* in the decades after the Russo-Japanese War did not question that in shaping the nomic disposition of the nation through what he called the "human-way" Oka was intermingling evolution with orthodoxy. Yet what these same readers would have been most struck by was the anthology's peculiarly compelling organicist logic that played health against decadence and decadence against health, thereby seeming to demand that developmental biology intervene in national affairs and adopt a redemptive role in revitalizing the higher individuality of the nation-state. Without erecting pedestals or approaching high altars, *shinkaron* insinuated itself into the precincts of orthodoxy simply by associating the macrocosmic destiny of the nation with the microcosmic life cycle of the individual person. Once the organic state was converted into a superorganism plagued by developmental disorders, evolution came to be identified with prospects for palingenetic cure, especially those offered by racial hygiene and eugenics.

Oka and the promoters of evolutionary biology did not, as Migita insists, step aside and wait for the Shinto ultranationalist orthodoxy to play itself out. Rather the regenerative vision of *Evolution and Human Life* proactively contributed an antidecadent, modernist mode of analysis to the continuing debate about national destiny. Though, as we will see here and there in this study, commentators and activists across the political spectrum condemned social Darwinism, they did so on Oka's terms, appropriating his organicism and reaffirming his critique of individualism as an engine of socially disintegrative anomy. In the epilogue we even suggest that Oka's attribution of

---

39 Ibid., 117–24, 164–98, 238–40. See Chapter 3, note 271.

degeneracy to an inherently anomic individualism may have provoked the Shinto orthodoxy to an organicist developmentalism of its own that called for "dying to the self and returning to the one."[40]

Oka's Background and Overview of Chapters

Before previewing the chapters ahead, something more needs to be said about Oka and his milieu. As should already be evident, I regard Oka's studies as a *ryūgakusei* (foreign-study student) in Germany as the defining experience of his career. Like so many of the over 1,200 other doctors, legal scholars, and fellow scientists who traveled to Germany in the critical years between the 1880s and the First World War, Oka accepted it as his duty to inculcate the knowledge he had retrieved from abroad as a means of fortifying the Japanese nation. His careers as a college instructor, research zoologist, education bureaucrat, and, finally, popularizer of evolutionary thought can all be seen as ways of fulfilling this calling. Though the sociopolitical essays that are the subject of this study were, in this spirit, ostensibly directed to the general reading public, their actual audience seems to have been the emergent stratum of cosmopolitan intellectuals of which Oka himself was a member—that is to say, the scientists, technocrats, legal scholars, journalists, medical practitioners, and literati who had been empowered through their socialization in modern universities, both at home and abroad. Oka's frequent contributions to *Chūō Kōron* (The central review) should be seen in this light: the premiere intellectual publication of the day, its pages served as the primary public forum for those who were bent on bringing their newly acquired expertise to bear on the ongoing development of the nation. Along with reaching out to the general public, Oka hoped to convey the imperatives of his organicist *shinkaron* to the cosmopolitan intelligentsia who read and contributed to this and similar publications.

It should also be noted that Oka's success in reaching this broad audience—and, indeed, becoming a widely recognized public intellectual for four decades—was a remarkable achievement given the personal tragedy he endured early on in his life. Born in Shizuoka during the first year of the Meiji era to a banking family and provided a privileged, polyglot education

---

40 Skya, *Japan's Holy War*, 268.

in the foreign quarter of Osaka by his father, a bureaucrat at the government mint, Oka, nevertheless, found himself a virtual orphan by the time he was a teenager. In quick succession, between 1879 and 1884, his entire nuclear family had succumbed to illness or accident—the most heart-wrenching of these losses being that of a younger sister who died from burns sustained when her kimono caught fire. Only thanks to the assistance of his banker relatives was Oka able to take up college preparatory courses in the capital, enroll at Tokyo University as a special student, and eventually pursue graduate studies in zoology first at Freiburg University under Weismann and later, as we have already mentioned, at Leipzig University under Leuckart. However, even after he returned to Japan, began to publish widely, married into a family highly placed in the Meiji bureaucracy, and, after a stint in Yamaguchi as a teacher at the peer school there, obtained the professorial position at the Tokyo Higher Normal School which he would keep until his retirement, personal calamity was not far behind. Cruelly echoing the summary loss of his parents and siblings, Oka's first two sons died prematurely of illness during the early years of his marriage. Distraught, he is said to have thrown himself in his work during his early career in order to cope with these losses.

Citing Oka's austere working conditions, punishing research regimen, and his grim intimations of permanent war some have concluded that these repeated misfortunes left him with a pessimistic disposition and that this largely accounts for his bleak conclusions concerning the eventual decline of humanity. However, his avid and persistent scientism suggests a more sanguine outlook, especially when it came to his enduring commitment to science education. His boosterism actually predated the popular works which he began to turn out with increasing frequency during the 1910s and 1920s. Most tellingly, in 1890, just before departing for graduate studies in Germany, Oka took it upon himself to devise his own Latin-based international lingua franca, Ji Rengo (Our language). Upon arriving in Europe and discovering that the Polish ophthalmologist L. L. Zamenhof had already created and begun distributing textbooks in Esperanto, Oka became the first Japanese to master this constructed international language. His enthusiastic promotion of the Esperanto movement in Japan was, like his fledgling efforts at Ji Rengo, pursued to help disseminate and inculcate a passion for the "new civilized knowledge" of modern science. This aspiration remained a constant throughout his long career. As we will see in upcoming chapters, many of Oka's initial readers felt he had revealed to them a novel and "fantastically wondrous world"—and given the colorful language and vivid illustrations that populated his texts even after he began prognosticating human degeneration there is every reason to believe he continued to share in this awe and excitement.

In this sense Oka really was a rationalist enlightener—however, his mode was not that of eighteenth-century philosophes, as Migita would have it, but of the biomedical specialists of a hundred years later whom Paul Weindling portrays as seeking to derive a transcendent "technocratic antipolitics" from corporatist biology. If notes of pessimism did creep into his oeuvre, they were partly an upshot of his goals for science education having been stymied by the Home and Education Ministries and undermined by the spread of state Shinto. Yet, ultimately, as we will argue, Oka's distinct *Lebensanschauung* must be seen a function of the declinist discourse that emerged from organicism toward the turn of the century being filtered through the imperatives of Meiji nationalism. Indeed, the main reason that this book will focus not on Oka the man but on the purport of his early sociopolitical writings is that the process of appropriating this discourse—and the regenerative logic built into it—has hardly been acknowledged, much less understood.[41]

As we have already intimated, the chapters that follow will be divided into three parts. The first part, "Organicism," addresses Oka's scientistic synthesis of the prevailing political philosophy of the organic state with notions of organic individuality derived from contemporary evolutionary biology. Chapter 1, "The Organic State: The Imperative of Ethical Life," begins by explaining the practical appeal for the Japanese oligarchy of organic theories of the state from German *Staatswissenschaften* (state science) and goes on to discuss how the imperative for a custom-based "ethical life" helped inspire the formulation of a unifying civic creed to accompany the promulgation of the Meiji Constitution. Out of the struggle to delineate the "*kokutai*"—national body or national organization structure—mentioned in this creed, two state-science approaches emerged: one reactionary, which longed for a static absolutist order based on fundamentalist renderings of

---

41   For more on Oka's biography, see Chapters 1, 2, 6, and the epilogue. Sketches of Oka's life can be found in Tsukuba, *Oka Asajirō Shū*, 430–55; and Watanabe, *The Japanese and Western Science*, 84–98.

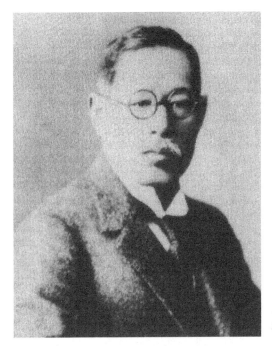

Figure 2. Oka Asajirō.
Source: Watanabe, *The Japanese and Western Science*, 85.

Shintoism, and the other reformist, which pursued a modern developmental state that employed technocratic expertise to adjust institutions, customs, and mores to the trends of the modern world. Oka Asajirō will be depicted as an adherent of this reformist statism, an outlook that was dominant at Tokyo Imperial University where he studied as an undergraduate in the late 1880s. The chapter concludes by contrasting the evolutionist political philosophy of the university's first president, Katō Hiroyuki, with Oka's later and more thoroughly organicist *shinkaron*.

Chapter 2, "Palingenetic Polypersons: Evolutionary Morphology and the Question of Organic Individuality," argues that Oka derived his biological correlate to the organic theory of the state from the scientific paradigm in which he received training as a graduate student in Rudolf Leuckart's Leipzig University laboratory in the early 1890s. Called evolutionary morphology, this paradigm featured an analysis of organic individuality that Leuckart and its author, Ernst Haeckel, used to explain the collective existence of colonial jellyfish and other superorganismic creatures. Not only would these "polypersons" serve as a model for moss animal nations and their "ideal group life," but Haeckel's stress on biogenetic law as the "palingenetic" force driving development at every level of organic individuality sets the stage for Oka's eventual appropriation of non-Darwinian theories. In the end, Oka, despite misgivings about Haeckel's speculative excesses, adhered to his organicist Darwinism and even sought to emulate the German's tremendous success in disseminating it among the general public.

Chapter 3, "Generative Scientism: Organicism beyond Reform," explores how unanticipated impediments to applying "corporatist evolutionism"—as Paul Weindling refers to Haeckel's evolutionary morphology—to the normative order (nomos) underlying sociopolitical arrangements triggers a radicalization in the use of organic examples from nature. Transcending the initial reformist scientism that simply attempted to fit customary nomoi to the atemporal interdependence exhibited within all forms of organic individuality, a new scientism emerges which seeks to use its knowledge of the epigenetic process of development to generate both new values and new men. Articulated initially in the so-called monist religion that Haeckel identifies in the healthy ontogeny of nation-states and civilizations as part of his response to the ultramontane reaction against scientifically based national reform, it is this historicist "generative scientism" which, especially in the hands of a cohort of younger biologists that includes Oka, will come to promote a programmatic modernist diagnosis of contemporary life as decadent and, therefore, in need of nomic-eugenic regeneration. By examining the first sociopolitical essay from *Evolution and Human Life* ("Good and Evil in the Animal World"), we will see that, despite an overtly reformist outlook, Oka's early efforts to "seek the foundations of ethics in ecology"[42] betrays latent generative features that will come to fore as he confronts the Shintoist version of the religious reaction against evolutionary theory.

Part II, "Metapolitics," explains how, in the context of the Russo-Japanese War, Oka's reformist scientism attempted to define the preconditions for biopolitical survival by treating the instinctual life of superorganisms as exemplars for the human nation-state. Chapter 4, "World War Zero," shows how Oka responded to the misguided humanitarianism of both the government and the anarchist-led peace movement with an evolutionary realpolitik that

---

42   Oka, Asajirō, "Seibutsukai ni okeru Zen to Aku" [Good and evil in the animal world], in *Shinka to Jinsei* [Evolution and human life] (Tokyo: Yūseidō Shuppan, 1968), 54.

depicted the apparent "national unity" (*kyokoku itchi*) during the war as evidence that Japan had cohered into a superorganism. We will suggest that Oka's biopolitical vision adumbrates similar analyses that would become common currency in Europe only after the First World War—namely, the imperative of a permanent total mobilization for perpetual war and the commitment to racial autarky as the proper metapolitical stance in an anarchic international arena. Indeed, Oka's construal of the ethnic nation (*minzoku*) as a distinct race will be seen to reflect Haeckel's ideas about human speciation, thereby contributing a scientistic rationale to later *jinshuron* (race theory) assumptions about the incommensurability of races and ethnicities.

Chapter 5, "The Human-Way: Nomic Instincts and the Transformation of Humanity," turns to the implications of this reform-oriented scientistic metapolitics for the internal, normative disposition of the national superorganism. After illustrating how, toward the close of the war with Russia, Oka was already advancing prescriptions for collective hygiene in order to dispel humanitarian qualms among biomedical practitioners about applying eugenics to the nation, the discussion directs its focus on the definitive expression of what we will call his soft organicism of interdependence: the internalization through Lamarckian use-inheritance of an altruistic "human-way" that renders national cohesion instinctual. These "nomic instincts" will not only get human nation-states to behave like collectivities of other gregarious creatures, but, by bringing the sociomoral disposition into alignment with evolutionary necessity through the transparency promised by biological science, introduce a monist rationale that creates a climate conducive to later totalitarianism.

The third and final part, "Regeneration," deals with how diminished prospects for implementing the metapolitical human-way pushed Oka to expand his organicist *shinkaron* into a more persuasive programmatic modernist vision that promised to overcome modern decadence, secure national destiny, and compete with religious cosmization through the eugenic rejuvenation of disappearing organic cohesion. Chapter 6, "Nomic Crisis," looks at how the fluidity and complexity of modern life in the period after the Russo-Japanese War was perceived by both Oka and reactionary statists as evidence of an ominous national dissolution. Both were particularly alarmed by individualism and the "social fevers" and subversive ideologies attendant to it. For reactionary statists the response to this corrosive menace was to secure the customary nomic foundations of the nation through aggressive promotion of the emperor-centered Shinto cosmology in local shrines and public schools. Inspired by the "reactionary Shinto ultranationalism"[43] of Hozumi Yatsuka, this state Shinto became for Oka as big a threat as the anomic society which was, during the "Darwin boom," misappropriating his evolutionism across the ideological spectrum. While the misuse of *shinkaron* by anti-imperial radicals, elitist technocrats, and ambitious egoists was a source of dismay, it was the invasive attempt by fundamentalist Shinto reactionaries to marginalize evolutionary science and insert their superstitious cosmological narrative at the center of the educational curriculum that impelled Oka toward generative scientism. A member of the Ministry of Education's textbook committee as part of his professorial duties at the Tokyo Higher Normal School, Oka lost two battles—in 1911 and again in 1918—to get the theory of evolution into elementary school textbooks. Due to these experiences he began to entertain a programmatic modernism that, in the manner suggested in "Ideal Group Life," matched the state Shintoist cosmology on its own turf.

Chapter 7, "Decadence and Destiny," describes how Oka's theory of decadence during the final years of the Meiji period advanced a regenerative vision that would use eugenic techniques to overcome nomic dissolution and secure future national health and power. Drawing tacitly on the non-Darwinian theory of orthogenesis that was closely affiliated with the biogenetic paradigm of Haeckel's evolutionary morphology, Oka classified humankind together with creatures who had come to dominate their habitat through the evolution of advantageous traits that subsequently overdeveloped, bringing on decline and eventual extinction. Like dinosaurs and saber-toothed tigers, humans evolved their advantageous traits—brains and hands—through predetermined life stages of healthy growth into robust maturity—but now these traits have overdeveloped, ushering in senescence and eventual extinction by undermining the cohesion of the collectivities that they had once rendered so dominant. For Oka, decline permeated the late Meiji setting: overdeveloped brains and hands had engendered a hypertrophied egoism that manifested itself in the dysgenic laissez-faire milieu as psychological exhaustion, physical degeneration, and nomic dissolution. To cope with this decadence and triumph in the battle with other advanced nations, which were

---

43   Skya, *Japan's Holy War*, 23–24.

becoming superorganismic invalids at an even faster rate, Oka proposed eugenic measures to rejuvenate an earlier stage of national hygiene. While specific initiatives could not yet be delineated until the nature of the hereditary mechanism had been settled, Oka's regenerative formula for defeating decadence, matching religion, and reviving healthy integration turned the organicist basis of corporatist evolutionism into a scientistic program, one that looked ahead to an alternate incarnation of life in a modern nation-state.

The epilogue, "Evolution and the National Body: An Unfinished Synthesis," suggests that even though Oka found his metapolitical evolutionism harder to inculcate than he had anticipated, it did, over the long term, prove much more congruent with modern experience than the reactionary Shinto orthodoxy of Hozumi. This greater suitability was, in fact, so pronounced that leading figures in the Shinto movement came to seek accommodation with defining features of organicist evolutionism. Not only did Hozumi's two most influential students attempt to reconceive the blood community of the family-state as something along the lines of a superorganism, but the living god at the center of this orthodoxy, Emperor Hirohito, befriended Oka, consulting privately with the zoologist on his research into marine specimens. According to Migita, the emperor even went so far as to paraphrase Oka's most inflammatory statements on the untoward consequences of governing through superstition, arguing that for a nation to remain viable in the modern world the ideological system must align itself to the nature revealed by evolutionary science.

Although scholars have tended to attribute the orthodoxy of early-twentieth-century imperial Japan to religious myths contrived by reactionary statists, these examples along with what we have said about Oka's generative scientism as a programmatic modernist attempt to reconstitute humanity and outdo religion points to something else: an indispensable role for biologically derived organicism in the constructions of imperial ideology. Far from being marginalized by the official Shinto cosmology, the palingenetic cure for decadence—a cure that involved reviving and optimizing the health and power of a natural body plagued by the anomy of egoism—may have been integral to the unfinished project of synthesizing science and Shinto orthodoxy into a single persuasive ideological account.

PART I

Organicism

The moss animal nations that Oka describes in "Ideal Group Life" did more than define his evolutionism—they served as a catalyst for his intellectual career, first as a scientist and later as a teacher and popularizer of evolutionary theory. It seems to have been at the Sanshiro Pond on the campus of the Tokyo Imperial University—one of the locations alluded to at the beginning of our introduction—that Oka first became acquainted with the curious physiology of these creatures. Not only would the dissertation, "Observations concerning Fresh Water Moss Animals (*Kokemushi*)," that he wrote for his degree in zoology at the university focus on *kanten kokemushi*, as he called moss animals, but the graduate studies he pursued in Germany eventually brought him to the Leipzig University laboratory of the renowned zoologist Rudolf Leuckart that specialized in examining the intricate structure of such "poly-persons" in the natural world. After returning to Japan, and publishing papers in this subfield of zoology, Oka obtained a position at another Tokyo institution also mentioned as a dwelling place of moss animals, Tokyo Higher Normal School. Oka would remain at the school until 1929, becoming, in his twilight years, a part-time instructor at both his old institution and the newly opened Tokyo University of Literature and Science until finally retiring in the early 1930s. The centrality of moss animals to Oka's career is testified to by the fact that his students, against his wishes, had the variety that he had discovered, investigated, and lionized posthumously renamed *Asajirella gelantinosa* in his honor.[44]

---

44 Oda, "Oka Asajirō Sensei no Ōmokage."

In this part we will explore how the scientific paradigm under which Oka obtained his scholarly training in Germany meshed with two other related influences to shape his evolutionism. This paradigm was that of evolutionary morphology, and it will be argued here that the question of organic individuality at the heart of this field of zoological investigation found resonance with the organic theory of the state, which had been embraced by the establishment Japan during Oka's student years, and scientism, which, as manifested in Ernest Haeckel's philosophy of monism and offshoot theories of racial hygiene and eugenics, was determining how evolutionary theory translated into sociopolitical applications in an era now dubbed by historians of science as the "eclipse of Darwinism." As we will see, the metapolitical vision that Oka intended to offer with his evolutionism was synthetic: it blended evolutionary morphology, organic statism, and monist scientism into an organicist amalgam that was supposed to underpin and modernize the existing sociopolitical order. The latter part of this study will reveal that it was also elements implicit in this organicism, most especially historicism, that enabled Oka to convert it from a straightforward reformist agent of statist modernization into something altogether more radical: the basis of a new overarching cosmology that could both critique and offer an alternative to the prevailing modern mode of existence that increasingly came to be diagnosed as decadent.

The appeal of organicism reflects what Kenneth Pyle calls the "realist patterns"[45] of the Meiji response to the intellectual and geopolitical thrust of the new imperialism. According to Pyle, the intense and prolonged interstate competition of the Sengoku (Warring States) era from 1467 to 1600 helped to shape a realpolitik logic that, into the late nineteenth century, continued to imbue the mutable set of attitudes, habits, and principles that comprised Japan's style of grand strategy. Organicism satisfied this strategic outlook because it seemed to identify the sources of power that would need to be appropriated and maximized in order to realize state interest in an anarchic arena of competing nations. Most immediately, this meant pragmatically emulating "Kaiser Wilhelm's empire," which "modern Japan's founders" deemed during "the last two decades of the nineteenth century in many

---

45   Pyle, *Japan Rising*, 41.

respects the most advanced power in the world."[46] Through its illiberal "protectionist and state-centric policies"[47] Germany had achieved the goal to which the Japanese oligarchs aspired: unification of an amalgam of small polities into an integrated and industrialized empire that stood poised to embark on an expansionist program in pursuit of autarky and regional hegemony. The organic theory of the state, which we will discuss in Chapter 1, was perceived to be intrinsic to this dawning success: in appropriating it to indigenous conditions the Japanese would be able to ensure sociopolitical cohesion, approximate German achievements in late development, and win international honor and prestige—which were needed to end the unequal treaties of the 1850s—by associating themselves with the cutting-edge Bismarckian monarchy of social reform.

Less immediately but perhaps more profoundly, organicism, especially in its scientific form, came to represent ineluctable trends of world development to which the realpolitik logic of Japan's national style demanded adaptation and accommodation. Pyle explains how political leaders "displayed a deep respect for the great impersonal forces of history and saw themselves maneuvering within the constraints of these great forces. They referred to the powerful forces controlling their environment as *sekai no taisei* (trends of the world), *jisei* (trends of the time), *shizen no ikioi* (natural forces) or *hitsuzen no ikioi* (inexorable forces), all terms denoting the dynamic force in human affairs impelling events that is beyond the ability of leaders to control."[48] Drawing on Kosaka Masataka's conclusion that, for the Japanese, "norms are considered to be created nature, not men,"[49] Pyle suggests that this meant conventions and institutional arrangements must be revised to align with such "trends and forces"—thereby limning a trajectory that could be understood as not only historical but cosmological. Divining and adapting to inexorable trends was the realpolitik formula for survival and prosperity.

In the late-nineteenth-century "world Japan entered,"[50] the understood "*sekai no taisei*" (trend of the world) was one of universal progress driven by the processes delineated by evolutionary science. According to Pyle, the strategically minded Meiji leaders quickly grasped this reality and "read-

46 Dickenson, *War and National Reinvention*, 22.
47 Ibid.
48 Pyle, *Japan Rising*, 51–52.
49 Ibid., 50.
50 Ibid., 6.

ily adopted the vocabulary of Social Darwinism and spoke of *jakuniku-kyō shoku* (the strong devour the weak) to describe the mores of international politics."[51] However, while Pyle is correct to assert that these leaders strove to socialize the state "into the prevailing norms of this new order"[52] as a means of ensuring national survival, he is wrong to suggest they simply appropriated a laissez-faire "social Darwinism" based on the survival of the fittest. Instead, they envisioned the struggle for existence as a conflict between nation-states, a stance which implied that the life within the nation was not to be a site of struggle but a harmonious order coordinated to support the larger entity. In other words, nation-states had to internally function as organisms in their own right in order to survive and thrive: they needed not only to restrict competition to the struggle against other national organisms but to instill in the members of the nation a predisposition to behave like body parts or cells—lesser selves that identified with and were utterly subordinate to the greater self of the state.

The "corporatist biology"[53] that German universities began to teach the growing numbers of Japanese *ryūgakusei* (foreign students) in the biomedical fields from the 1880s onward both shaped and helped lend scientific credibility to this outlook.[54] Oka Asajirō was one such foreign student and in Chapter 2 we will see that evolutionary morphology, the research program in which he received training, offered a "biological synthesis of Darwinism with cell biology and embryology."[55] Promoted vigorously by its founder, Ernst Haeckel, this "organicist Darwinism"[56] became the basis of "an organicist consensus by the 1890s" in which "Darwin's most original contribution to evolutionary theory, that of natural selection, was often lost from sight."[57] It was this organicist evolutionism that came not only to stand

---

51   Ibid., 78.

52   Ibid.

53   Weindling, *Health, Race and German Politics*, 45.

54   Hoi-Eun Kim thoroughly documents the interaction between the burgeoning Meiji biomedical community and German science in his recent *Doctors of the Empire: Medical and Cultural Encounters between Imperial Germany and Meiji Japan*. According to Kim and William Johnston, Rudolf Virchow's *Cellular Pathology* remained the basis of medical training at Tokyo University during and after the time Oka was a student. This is significant not only because Ernst Haeckel was a student of Virchow, but also because he derived hierarchy of organic individuality from Virchow's system. See Kim, *Doctors of Empire*, 127–28; Johnston, *The Modern Epidemic*, 168; Weindling, *Health, Race and German Politics*, 38–39.

55   Weindling, *Health, Race and German Politics*, 27.

56   Ibid., 47–48.

57   Ibid., 27.

for the inexorable forces of nature and trends of the world but, by portraying human nation-states as *Gesamtpersons*[58]—that is, "total persons," overindividuals, superorganisms, corms, or, in Oka's parlance, "ideal" or "consummate groups"—pointed the way, as we will see in Chapter 3, to comprehensive scientistic extrapolations of examples of organic cohesion in nature onto human affairs. The physiological integration of organisms would become an indicator of health and, by extension, an ultimate measure of value. In the end, the epigenetic unfolding of the organic process would aspire to religious-like authority, a final cosmological trend that both captured the system of norms (nomos) and offered a means to manipulate national life so it could be regenerated back into a future semblance of original health.

As we will see in Part II ("Metapolitics") and Part III ("Regeneration"), Oka's move from a reformist metapolitics to a totalistic vision of national destiny that imagined the eugenic production of new human beings was provoked by the difficulties he would encounter in inculcating his evolutionary conception of interdependence. Such "soft organicism," he would decide, was not sufficient to deal with the anomy that modern life had brought on and, as a result, he would, following the lead of Haeckel and members of the eugenics and racial hygiene movement, expand his organicism into a fully developmentalist, temporal cosmology—a "hard organicism" that more consistently embodied the ontology of embryology and cell biology. Our third chapter will dub this more vigorous and invasive imposition of organic processes of growth onto human affairs, "generative scientism." Coupling norm-generating values of health with eugenic techniques of regeneration, this programmatic outlook will enable the *shinkaron* of *Evolution and Human Life* to move beyond mere reform and compete with the emerging orthodoxy that had its own theocratic formulae for restoring cohesion and reversing national dissolution.

---

58 Ibid., 30–31.

CHAPTER 1

THE ORGANIC STATE:
THE IMPERATIVE OF ETHICAL LIFE

Religion and morality together try to prevent wrongdoing before it occurs.
OKA, 1907[59]

Oka's selection of the superorganism as a moral-political exemplar was not a matter of happenstance. The developmental state that the Meiji oligarchs constructed to achieve their goal of a "rich nation, strong army" relied predominately on a state-science tradition that featured the Hegelian concept of the nation-state as an organism as its basis. A pragmatic means to promote strength through unity and to preempt dissent, this organic theory set the parameters for Japanese political debate until 1945. It was during the years that Oka Asajirō was an undergraduate at the Imperial University in Tokyo, which had been set up to groom the "universal class" of bureaucrats who would administer this state, that signs began to appear that the modern society that was coming into existence with the new constitutional order might, in fact, undermine national cohesion. In response, this statist intelligentsia, in the lead-up to the promulgation of the Meiji Constitution in 1889, resorted to emphasizing a central feature of state science—the imperative for *Sittlichkeit* or "ethical life"—in order to counteract dissolution and fuse society and state into a single entity.

Rooted in customary practice, ethical life, as conceived by this Hegelian tradition, tried to engender cohering tendencies within civil society not through external, abstract mechanisms but via the internalized, concrete bonds of community which were conceived as emanations of an underlying

---

59   Oka, "Risōteki Dantai Seikatsu" [Ideal group life], 71.

ultimate reality. An ontologically grounded credo would perform the work of englobing the disparate elements of the national society in a manner that brought them into concert with each other and the interests of the state. The nation-state would behave like an organism with the specialized parts, which had differentiated in the process of historical growth, voluntarily re-embedding themselves into the national body. Not only the administrative mechanism used to promote strength through unity but the imperative for an ethical credo that resonated with pretheoretical cultural practice accompanied this organic or fused state.

Out of the attempt to delineate such a credo and establish its ontological ground two sets of statist responses arose in the 1890s. On the one hand, a reactionary group took a fundamentalist approach that grounded the credo in religious ritual and legitimation and construed the organic or fused state as absolutist. On the other hand, a more loosely defined reformist group took a scientific approach that grounded national doctrine in the investigation of developmental trends and construed the fused state as a technocratic order. While the reformists would eventually include a subfaction that famously questioned the place of sovereignty in the constitutional arrangement, the more basic conflict was between those who wanted to preserve statist unity by returning to an unchanging past and those who wanted to realize the same ends through an indigenous co-option of world historical developments—a process of adaptation that Itō Hirobumi called the "normalization of trends."[60]

In this chapter we will situate Oka's early career within this reformist approach to the question of the state's ethical life. After describing organicist state science and the centrality of ethic life (*Sittlichkeit*) to the *Modell Deutschland*[61] that the Japanese appropriated through their German advisors (such as Lorenz von Stein), we will address how the attempt to craft an ontologically grounded national doctrine around the nomos of the *kokutai* (national body) produced the two approaches to which we have alluded. Oka's studies at Tokyo University in the late 1880s were undertaken against the background of this concern for grounding and stabilizing the customary ethical basis for nationalism and social cohesion. Though his use

---

60 Pyle, "Meiji Conservatism," 123.
61 Lehmbruch, "The Institutional Embedding of Market Economies," 60.

of superorganisms will be shown to have been foreshadowed in the writings of the most prominent of the reformist statists, Katō Hiroyuki, Oka's thorough scientific training in corporatist biology brought with it a more complete organicism that regarded wholes as prior to and more than an aggregation of constituent parts. In his *shinkaron* egoism—individualism that would not subordinate itself to the organic state—became the source of dissolution and the "way" grounded in nature—his version of ethical life—was devised to reembed individuals in the state organism. Internalizing this way through instinct will be his formula for achieving the ethical life necessary for a viable organic polity.

THE USES OF ETHICAL LIFE

For the Meiji oligarchs the lure of organicism was the practical solution it offered to a primary problem of the era: how to preempt the sociopolitical disunity that seemed destined to accompany modernization. Faced with the challenges of followership but also aware of the social problems that had come to plague the front-running industrialized nation-states, Itō Hirobumi, Yamagata Aritomo, and the fellow former samurai that had founded the new order quickly came to regard the People's Rights Movement of the early Meiji era, which was agitating for liberal democracy, as the local manifestation of what Itō called in 1880 a "general trend sweeping the whole world." "A tremendous force" that would eventually transform nearly all governments, this trend had started with the French Revolution and often brought about "violent disturbances" in the "change from new to old," some of which "lasted to this very day." According to Itō, the only way to prevent such disturbances—which would prove fatal to a nation such as Japan encircled by hostile powers with which it was desperate to catch up—was to get out in front of this trend and control it by channeling otherwise unruly democratic impulses toward nationalist ends: "An enlightened ruler and his wise ministers would control and divert the force towards a solidifying of the government. To achieve this, all despotic conduct must be abandoned, and there can be no avoiding a sharing of the government's power with the people."[62]

---

62 Pyle, "Meiji Conservatism," 122–23.

Though they had the emperor issue an imperial rescript in 1881[63] promising a constitution by the end of the decade, the oligarchs never intended to erect a political order with power sharing along liberal democratic lines. Instead, they deliberately rejected the Western liberal prioritization of social contracts and individual natural rights and turned to what Kenneth Pyle calls the "conservative reform tradition of German political-economic theories."[64] In particular the formulas for nation-building advanced by German *Staatswissenschaften* (state science) and related organicist economic doctrines promised to supply preemptive solutions to the problems that seemed destined to threaten Japan's very survival: social-political integration, late development and imperialist competition. In 1889 the emperor handed down a constitution to the people that would enshrine this German alternative to liberal pluralism and set Japan on the course of a bureaucratic statism that influences its politics to this day.

To begin writing this constitution Itō returned to Europe and sought out the advice of Lorenz von Stein, Rudolf von Gneist, and other leading state-science theorists.[65] A Hegelian who had investigated the emergence of socialism and communism in France between 1789 and 1830, Stein's approach was especially conducive to Itō and the other oligarchs. Not only had Stein received the Iwakura mission back in 1873, but he kept up a correspondence with fifty Japanese contacts during his lifetime.[66] In 1882, after meeting personally with Otto von Bismarck and studying under one of Stein's close colleagues, Von Gneist, Itō spent six weeks in Vienna with Stein himself, sitting for seventeen private lectures on German constitutionalism, social classes, political parties, social reforms, elections, and the Prussian-style civil service.[67] Itō also arranged for Stein to lecture the Meiji emperor, which he did by giving a series of presentations to Fujinami Kototada, the imperial chamberlain, "as if he were talking to the emperor in person."[68] The chamberlain then returned to Japan and, over the course of thirty-three evenings, repeated what he had learned to his imperial majesty.

63 Pittau, *Political Thought in Early Meiji Japan*, 92.
64 Pyle, "Meiji Conservatism," 123.
65 See Martin, *Japan and Germany in the Modern World*, 33–36; Lehmbruch, "The Institutional Embedding of Market Economies," 52–56, 60–62; Coker, *Organismic Theories of the State*, 66–73; Cumings, "Webs with No Spiders," 87–90. For Stein's political writings, see Von Stein, *The History of the Social Movement in France*.
66 Lehmbruch, "The Institutional Embedding of Market Economies," 61.
67 Ibid., 60.
68 Nishiyama, "Lorenz von Stein's Influence on Japan's Meiji Constitution of 1889," 54.

Stein's state science possessed such tremendous appeal to the oligarchs due to its formula for preempting the enervating antagonisms that followed the twin revolutions of industrialism and participatory government. In Stein's historicist schema these antagonisms were inevitable: he "saw the development of industrial capitalism as creating acquisitive instincts that if unchecked would lead to the dominance of the bourgeoisie"[69] and a showdown with other classes. To neutralize these threats he advised setting up a transcendental institutional power, a "monarchy of social reform,"[70] that would work to advance the interests of the nation as a whole. This apolitical bureaucracy would function above the friction of parties and other factions. It would also use its executive authority to steer market forces toward national aims and to reconcile the latently revolutionary working class to the political economy through the distribution of welfare benefits. The economy, the arena where "acquisitive instincts" might provoke social eruptions, would be embedded safely within the state.

Seeing it as particularly alluring to Northeast Asian nations as a result of their long histories of bureaucratic leadership, Bruce Cumings has referred to this conception devised by *Staatswissenschaften* as a "fused state."[71] According to this *Modell Deutschland*, the modernization goals of late-developing nations could be achieved if enlightened ministers acted in the interests of the nation-state and worked proactively to ensure social harmony and stability. State and society would be fused into one, an organic whole devised by transcendentally positioned bureaucrats who would protect the communitarian harmony that industrialization, global markets, and bourgeois individualism promised to leave in tatters.[72] Such a model must have seemed particularly appropriate because of the successful unification and ascendancy of the Second Reich after centuries of inner division. To former samurai raised in the final years of the fractured Tokugawa polity, the achievements in education, science, technology, diplomacy, local administration, philosophy, military affairs, institution building, and social reform that typified Bismarck's regime made the adoption of this fused state

69 Pyle, "Meiji Conservatism," 123.
70 Lehmbruch, "The Institutional Embedding of Market Economies," 60–65.
71 Cumings, "Webs with No Spiders," 88.
72 Pittau, *Political Thought in Early Meiji Japan*, 187.

approach—to which, in large measure, they attributed its successes—seem imperative.[73]

In essence, the fused state of state science is Hegel's organic polity updated in light of the class antagonisms, political revolutions, industrial innovations, and scientific advances that characterized the mid-nineteenth century. In his *Philosophy of the Right*, "Hegel constantly refers to the nation-state as an organism."[74] For instance, in the third part of the book he describes "the constitution of the state as "in the first place, the organization of the state and the self-related process of its organic life, a process whereby it differentiates its moments within itself and develops them to self-subsistence. Secondly, the state is an individual, unique and exclusive, and therefore related to others."[75] What qualified it as an organism and not just a machine or dead mechanism acted on externally—which was how idealists viewed liberal, natural right regimes founded on the social contract—was the inner teleology of this "self-related process": this served as a shared overarching purpose that bound the differentiated parts together and subordinated them to the interests of the polity as a whole—the integrated organic "individual, unique and exclusive." Hegel portrayed this communitarian glue as the ethical life (*Sittlichkeit*) of the nation-state, and it was conceptualized in a manner intended to keep one particular element within that nation-state in line: civil society—that is, the *bürgerliche Gesellschaft*. It was this stratum of aspiring laissez-faire liberal individualists that the French and industrial revolutions had brought into being and who were now "sweeping the whole world."

The state-science tradition Hegel founded warily eyed this bourgeoisie and the unregulated commercial arena it desired. He and his followers believed such supposedly autonomous individuals misconstrued the nature of freedom, regarding their personal achievements as due solely to their own efforts and not, as was really the case, to the fortunate consequence of having been embedded in a community that facilitated the actualization of personal potential. Having overlooked their historical debt to community, these "autonomous" individuals not only treated the intricate web of norms,

---

73 Dickenson, *War and National Reinvention*, 22; Lehmbruch, "The Institutional Embedding of Market Economies," 59–68.

74 Beiser, *Hegel*, 239.

75 Hegel, *Philosophy of Right*, 174.

conventions, and laws (nomos) as something to be negotiated and constructed from scratch according to self-interest, but they never settled on an ontological substructure to undergird this fragile nomos. Without a stable and coherent customary world in common, such a civil society threatened to become a mere mass of disconnected individuals—something latecomers to industrialization could especially ill-afford. The organic state would prevent this debilitating fragmentation and atomization by "englobing" individuals, families, and the state with ethical life—an inner teleology that would fuse and coordinate these facets of the nation-state into a single living entity. The nation-state would thereby achieve a higher individuality once its constituent parts were animated with a collectivist ethos. In Stein's rendering this "supraindividual" was imagined as a "personality." In his words, these personality-possessing states were to be thought of as "independent organisms endowed with their own form, content, and independent destiny for the whole."[76]

This Hegelian provenance is important in the Japanese context because the ethical life of the organic state did not simply meet the practical aim of achieving unity by coordinating society in support of the polity. It simultaneously established national goals as the overarching purpose for life by granting the state status as a metaphysical ground. In other words, even as the mechanisms of the organic state unified the people it also provided them with a horizon of meaning that forestalled the anomy which the oligarchs so feared. For all the exhilaration of *bunmei kaika* (civilization and enlightenment) in the 1870s, the prospect of a national society in which norms, conventions, and laws were open to negotiation and in which the nature of ultimate reality was left indeterminate was both disorienting and dangerous for a nation struggling to maintain its autonomy against ominous external threats. Though scholars today tend to downplay the metaphysical aspect of the Hegelian political philosophy, it was, in fact, a solution to the practical problems of encouraging development and preventing degeneration into anomy that the organic state offered along with its bureaucratic efficiency. Hegel's conception accords ontological significance to the state, for, as Charles Taylor explains, "the public life of the state has this crucial importance for men because the norms and ideas it ex-

---

76 Coker, *Organismic Theories of the State*, 68.

presses are not just human inventions. On the contrary, the state expresses the Idea, the ontological structure of things … the formula of rational necessity underlying man and his world."[77] While it is doubtful that they became thoroughly versed in Hegel's metaphysics, the ontological heft of his conception of the state—the religion-like norm-engendering cosmic role he assigned it as "the world-spirit marching through history"—does not seem to have been lost on Itō and the other oligarchs. For them the practical goals of the constitutional system coincided with ideological ones: fusing society into an organic whole went along with defining the ontological horizon that validated the consensus-based normative sociopolitical order and thereby prevented anomy.

This comingling of practical and ontological ends would produce a complex legacy. Led in theory by a transcendental cabinet, Japan's bureaucratic monarchy of social reform did indeed come to feature a highly successful program for national development: a powerful civil service, a centralized system of local administration, and a market economy that was "institutionally embedded" in the activist state,[78] all of which facilitated integration, modernization and nation-state survival. However, what seemed less certain was the potential for such an ostensibly secular state to organically envelope its subjects within a new horizon of meaning that coordinated their plans and projects with those of the nation as a whole. During the 1880s ideological agents both inside and outside the government were fearful that the coming constitutional order would empower an anomic civil society and thereby destroy national unity. As a consequence they put considerable effort into "denaturing politics," depicting it as merely self-interested and therefore something illicit, "unpalatable,"[79] and in direct opposition to the "nonpartisan neutrality" that a proper government should exhibit. By the end of the decade "a commonplace perception" had emerged that there was a "need for social-moral bonds to draw the country together under its new constitution."[80] A "civic creed"[81] was required that would, as Yamagata put it in his "line of advantage" speech, "unite the minds of the people"[82] and make

---

77 Taylor, *Hegel*, 386.
78 Lehmbruch, "The Institutional Embedding of Market Economies," 61–68.
79 Gluck, *Japan's Modern Myths*, 60.
80 Ibid., 110
81 Ibid., 127.
82 Ibid., 119.

devotion to the nation "second nature."[83] It was with a mind to not only forging such a social morality that would establish a sense of nation but placing this ethos on firm ontological foundations that Itō Hirobumi inserted the "main tenet" of what would become "state Shinto" in the first article of the Meiji Constitution: "[T]he Empire of Japan shall be reigned over and governed by a line of Emperors unbroken for ages eternal."[84]

Along with Article 3 which described the emperor as "sacred and inviolable,"[85] this initiative to foster an aura of permanence around the new nomos by implicating it in a cosmic framework was carried out against the council of Itō's trusted advisor on the constitution, Herman Roesler. In keeping with Stein's Hegelian state-science outlook, Roesler believed the organic state should be ontologically shored up by fitting it within the developmental trends of history. Thus, he wanted the first article to stress the continuity of imperial rule, reading "the Japanese Empire is one indivisible constitutional monarchy."[86] If Itō had learned anything from his German teachers it was that one had to "control the trends" and "set the pace of progress"[87] in order to preempt subversive pluralism. However, Itō had also drawn his own conclusions about the need for religious legitimation from his exposure to contemporary Europe. At the beginning of deliberations on the draft of the new constitution he argued that "[i]n Europe, religion is the foundation of the state. The feeling of the people is deeply penetrated by and rooted in religion. In our country, however, the religions represent no important force. In our country what alone can be the foundation is the Imperial House."[88] Although it rubbed against the rationalist sensibilities of Roesler, this call for sacralization did not represent a break with organic theories of the state. Indeed, Itō and the other oligarchs, in paying reverence to an ontological pivot or axis[89] of the nation were closer to the original pre-Bismarckian formulators of the organic theory, who longed for national unity amid division, than Stein, Roesler, and other contemporaries who took such unity for granted after 1870.

---

83 Ibid., 118.
84 Skya, *Japan's Holy War*, 44.
85 Ibid., 45.
86 Ibid., 44.
87 Pyle, "Meiji Conservatism," 123.
88 Skya, *Japan's Holy War*, 44.
89 Pittau, *Political Thought in Early Meiji Japan*, 177.

This attentiveness to the function of metaphysical grounds in the organic state can be seen in how the civic credo that the oligarchs contrived along with the constitution was designed to serve as a *Sittlichkeit* in the Hegelian sense—an englobing, customary, communitarian, lived-ethos that would fuse state and society into a single entity. The culmination of a decade-long discussion on the need for customary nomic foundations, an Imperial Rescript on Education, promulgated in 1890, articulated the cosmically grounded "Way" for subjects to follow. To anchor this "Way" in the ontological order, the diverse compilers of the Rescript, in keeping with Aizawa's Mitogaku writings of the 1820s, construed the imperial line "unbroken for ages eternal," cited in the constitution, as Japan's *kokutai*—national essence, body, or structure—"coeval with heaven and earth."[90] This construct satisfied not only traditionalists such as Motoda Eifu who desired a national doctrine on a Confucian basis, but, more importantly, Hegelian-trained state theorists such as Inoue Kowashi who regarded the concept of *kokutai* as a manifestation of Japan's ethnic heritage, a product of nonreligious "national classics" that could play the same role as the "science that in the West is called 'philosophy.'"[91] Though "mixed and homogenized" this civic morality, which some in the press called "*kokutai-ron*,"[92] met with a positive and even "matter-of-fact" reception, mainly because it managed to express, as *Sittlichkeit* was meant to do, a "familiar code of customary morality."[93] Attuned to the cultural background and invoking metaphysical grounds, the "Way" mentioned in the Rescript was geared to turning the largely pretheoretical "ethical life," embodied in norms and conventions, into a unifying "sense of the nation."[94]

REFORMIST STATISM

The fusion of state and society envisioned by the crafters of the new constitution did not ever materialize. This "ambiguous document,"[95] as Joseph Pittau called it, did anything but avoid the pluralism and anomic contestation that it had been designed to preempt. Instead of promoting harmony,

90 Pyle, "Meiji Conservatism," 126.
91 Gluck, *Japan's Modern Myths*, 123.
92 Ibid., 125–26.
93 Ibid., 127.
94 Ibid., 112–13.
95 Pittau, *Political Thought in Early Meiji Japan*, 1.

the constitution resulted in gridlock. The Diet, which opened in 1890, had been conceived as playing a "mediating" role in the state, meant to siphon off discontent in harmless debate while helping to project an illusion of accountability needed for subjects to participate in the government's plans and projects. The one concession to legitimate accountability granted by the constitution was the power of budgetary oversight: failure to win the approval of the lower house meant a reversion to the budget of the former year. Against the background of ever-increasing outlays needed to support imperialism in the 1890s, this loophole enabled elected members to hold the transcendental bureaucracy hostage to their demands. In particular, liberal-oriented former oligarchs, many of whom had been ousted from the government in 1881, won election to office, formed parties, and began the long process of trading budgetary support for policy concessions, bureaucratic positions and, eventually, cabinet posts. However, in the very first years of the Diet these parties used their veto discretion over the budget in a manner that directly appealed to their constituents: to try to lower taxes. The oligarchs responded to these tactics by repeatedly dissolving the Diet, doing so a total of six times between its opening in 1890 and the Sino-Japanese War which began in 1894.

These "implacable hostilities between the oligarchy and the parties"[96] led, according to Walter Skya, to "mounting fears among the intellectual and political elite that the country was steadily descending into political chaos."[97] The immediate response to the appearance of this seemingly uncoordinated civil society was to reinterpret the civic creed of the Rescript on Education as enunciating a "collective patriotism"[98] that would morally obligate subjects to the state. Enlisting the Todai philosopher Inoue Tetsujirō (1855–1944) as an author, the Ministry of Education in 1891 printed and distributed four million copies of an official commentary on the Rescript. Inoue had spent 1884 to 1890 in Germany studying idealist philosophy and entertained grandiose ambitions to construct an intellectual system that would encompass both Western and Eastern traditions.[99] Along with fears of internal political disorder, his commentary was writ-

---

96 Pyle, *The Making of Modern Japan*, 162.
97 Skya, *Japan's Holy War*, 49.
98 Gluck, *Japan's Modern Myths*, 130.
99 Ibid., 129. See also Inoue, *Chokugo Engi*.

ten in response to the sense of an emerging international crisis brought on by the Russian empire's eastward railroad construction and growing friction with the Qing over Korea. A founding member of the Oriental Society that, in the face of threats from Tsarist Russia and Qing China, promoted an aggressive foreign policy that included treaty revision and imperial expansion on to the Asian continent, Inoue interpreted the ethos of the Rescript as preparation for a coming national emergency: "If we do not unite the people, fortifications and warships will not suffice. If we do unite them, then even a million formidable foes will be unable to harm us."[100] According to Carol Gluck, Inoue's collectivist patriotism sought to achieve this unity by wedding "Confucian analogies of ruler to father and Western organic theories of the state."[101] The result was a rudimentary formulation of what would become a central feature on the Japanese ideological landscape: the conception of the nation as a family-state.

Though grounded in the national heritage, Inoue's civil morality was intended to be secular. In Gluck's view he and many other Meiji intellectuals with his background kept a "scientific" distance from religion.[102] In Inoue's case this extended to open hostility toward Japanese Christians whom he publicly accused in 1892 of "nonnationalism"[103] for their divided loyalties. In his account of European history, nationalism (*kokkashugi*) had been initially developed by the rationalist Greeks and Romans and modern science had only been able to reemerge due to the decline of Christianity. Japan possessed a "civilizational advantage" because it was "free of any religious affiliation" and could therefore "conduct a pure form of moral education."[104] It was from this perspective that Inoue not only offered utilitarian explanations of the Rescript's collective patriotism but argued that Japan alone possessed the spirit of modern scientific progress in the East.

In his essay on "Meiji Conservatism," Kenneth Pyle contends that Inoue's rational and utilitarian arguments, despite their wide dissemination, were of limited effectiveness and that it was actually Kuga Katsunan's views from the same period that provided a more viable framework for preserving the kind of civic virtues imagined by the Rescript. Part of a younger gen-

---

100 Ibid., 130.
101 Ibid. See Inoue, *Kyoiku to Shūkyō no Shōtotsu*.
102 Ibid., 134.
103 Ibid., 132–33.
104 Ibid., 134.

eration of fellow journalists and publicists who were questioning the universality of Western civilization amid heated debates over treaty revision, Kuga (1857–1907) presented the "common sentiments"[105] necessary for international competition as a manifestation of "the historic, that is to say, organic relationship between the nation and the individual."[106] In Kuga's ethnic nationalist construal of what looks very much like Hegelian organicism, each nation had its own essence or roots from which it gradually developed a unique trajectory of growth. Provisions of the Rescript, such as "loyalty of all to the Imperial Throne," constituted "historic customs of the Japanese people, the basic elements that support her society"[107] and Kuga imagined social progress unfolding in keeping with the national essence. Worried that Japan would agree to a wholesale adoption of Western legal codes in order to bring the unequal treaties to an end, Kuga and Miyake Setsurei were adamant that their countrymen abandon the universalist attitude from the *bunmei kaika* era which stipulated Japan must follow the historical development of the West. Instead, Japan should nurture and cultivate its own nomic foundations in the spirit of *kokusui hozon* (preservation of cultural essence).[108]

This assertion of ethnic particularism was not, however, a disavowal of the developmental ontology that underlay "Civilization and Enlightenment." On the contrary, Kuga believed that "world civilization progresses through the competition of different cultures."[109] In Europe a culture which "derived from the people" in "the cities and villages"[110] had made enormous contributions to world civilization that the Japanese could not help but admire: "We recognize the excellence of Western civilization. We value the Western theories of rights, liberty, and equality; and we respect Western philosophy and morals. We have affection for some Western customs. Above all, we esteem Western science, economics, and industry."[111] This high esteem, however, should not lead to an indiscriminate appropriation that transformed Japanese into "naturalized Westerners."[112] Rather Japan

---

105 Pyle, "Meiji Conservatism," 112.
106 Ibid., 110. For Kuga's writings, see Kuga, *Katsunan Bushū*.
107 Ibid., 110–12.
108 Ibid., 116.
109 Ibid., 115.
110 Pyle, *New Generation in Meiji Japan*, 95.
111 Ibid., 94.
112 Ibid.

needed to "hold steadfast" to its "special character [*honryō*]"[113] and open its own path to development. While it was certainly necessary to adopt aspects of Western culture that promoted the nation's welfare, Japan's own culture "emerged from the patronage and leadership of the imperial court"[114] and it was on the basis of this continuity, "the evolution of things [that] joins past and present,"[115] that Japan could match the accomplishments of the West. It would not only compete with advanced nations, but participate in the progress of "world civilization" through the actualization of the imperial-based national essence.

The reformist approach to statism that we introduced at the start of the chapter begins from this premise that Japan's destiny ultimately depended on fitting its own modern advancements into an overarching global (or cosmic) trend of development. Rationalist in outlook, these reform-minded statists regarded the *kokutai* as an organizational structure, "a general name," as Itō explained, "for the land, people, language, clothing, shelter, and institutions of state." According to this view "it was only natural that it change with the times."[116] While some, such as Kuga, believed this change had to be indigenously impelled, and others saw Japan following in the footsteps of a universal Western progress, both perspectives shared the basic conceit that institutions had to go through an evolutionary process of adjustment, improvement, and self-realization in order to remain viable in a global order that was itself developmental.

Though Pyle wants to depict the indigenous version of this developmentalism as conservative and distinguish it from the universalist version that he associates with the rationalism and liberalism of *bunmei kaika*, both were in fact reformist.[117] That is to say, they envisioned deploying the techno-

---

113 Ibid.

114 Ibid., 95.

115 Ibid.

116 Gluck, *Japan's Modern Myths*, 145.

117 The problem with projecting a liberal-conservative schematization on Meiji history is not just the Eurocentrism of this move but that doing so tends to segregate any attempt to preserve sociopolitical cohesion from progressive visions of national development. In the mode of not only reformist statists but the biomedical technocrats in Germany who were his teachers, Oka embraced both traditional unity and future-oriented growth. In a sense, Oka's programmatic modernism (see Chapter 7) was a reconciliation between these two impulses which had existed from the beginning of the Meiji era among scientifically oriented nationalists: regenerating the nation entailed returning to an earlier moment of healthy cohesion and replaying the present and future in a manner that claimed the positive advances of modern life. In short, progressivist developmentalism can be employed to rejuvenate past arrangements—not overcome them—in a manner that defies the liberal versus conservative dichotomy.

cratic powers of the organic state to bring society in line with developmental trends. Dismayed by the gridlock of the 1890s, they looked to trained bureaucrats to rationally analyze, manage, and direct these trends. From the perspective of such developmental statism the constitution's "sacred and inviolable" portrayal of the emperor was a useful stabilizing measure that could, perhaps in makeshift fashion, effectively establish *Sittlichkeit* because of its genuine roots in tradition. Whether or not they invoked the concept of *kokutai*, these secular reformists conceived the organizational structure within which the nation's ethical life was enmeshed as the "product of a long evolutionary process and capable of change and development in the future."[118] Attuned to both universal and indigenous trends and relatively open to innovations from without that promoted unity and strength, educated technocrats would steer the development of the "national body" [*kokutai*] by modernizing the organic state from within. Though the imperial house was "an unchallengeable and invulnerable centerpiece of the government,"[119] it was understood that the nature of this cornerstone of moral authority would evolve in concert with the modernization process. The *kokutai*, in other words, was mutable—and it was the task of trained servants of the state to divine internal and external trends and engineer adjustments that would fortify the nation-state through the integrating ethical authority of the imperial institution.

The attitude of reformist statism shaped Tokyo Imperial University (Todai), the institution set up not only to create this "universal class"—which is how Hegel referred to such civil servants—but to systematically appropriate modern knowledge. The effort to import such knowledge, especially in the sciences, began in earnest in the aftermath of the Iwakura Mission at, among other places, Kasei Gakkō, one of the institutional predecessors of what became Todai. Led by Katō Hiroyuki, the one-time tutor of the Meiji emperor and eventual member of the Privy Council and House of Peers, who, as we will explore in a moment, provided a precursor to Oka's evolutionism, Todai started to hire foreign experts and offer lecture courses in a wide variety of academic fields. By the 1880s the university was reversing the process, sending increasing numbers of graduates abroad to retrieve the knowledge

---

118 Pyle, "Meiji Conservatism," 125.
119 Ibid.

needed for Japan's modernization.[120] State science, which we discussed earlier in the chapter, garnered particular attention at the university from the time of Itō's studies under Stein in 1882. However, it was not only the philosophical content of Hegelian state science but the need by the oligarchs to legitimate "the bureaucracy" as "the primary structure of political leadership"[121] that scientific learning and technocracy became deeply interwoven at Todai. Worried that the factional basis of their own power undermined their claims to act for the public interest, the oligarchs sought to perpetuate the statist order they were creating by establishing a civil service comprised of experts who had risen meritocratically through educational system. Though entry into the higher echelons of the state ministries was based on civil service examinations and, thus, technically open to all, the reality was that the "advanced legal education"[122] needed to pass these rigorous tests accorded an overwhelming advantage to Todai graduates. Even after special exemptions for Todai students had been lifted in the early 1890s, graduates of this rarefied public institution "retained a considerable degree of exclusiveness"[123] in qualifying for the civil service and by the end of the Meiji era they "dominated the upper bureaucracy."[124] The situation was so extreme that contemporaries complained that "the university was no longer worthy of the name and should call itself a *Kammerschule* or Bureaucrat Training Institute."[125]

This statist orientation at the university both influenced and was reinforced by academic fields outside the study of law. In particular, students were given access to not just expert knowledge of developmental trends but a presentation of these trends which, like the state-science theories we have already touched upon, attributed them to the process of organic growth. Partly a spillover into other disciplines of organic theories of the state, but mainly a product of an era in which biomedical examples were being scientistically extrapolated on to other fields of investigation—a phenomenon we will explore in detail in the coming two chapters—this organicism offered reformist technocrats analytic tools to realize the cohesion of ethical life and manage the trajectory of growth. Organicism also allowed these sec-

---

120 Kim, *Doctors of Empire*, 54–101.
121 Silberman, *Cages of Reason*, 221.
122 Ibid., 206.
123 Ibid., 205.
124 Gluck, *Japan's Modern Myths*, 55.
125 Ibid.

ular rationalists to paper over the difference between the indigenous and universalist approaches to development. Through the organic conception of progress, in other words, a nation or a society, just like an individual organism, would complete the universal process of reaching maturity but do so according to its own self-generated pattern of growth. The unique features of the nation's heritage would neither mimic nor stand completely at odds with the overriding progressive movement of the world. Instead they would become the basis by which the nation participated and even reaffirmed this progress—but only on its own terms and according to its own timetable.

Along with the statist philosophy articulated by Katō Hiroyuki, whom we will turn to shortly, perhaps the outstanding example of this blend of organicism and reformist statism at Todai was Japan's first major academic economist, Kanai Noburu (1865–1933), whose work led to the dissemination of German economic thought throughout the Japanese bureaucracy from the 1890s onward. Directly inspired by Bismarckian social policy, Kanai returned from his student years in Germany in 1890 to introduce the doctrines of the German Historical School of Economics to Todai. Rejecting laissez-faire and its universalist presumptions, the school portrayed each nation as embodying a unique social harmony that was the outgrowth of its historical roots. Kanai echoed his German mentors—and, indeed, Stein and his Japanese protégé—in believing that preventive action on the part of the state was required to preserve this organic cohesion. Despite the indigenous roots of growth, the overriding universal developments embodied by self-interested individualism, class divisions, and even social revolutions would inevitably come to Japan's shores with the spread of industrialism and the market economy. However, using their historical foreknowledge, informed bureaucrats could preempt these developments by guiding thought in a "positive and harmonious direction" and building social solidarity between classes with Bismarckian welfare measures. What Kanai hoped to establish was a "socially cooperative life based on intimate relations of mutual help and interdependence."[126]

In the aftermath of the Sino-Japanese War of 1894–95, Kanai's disciples, who had formed a widely influential professional organization known

---

126 Pyle, "Meiji Conservatism," 132; Pyle, "Advantages of Followership"; Lehmbruch, "The Institutional Embedding of Market Economies," 62.

as Shakai Seisaku Gakkai (Society for the Study of Social Policy), and others of a Listian predisposition began to conceive of these untoward universal trends as forms of decadence. The term they used to describe this decadence was biomedical: it was a *bunmei byō* or "civilization sickness." This slogan would come to stand for the *shakai mondai* (social problems) that were thought to be plaguing Western industrial societies during this era, problems that included class antagonism, labor hostilities, materialism, decadence, ideological radicalism, decline of cooperativism, and the destruction of rural village life. By the turn of the century a consensus existed among reformist bureaucrats that Japan's status as a late developer presented the nation with the chance to circumvent the "sad and pitiful" troubles that had attended the advent of industrial society in Europe. As Kaneko Kentarō stated: "[I]t is the advantage of the backward country that it can reflect on the history of the advanced countries and avoid their mistakes."[127] By acting beforehand to forestall the spread of the *bunmei byō* contagion, Japan's reformist bureaucracy could preserve the political hygiene of the organic state.[128]

As we will explore in the coming chapters, implicit in this historicist anticipation that unregulated modernization would eventuate in "civilization sickness" is an association of decadence with the breakdowns of norms and conventions—that is, with the prospect of anomy. Organicism's answer to anomy was to posit an integrating counterforce within the potentially atomized civil society that modernization had begun to produce: even as the life of the nation differentiated with the move to industrialization and urbanization, this internalized force would prevent it from turning into a mere mass by compelling its members to cohere into a single body. Through such a "unity-in-difference" the society could take advantage of the benefits of modern specialization without abandoning the concrete relations that were thought to ensure moral, political, and spiritual solidarity. Hegel's *Sittlichkeit* or ethical life supplied this integrating imperative in the state-science thought that Japanese appropriated to train future administrators of the organic nation-state. What the diagnosis of *bunmei byō* reveals is how prone this organicist diagnosis of decadence as a differentiation-without-unity was to a regenerative logic—one in which the cure of present disunity in-

---

127 Pyle, "Meiji Conservatism," 135.
128 Ibid., 129–46; Lehmbruch, "The Institutional Embedding of Market Economies," 59–68.

volved proactively instilling ethical life or its equivalent into the atomizing masses. By using the state to enact preventative measures Japan could overcome decadence and exploit its advantages as a follower country.

EXTREME MEASURES: REACTION VERSUS REFORM IN JAPANESE STATISM

If reformist statists looked to preserve the cohesion of the "national structure" by nurturing its organic development in a manner that forestalled decadence, the reactionaries adopted an opposite approach. For them change itself signaled decay, and it had to be resisted in order to preserve an integrating ethical life. Their *kokutai* was not mutable but a permanent essence, shrouded in mystification and grounded in an unchanging ontological fundament. In order to constantly replenish this national structure and access the cosmology from which it emanated, ancestor worship—the indigenous ritual practice that had allegedly always occupied the core of Japanese communal life—needed to be maintained. At Todai the German-trained head of its law school in the late 1890s, Hozumi Yatsuka, turned this spiritual insight into a reactionary theory of the nation as a family-state. By ritually fusing individuals back into an imagined primordial blood community Hozumi believed this family-state would restore an absolutist order and overcome the political gridlock and social dissolution brought on by modernization and the excesses of constitutionalism.

Hozumi's reactionary statism, especially as laid out in his major work, *National Education: Patriotism* of 1897, articulated the aspirations of a resurgent Shintoism in the wake of the constitution and the Imperial Rescript on Education.[129] Along with the invocation of *"waga kōso kōsō* [our imperial ancestors from Amaterasu and Jimmu through the unbroken line of historical emperors]"[130] in both documents, the depiction of the imperial house as "coeval with heaven and earth"[131] in the Rescript encouraged Shintoists to believe they could regain their proper central station in affairs of state. Though the Meiji state had at its inception briefly attempted to revive the ancient unity of rites and governance (*saisei itchi*), the secularizing policies

---

129 For Hozumi's original text, see Hozumi, *Kokumin Kyouiku.*
130 Gluck, *Japan's Modern Myths,* 139.
131 Pyle, "Meiji Conservatism," 126.

of *bunmei kaika* (civilization and enlightenment) in the 1870s disestablished Shinto as a national teaching. In the 1880s Shinto had been accorded an ambiguous status as imperial rites of state which were understood as separate from religion. Not only the association in the Rescript of civil morality with the *kokutai* but the suggestion by one of its reformist compilers, Inoue Kowashi, that Shinto rites comprised "the source of custom" and "the foundation of the nation"[132] emboldened the Shinto priesthood to lobby for a revival of the Department of Shinto (Jingikan) with full government support and recognition of Shinto's official religious function. By 1900 a Shrine Bureau had been created in the Home Ministry and, though Shinto still had not regained its religious status, it had won preferential administrative treatment which, as we will see in Chapter 6, would expand exponentially after the Russo-Japanese War.

How the Rescript was incorporated into school life added further impetus to this Shintoist momentum in the 1890s. The Rescript was not just recited at schools but a whole ritual apparatus was created around it. Though not officially Shintoist, the placement of the Rescript—and the official imperial portrait that was disseminated to schools along with it—in a sanctified space resonated with Shinto practice and turned the school events where it was read out to instill loyalty and patriotism into the equivalent of religious rites. Like the Shintoists, Hozumi seems to have regarded the establishment of these rituals, which celebrated the unbroken line of the *kokutai*, as an opportunity to convert the emerging civic credo into the central component of his reactionary version of the organic state. Although sharing the concerns over patriotism and the national essence, he presented the family-state, which the reform-oriented Inoue had spoken about in 1891, in distinctly theocratic terms that rendered the *kokutai* an immutable manifestation of a timeless and eternal ontology. In place of the investigation and management of trends, reactionary statism promoted ritual gestures to a sacred reality as the means to establish the integrating social morality required for a cohesive organic state.

In order for his fundamentalism to still count as *Wissenschaft*, Hozumi placed a quasi-biological tribalist construct at the crux of this state theory. The *kazoku kokka* or family-state was thought to be united genealogically into

---

132 Gluck, *Japan's Modern Myths*, 139.

a blood community. This *"kokuminzoku"* or *"Volksstaadt"* (people's state)[133] took on the aspect of a literal extended family with the people (*kokumin*) having been born to branch lines of a central imperial stem-line that sprang from divine ancestors. All Japanese were part of the same *völkisch* or ethnic group because they constituted "blood relations of the same womb."[134] Despite these genealogical origins, this family-state did not affirm the organic process of development. The current head of the imperial stem-line, the emperor, was a descendent of hallowed ancestors but not in the evolutionary sense. Rather, he and, indeed, all previous emperors from Jimmu onward in the lineage were reincarnations of the Sun Goddess: "[T]he emperor is Amaterasu Ōmikami existing in the present."[135] The family-state had not developed but remained the same. This is what was meant by the immutable *kokutai*: the patriarchal structure of a father-emperor ruling over his docile child-subjects had been reborn and would be reborn again in its original form with each succeeding generation. Japan has always been a national household, one in which "the family is a small state" and "the state is a large family."[136]

Ancestral rites were critical to sustaining the absolutist relations of this household because they prevented members of the nation from separating out and embracing an independent moral existence. This is what had undermined, in Hozumi's account of world history, all of the other ethnic states: universal ideals that portrayed humanity as a single community had encouraged private morality apart from the interests of the *Volksstaadt* and this had permanently and fatally weakened the sacredness and stability of law and political authority. Hozumi was particularly alarmed by the Enlightenment-inspired "fads of the decadent West" which would "contaminate the purity of the blood of our ancestors and destroy the wholeness of their customs and religion unwittingly in the name of social change."[137] To combat this corrosive threat which was most pronounced in the spread of individualism, Japanese must see themselves as a blood community of worshipers. By paying ritual homage to their common divine progenitor, the Sun Goddess, they could keep the primordial blood-ties of the eternal *kokutai* alive in the present.

133 Skya, *Japan's Holy War*, 57.
134 Ibid., 56.
135 Ibid., 71.
136 Ibid., 64.
137 Ibid., 75.

The ideological potency of this tribalist concept can be attributed to what Peter L. Berger calls "cosmization." Berger portrays cosmization as the means through which "inherently precarious and transitory constructions of human activity are ... given the semblance of ultimate security and permanence"[138] by "bestowing upon them an ultimately valid ontological status, that is, by locating them within a sacred and cosmic frame of reference."[139] In the case of the family state, Hozumi manages to simultaneously locate the "national body" in two overlapping frameworks of ontological legitimization.[140] On the one hand, the blood relationships, the consanguineous ties that bind members of the state together, justify the tribal order as a manifestation of nature: "Our family state is a racial group. Our race consists of blood relatives from the same womb."[141] On the other hand, the ancestral *kami* or god that gave birth to the nation and survives in the present elevated the family-state to a sacred plane and thereby legitimated hierarchical relations within it. As Hozumi explains: "the ancestor of my ancestors is the Sun Goddess. The Sun Goddess is the founder of our race, and the throne is the sacred house of our race. If father and mother are to be revered, how much more so the ancestors of the house; and if the ancestors of the house are to be revered, how much more so the founder of the country."[142]

The aura of religious reverence attending to this double cosmization was intended to render national morality unassailable and, just as importantly, leave individual subjects with no other choice but to assent. Karl Popper called tribalism's "lack of distinction between the customary or conventional regularities of social life and the regularities found in nature," which "often goes together with the belief that both are enforced by supernatural will," as "the magical attitude toward social custom."[143] With norms and conventions rendered sacrosanct, the "right way is already determined" and the individual rarely finds himself "in the position of doubting how he ought to act."[144] It is to this premoral and, indeed, prepolitical world that Hozumi

138 Berger, *The Sacred Canopy*, 36.
139 Ibid., 33.
140 For a provactive discussion of a possible combinatory paradigm based on hierarchical inclusion during the Meiji Era see Josephson, *The Invention of Religion in Japan*, 23–29, 94-163.
141 Minear, *Japanese Tradition and Western Law*, 74.
142 Pyle, "Meiji Conservatism," 126.
143 Popper, *The Open Society and Its Enemies, Volume 1*, 172.
144 Ibid.

wants to return—a world in which imperial subjects docilely obey the divine, racial *pater familias*, the *tennō*:

> The family state has basically only one meaning: it is that one family forms one state, and one state forms one family; that together they worship parents and ancestors; and that under the protection of their spirits the sons and grandsons come together and fulfill a common life of familial love. The position of the father in the family is that of the spirits of the ancestors; in the present life the father takes their place and protects the sons and grandsons. To be obedient to the family head is to be obedient to the spirits of the ancestors. The throne in the nation is the location of the spirits of the imperial ancestors; and the present emperor sits on the throne in the place of the imperial ancestors and rules the racial descendants beloved of the imperial ancestors. For the race to be obedient to this power is to be obedient to the spirits of the imperial ancestors. The state is a great family; the family is a small state: this is the great basis of the founding of our racial state, and here is the source of our *kokutai*.[145]

Although Walter Skya claims that this schema derives from Hozumi's exposure to absolutist political philosophy, an equally significant source is the Hegelian system in which Hozumi received his academic training. Even if we do not fully accept Popper's verdict that "Hegelianism is the renaissance of tribalism,"[146] Hegel's presentation of the state does—as Itō Hirobumi had perhaps discovered—make available powerful rationales for both absolutism and *völkisch* nationalism which can and have been lifted from the wider context of his political thought. In particular, Popper sees the "so-called organic or biological theory of the state"[147] as facilitating a tribalist reaction to the anomic "abstract society" of deracinated individuals that modernity produces. Whether or not directly inspired by Hegel's ethical life (*Sittlichkeit*), Hozumi's ethos of *kōdōshin*, the "desire of two or more independent elements to become one," was intended to yield an "ideal person" who aspired to "total assimilation into the society, which was a higher organic totality."[148] Such complete transparency to the whole was in keeping with the organic nature of

---

145 Minear, *Japanese Tradition and Western Law*, 80.
146 Popper, *The Open Society and Its Enemies, Volume 2*, 30.
147 Ibid., 173.
148 Skya, *Japan's Holy War*, 69.

reality itself, which Hozumi understood by the concept of *gōdō seizon*, fusion or amalgamated existence.[149] Though he quickly dismissed it as a mere addition to a more basic "ethnic, patriarchal concept of the state," Walter Skya's summary of Hozumi's organic theory of the state backs up what Popper says about tribalist reactions to liberal "open society" and their potential for anomy: "Hozumi's ideas here on the state and society were totalistic; he considered any theory of state and society that did not advocate the total integration of the individual into society as within the orbit of liberal thought."[150]

As we will see in the coming pages, this prescription of totalistic assimilation of individuals as the remedy for the "complicated society" of the Meiji era served not only as a political and ontological curative, but a historical one as well. In Hozumi's case, the disease to be cured was change. What made his Shinto ultranationalism into a reactionary doctrine was the belief that the ethnic, patriarchal national body (*kokutai*) represented a primordial tribal particularism that must be preserved in its original form. The family-state, as embodied in the imperial house, continually revived the *kokutai* because "the emperor is Amaterasu Ōmikami existing in the present."[151] By worshiping and obeying the emperor, totally assimilated imperial subjects reaffirmed their physical and spiritual bonds to the immutable divine ancestor. The present age only secured legitimacy as the never-ending rejuvenation of this apotheosized static past.

In the epilogue we will see that, along with its denial of human invention, the hierarchical, absolutist aspects of this doctrine would lead to a crisis that caused its transformation into an ideology with mass appeal. Our focus here and in the coming chapters, however, is still the late Meiji period and during this time its influence was immense. Not only did Hozumi mentor a generation of other fundamentalist constitutional scholars at Todai, but he would help inspire, as we will describe in Chapter 6 when we return to his contribution, an aggressive social program enacted by both state ministries and nonstate actors,[152] to shape the binding ethical life of the nation-state. According to Kenneth Pyle, by 1900 a "powerful conservative orthodoxy"[153] based on reactionary ideas had taken hold.

---

149 Ibid.
150 Ibid., 70.
151 Ibid., 71.
152 Gluck, *Japan's Modern Myths*, 186–204.
153 Pyle, "Meiji Conservatism," 142.

Those with reformist proclivities recoiled from this reactionary turn. Moderates such as Kuga Katsunan and Miyake Setsurei wanted to modernize and industrialize on the basis of indigenous roots and were dismayed that their notion of *kokusui hozon* (preservation of the national essence) had been warped into a rejection of reform and a stigmatization of change. In Pyle's view, the absence of a social constituency for *bunmei kaika* meant that once oligarchs placed "the full weight of their power behind the new conservative tide"[154] reactionaries were dealt the upper hand. Even though a dual strategy for dealing with *shakai mondai* was adopted that paired a reformist early social policy with the propagation of a collectivist ethic, the imperative for national unity granted special impetus to reactionary formulas for countering the inevitable internal changes of the early twentieth century. In Pyle's words, "Meiji conservatism had set a pattern for handling the problems of industrial society that tended under these circumstances to lead to more and more extreme measures."[155]

Our analysis differs from Pyle's in that it questions whether "conservatism" was really the source of the extreme measures to which he alludes. While he is correct to split off the reactionary conservatives, his decision to label those who wished to use the state to steer development and prevent discord as "conservatives" enforces an artificial distinction, one that inappropriately divides liberals, rationalists, and those who continued to invoke universal developmental trends from the construction of civil morality—that is, a unifying nomos lent stability by an underlying cosmic substrate. This, I believe, represents a fundamental misreading of the *Staatswissenschaften* (state science) thought that became current in Japan—and especially at Todai—from the 1880s onward. As we have suggested, ethical life (*Sittlichkeit*) was integral to Hegelian conceptions of the organic state which were not necessarily conservative, liberal, or reactionary. All three approaches could and did promote civic creeds which were based in customs—and they did so to foster the organic integration of differentiated individuals into the greater self of the nation-state. The real point of contention was not the appropriateness of this organicist model but the means of overcoming anomy-as-decadence and achieving unity. For reactionaries

---

154 Ibid., 143.
155 Ibid., 146.

working within this general statist framework, cohesion would be achieved by enforcing an immutable nomos, one which manifested an unchanging mystical cosmology. Hozumi and the state Shintoists would use the language of the Imperial Rescript on Education and the Meiji Constitution to stabilize an absolutist sociopolitical order under which imperial subjects would cohere into one out of submission to theocratic authority. As Walter Skya argues, such an ossified, top-down form of authoritarianism was never really politically viable over the long term and even those Hozumi personally taught would be eventually forced to devise radical adjustments to render it relevant to members of a modern society.[156]

In contrast, for the more loosely defined reformists—whose statism can actually be said to have predated that of the reactionaries—realizing cohesion meant simultaneously divining and fostering developmental trends. As we have suggested, this reformism ran the full spectrum from, on the one side, simply fitting indigenous developments into the preestablished pattern of universal progress, to, on the other side, nurturing native customs and institutions along their own largely distinct path of growth. However, in each case it was clearly understood that there was something like an overarching cosmology of global progress according to which indigenous developments would be judged and have ultimately to contribute. Equally important is the fact that organicist conceptions, especially those supplied by the state-science tradition that had come to define political theory at Todai, tended to blend the particularistic and the universal, often presenting the transition from indigenous growth to universal progress as seamless. Though for some of these reformists integrative *Sittlichkeit* required nurturing the customs and ideas on offer in the Rescript, for others it was more important to delineate correlates in a modern scientific idiom.

We have already seen an example of the former in how economists at Todai trained in the organicism of the Historical School proposed thought guidance for the incipient *shakai mondai* that their theories anticipated. In the coming chapters we will find that Oka's evolutionism offered an example of the latter option: a binding social morality within the developmental order described by modern science that served as an equivalent for the "way" mentioned in the Rescript. Oka's "way"—or, as he called, the "hu-

---

156 Skya, *Japan's Holy War*, 156–57.

man-way" (*jindō*)—came, in fact, to be preoccupied, much like *shiso zendō* (thought guidance) with decadence, and eventually would become a rationale for invasive state initiatives devised to reverse dissolution and restore nomic unity. It was, we will suggest, such responses to decadence first envisioned by reformist statists that set the stage for "extreme measures" in the future. While reactionaries also deplored decadence, their efforts to turn back to a healthy and harmonious past amounted to reinforcing traditional customs and concepts in the hopes of preserving the sociopolitical hierarchy. As Skya argues, this reaction not only proved ineffective but it provoked radical reimaginings of social morality in the years to come. While Skya has in mind what calls "radical Shinto ultranationalists" who attempted to excise the familialist aspects from Hozumi's version of the *kokutai* in order to devise a totalitarian ideology, it can also be said that Oka's *shinkaron* began to reach for its own total solutions to the problem of degeneration into anomy due, in large part, to the inadequacies of the "way" that reactionaries were trying to inculcate in the school system. The eugenic vision of ethical life that Oka comes eventually around to articulating in *Evolution and Human Life* represents perhaps the most vivid example of the "extreme measures" that emanated from the reformist critique of decadence.

KATŌ AND OKA

The year of Oka's arrival as an undergraduate at Todai—1886—was also the year in which the college was designated as an imperial university. This new status had in no small measure to do with the promulgation of the new constitutional order at the end of the decade which would require, as we have already discussed, scholar-bureaucrats versed in state science. Not coincidentally the president of the university, Katō Hiroyuki, had turned away from liberalism when the promise of a constitution had been made at the start of the decade and began to codify a statist political philosophy of his own. As we will soon explore, his reformist statism drew directly on contemporary evolutionary theory and, thus, set a precedent for Oka's later efforts. Yet before turning to Katō it will be necessary to fill in Oka's early biography in order to suggest how his version of reformist statism could come to combine knowledge of universal development with a binding ethical life or social morality.

An 1890 graduate of Todai, Oka was a product of its intellectual milieu and an example of these proestablishment reformists who were bringing a pragmatic and rationalist developmentalism to bear on the same nation-state that reactionaries would soon try to turn into a tribalist theocracy. Oka was, in fact, groomed for Todai from an early age. After the restoration his father, Oka Shūkō, who hailed from a family of bankers in what is now Shizuoka-ken, was assigned an official post in 1870 to run the government mint in Osaka. An enthusiast of *bunmei kaika*, the older Oka moved his family to the foreign quarter and insisted his children be raised as polyglots, reportedly teaching his second son, Asajirō, the ABCs from the time he was only six or seven days old. Asajirō was proficient enough by his twelfth year to enter Osaka's School for English. This early facility for foreign languages became a theme in Oka Asajirō's life: he eventually came to study twelve foreign tongues and publish over a hundred articles in European languages. He even attempted to devise his own international language, Ji Rengo, while still a university student in order to facilitate the spread of science. In later years he was an early proponent of Esperanto in Japan.[157]

Despite these promising early prospects, Oka's youth would later turn tragic. By the age of sixteen he had lost his entire nuclear family due to a series of illnesses and accidents—the most horrible of which involved a younger sister who burned to death after her kimono caught fire during a trip to the family's ancestral home in Shizuoka-ken. Fortunately, his extended family seems to have come to his aid and he was able to enroll first at the preparatory school connected with Todai and eventually as a special student in the zoology section of the college of science at the university itself in 1886, the year the school received its designation as an Imperial University.[158]

Oka would become only the fifth student to graduate from the zoology section. Written in English, his graduation thesis of 1889 was entitled "Observations concerning Fresh Water Moss Animals (*Kokemushi*)." Not only would its object of investigation come to serve, as we saw in the introduction, as the basis of the scientistic essays in *Evolution and Human Life*, but the question of organic individuality, which the thesis explored, most likely

157 Oda, "Oka Asajirō Sensei no Ōmokage"; Watanabe, *The Japanese and Western Science*, 84; Tsukuba, "Kaisetsu" [Commentary], 430–63.

158 Ibid.

accounts for why Oka pursued his graduate studies at perhaps the most highly regarded laboratory where such questions were investigated in the late nineteenth century: the zoological research institute at the University of Leipzig.[159] The founder and head of the institute, Rudolf Leuckart, had mentored Charles Otis Whitman, an American zoologist who taught for two years at the Tokyo University in the early 1880s, and Iijima Isao, one of Oka's professors during his undergraduate studies. We will extensively deal with the expert knowledge he gleaned in the next chapter.

Upon returning to Japan Oka further cemented his already significant ties to the establishment. In 1896 he had married Iwamura Tsukiko, the daughter of a high official in the Meiji government, and his position at the Tokyo Higher Normal School would serve to further deepen his association with the state.[160] Not only was the college involved in preparing middle and normal school teachers for public school assignments but it worked closely with the Ministry of Education, compiling official textbooks and conducting educational conferences.[161] As a result, Oka was part of a committee for teacher certification within a year of coming to Tokyo, a position he held for the remainder of his career. Even more significant was his inclusion by the Ministry of Education on a commission that was formed in 1904 to put together the first nationally authorized science textbook for use in elementary schools. Oka was chosen to the commission due to the educational ideas advocating teaching science to children that he had put forth in his 1901 book entitled *Education and Natural History*. As Migita argues, Oka indubitably viewed the textbook commission as a vehicle to realizing his plan of educating the Japanese public in evolutionary science, and doing so in a way that would replace superstition. The exclusion of any mention of evolution not only in the initial 1911 version but in all subsequent editions of the elementary school science textbook upon which Oka worked (from 1904 to 1919) would turn out to be, as we will see, a pivotal disappointment in Oka's life.[162] It ultimately pushed him to emphasize the historicist aspects of evolutionism and suggested that national hygiene could only be regained by regenerating an earlier epoch of collective health.

---

159 Watanabe, *The Japanese and Western Science*, 84–85.

160 Tsukuba, "Kaisetsu" [Commentary], 430–63.

161 Migita, *Tennosei to Shinkaron*, 34.

162 Ibid., 108–11.

The same year that Oka began work on the textbook commission he published the book that would transform his life: *Lectures on Evolutionary Theory*. Written in a lively and entertaining colloquial style, its pages replete with aphorisms and full of illustrations, this primer not only became an instant runaway best-seller but remained a highly popular book through the Second World War, appearing in fourteen editions. Its audience seems to have encompassed the entire reading public, ranging from literary intellectuals,[163] political activists, state ideologues, to schoolboys, housewives and the young Prince Hirohito. Migita regards it as largely responsible for the "Darwin boom" of the late 1900s that culminated in the "Conference to Commemorate Darwin" and the "Darwin Festival,"[164] both of which celebrated the hundredth anniversary of Darwin's birth in 1809. By the 1920s, according to Imanishi Kinji, *Lectures on Evolutionary Theory* and Nishida Kitarō's *An Inquiry into the Good* were the two books that students entering universities consulted to obtain a "cultural education."[165] Tsukuba reports that the book was the one item which returnees from Manchuria after the Second World War wished they had been able to bring back with them.[166]

Evolution and Human Life, the work that is the focus of this study, was comprised of the widely read articles, essays, and lectures that Oka began to produce as his reputation was being established by *Lectures on Evolutionary Theory*. As we will come to understand in the following pages, what this best-selling anthology laid out was a biological correlate to the organic state. While the full range of the geopolitical imperatives that preoccupied the statist-oriented establishment intelligentsia find their way into his treatment, one stands out above all others: the need to articulate and inculcate a communitarian ethos that would collect the disparate, individuating elements of the nation into an anomy-dispelling, strength-projecting organic entity. The culmination of ethical life, this organism would not only consanguineously unite the people into a true ethnic nation but provide an ontological framework that would internally shape the cognitive responses of individuals and render the nation-state impervious to anomic dissolution. Hozumi's tribalism was attempting to achieve this unassailable unity by propagating a state

---

163 Matsunaga, "Evolutionism in Early Twentieth Century Japan," 221.
164 Migita, *Tennosei to Shinkaron*, 29–30.
165 Ibid., 72.
166 Tsukuba, "Kaisetsu" [Commentary], 430–63.

religion and Oka, like his fellow reformists, hoped to counter this reactionary gambit by using his expert knowledge to attain some of the same ends through scientific means. In keeping with what appear to be Itō's original intentions for the Meiji state, Oka's vision amounted to a metapolitics that imagined technocrats employing evolutionism to modernize the political order that the constitution had set in place. The expedient fiction of the sacred and inviolable emperor would not be overthrown but, much like the cells and various organs that comprised the state organism, englobed with an ethical life delineated by evolutionary science. As we will see, this internalized, self-regulating ethos came to be identified by Oka with social instincts.

To clarify Oka's status as an establishment-oriented reformist and begin to distinguish the regenerative features of his *shinkaron*, we can compare and contrast him to his forerunner in enunciating a biological correlate to the organic state: Katō Hiroyuki (1836–1916), the first president of Todai and a figure Irokawa Daikichi has called—perhaps due to his having tutored both the last shogun and the Meiji emperor—"the archetypically establishment scholar."[167] Beginning his career as a student of Dutch studies, Katō served in the shogunate's Institute for Western Studies and became the first Japanese to master the German language. His tenure as president of Todai saw, among myriad other accomplishments, initiatives to begin integrating the university into the international scientific community. For our purposes his work promoting biology and evolutionary science, both as an administrator and as a scholar, is of particular significance. This work began with the hiring, in 1877, of the Harvard-trained zoologist Edward Morse. Morse gave lectures on Darwinism at the school and the year after his arrival a Todai biological society, Tokyo Daigaku Seibutsu Gakkai, was founded.[168] In 1879 Morse was succeeded by his compatriot Charles Whitman, who would in subsequent years gain renown at the University of Chicago and establish the oceanographic institute at Woods Hole on Cape Cod. Whitman had been trained in Germany and evidently his harsh criticism upon leaving Todai in 1881 prompted Katō to work harder at build-

---

167 Irokawa, *The Culture of the Meiji Period*, 62.

168 Watanabe, *The Japanese and Western Science*, 41–45; Shimao, "Darwinism in Japan," 93. Yajima Michiko claims that evolutionary theory was first introduced to Japan not in 1877 by Morse, but in 1873 by the German biologist Franz Hilgendorf (1839–1904) at the Tokyo Medical School. See Yajima, "Hilgendorf Predated Morse."

ing foreign connections.[169] During the 1880s there was, as we saw earlier, an upsurge in the number of students sent abroad and to study in Germany, in particular. Oka's embrace of evolutionary morphology, the scientific paradigm we will describe in the next chapter, can perhaps be attributed to students of Morse, Ishikawa Chiyomatsu, and of Whitman, Ijimi Isao, having returned to teach on the Todai faculty after completing graduate work in Germany under world-renowned zoologists. It is no coincidence that the two zoologists in question, August Weismann and Rudolf Leuckart, would become Oka Asajirō's teachers when he traveled to Germany in the early 1890s, with the latter regarded by Oka as a mentor.

Katō began to espouse an evolutionist political philosophy in the early 1880s after a very public turning away from his earlier thought which had, in the spirit of *bunmei kaika* liberalism, attempted to fend off nativism with a conception of the *kokutai* based on natural rights and contract theory. Katō's conversion or *tenkō* was announced just prior to the promise of a constitution—and in the same manner that Itō Hirobumi returned to Europe in search of a political vision that could tame civil society, so Katō renounced his earlier liberalism and embraced an organic form of statism.[170] By Katō's own account it was his encounter with the description of evolutionism in *Sittlichkeit und Darwinismus* (Ethical life and Darwinism) by the Austrian Bartholomaus von Carneri in June of 1880 that convinced him that "we are not 'endowed' with rights; we acquire them" and "that our individually acquired rights are inextricably tied to the fortunes of our country."[171] Carneri was not the ultimate source of Katō's evolutionism but instead he relied on a central intellectual figure of Wilhelmine Germany with whom Carneri and Friedrich Helwald[172]—another writer from the period that Katō frequently cites—were in frequent contact. This was Ernst Haeckel (1834–1919),[173] the Jena University zoologist who, according to Stephen Jay Gould, was not only "the chief apostle of evolution in Germany" but a figure that may have been "even more influential than Darwin in convincing the world of the truth of evolution." His impact beyond the sciences was even more profound: Gould cites a contemporary of Haeckel stating that "there are not many personali-

---

169 Watanabe, *The Japanese and Western Science*, 44; Bartholomew, *The Formation of Science in Japan*, 94–96.
170 For Katō's writings, see Katō, *Katō Hiroyuki no bunsho*.
171 Pittau, *Political Thought in Early Meiji Japan*, 119.
172 Di Gregori, *From Here to Eternity*, 376–92, 427–28.
173 Davis, *The Moral and Political Naturalism of Baron Katō Hiroyuki*, 114.

ties who have so powerfully influenced the development of human culture—and that, too, in many different spheres—as Haeckel."[174] As will be illustrated in subsequent chapters, Haeckel's influence would prove decisive not only for Katō, but for Oka Asajirō as well.

The political philosophy that Katō crafted out of Haeckelian evolutionism and the ideas of related German thinkers was a biological version of reformist statism. It, in other words, sought to align the organic state with the universalist patterns of development described by Haeckel's evolutionary science. However, like many organicist theories, trends of indigenous growth and the overriding progressive ontology were often blended together. As a result, Katō grafted features of tribalist thought, including reactionary notions of the imperial sovereignty based on the *kokutai*, into his evolutionary vision. Serving the government official more than the genuine scholar, Katō's reformism constituted the kind of metapolitics that, as we will show in Part III, Oka's more thorough organicism will be compelled to supersede.

Katō's investment in a universal developmental order is on display in how he builds up his vision of the nation-state. First in his *New Theory of Human Rights* (*Jinken Shinsetsu*) of 1882 and ultimately in his *The Struggle for the Rights of the Strong* (*Kyōsha no Kenri no tame no Tōsō*), which appeared in 1893 in both German and Japanese, Katō recounted how the ego drives inherent in cells eventually evolved into the social organism of the nation-state. Clearly drawing on Haeckel's global best-seller of 1868, *The History of Creation*, which delineated how all of living nature was derived from a hypothetical, soul-possessing unicellular creature he called the *monera*,[175] Katō's account begins with individual cells unconsciously cooperating in response to outside pressure and forming multicellular organisms. This cooperation represents the origins of ethics: not only are good and evil defined according to what benefits and harms such organisms, but the cells adapt in such a manner that they are able to attain indirect ego fulfillment through altruistic conduct toward the organic whole. At the level of individual organisms, including human beings, this process of evolutionary ethics repeats itself, with individuals forming altruistic bonds with others—first through emotional ties to their kith and kin and later through more expedient connec-

---

174 Gould, *Ontogeny and Phylogeny*, 77.
175 Haeckel, *The Riddle of the Universe*, 257.

tions to the larger community. In his summary of Katō's "theory of the natural origins of nations," Winston Davis explains how nation-states, which represent the next echelon of individuality, evolve from this process among humans:

> Typically, what happens is this: At some point in time individuals discover they cannot fulfill their own ego drives by living separately. Even though they are not naturally cooperative, their 'specific natures' enable them to lead a cooperative life and form a larger group if and when it furthers their own interests. Generally, however, these groups are not begun by individuals, but by small kinship groups. The state evolves out of the natural aggregation [shizenteki shūgō] of these families, each family being composed of ego-driven individuals. Just as incorporation in multi-celled organisms enables the individual cell to fulfill its ego drives, so the formation of the state allows the multi-celled individuals that compose it to fulfill theirs. In both cases, the creation of the higher, more complex organism is an unconscious process.[176]

Such nation-states exemplify, according to Katō, the "highest *Über-organismus*,"[177] or superorganisms, in the natural world. Katō's Japanese term for superorganism was *yuetsuteki yūkitai* and he employed the term quite literally: a proper nation, such as Japan, was an actual biological organism, a "natural nation" [*shizenteki kokka*], not a merely "artificially constructed legal person [*jin'iteki naru hōjin*]."[178] Implicit in this portrayal was Katō's Lamarckism, which enabled moral conduct and habits to become a permanent, inheritable physical endowment in the form of acquired traits. More explicit is something we will discuss at length in our next chapter: Haeckel's hierarchy of organic individuality. Haeckel was, in fact, also a Lamarckian and Katō's depiction of the nation-state cementing physical bonds through altruistic behavior in order to achieve the supreme example of organic integration in living nature, the *Über-organismus*, plainly derives its conception from Haeckel's *History of Creation*.

It turns out, however, that the process of incorporating "small kinship groups" into the nation's "natural aggregation" involved more than just altruistic assimilation in Katō's account. The birth of the nation also depends

---

176 Davis, *The Moral and Political Naturalism of Baron Katō Hiroyuki*, 69.
177 Ibid., 38.
178 Ibid., 71.

on the dominance of the strong over the weak. Employing a circular reasoning which claims that the strong possess special rights to freely exercise their power because they are powerful, Katō argues that ultimate unity is enforced within the nation when the strong leaders of kinship groups subordinate weaker members in response to outside threats. As Davis explains: "[T]his external competition creates, internally, leadership in society. Nations come into being after tribal chiefs enslave the weaker members of their own communities. The resulting unity gives these communities the ability to subdue adversaries and incorporate them in expanded federations or empires. Eventually, the chief turns into a king and the nation is born."[179] The role that this dominant tribal chief turned king comes to play in the national superorganism is very specific: he is the "controlling organ" [tōchi kikan], also cryptically referred to by Katō in German as the *Denkcentrum* or thought center, the state executive function. Other aspects of the nation-state are conceptualized as cells or "assisting organs" [hojosha taru kikan] and Katō makes their subordinate function quite clear: "As the auxiliary organs of the state the people have the duty and the right to be controlled by their leaders; and leaders have the duty and the right to control the people who are their own auxiliary organs."[180]

In the Japanese context this "controlling organ" theory of the state would seem to anticipate Minobe and his antireactionary organ theory—except that Katō himself is explicit that his evolutionary approach was meant to "buttress the doctrine of imperial sovereignty [shutaisetsu]."[181] In fact, the reasoning he employs and the conclusion he arrives at come closer to Hozumi's tribalist absolutism than an "organ theory." As Davis summarizes: "Japan's 'patriarchal sovereignty' rests on a natural, filial relationship between the emperor and his subjects. The imperial family is the stem family (sōka) of the people who, in turn, constitute the branch families (shizoku) of the imperial line. This unique parent–child relationship means that in Japan, devotion to the emperor and to the nation is one and the same thing. Following the standard nationalist line, Katō held that the emperor *was* the nation."[182]

---

179 Ibid., 69.
180 Ibid., 73.
181 Ibid., 71.
182 Ibid., 71–72.

What devotion to this quasi-absolutist controlling organ entailed for the cells was embracing their auxiliary status and completely identifying their own self-interests with the higher self of the patrilineal superorganism. "As cells in the body of the nation, individuals fulfill their own 'specific natures' by devoting themselves to the health and happiness of the nation. This is the greatest of their duties. Even if they are unaware of it, they will naturally tend to act this way. On the other hand, because good moral relations between individuals indirectly benefit the state, interpersonal benevolence is the same thing as loyalty or patriotism [*chūkun aikoku*]."[183] Such duty is the *Volksmoral*, Katō's equivalent to Hegel's ethical life. Yet it must be emphasized that for Katō, as it was for Hegel, this ethical life of the *Volk* was not passively imposed upon the cells and organs of the nation-state. Rather it was a morality "artificially selected" by the strong—"tribal chieftains, kings, religious leaders, or wise men"—and then actively "self-selected"[184] by individuals. The strong expediently "encourage, supplement or reform the morality (or religion) that has already evolved, giving it a new shape that enables society to survive and prosper" while cell-like individuals proceed by "selecting those appetites that will benefit society and overcoming those that will not."[185] In Katō's "cellular theory of society" the "exemplary person" was one who was "ready to engage in self-sacrifice for the well-being of the whole."[186] It was such a self-selecting ethical stance that Katō construed as a form of individualism—one which has been "thoroughly imbued with the values and ends of the 'macromulticelled organism,' that is, the nation-state."[187]

Katō's stress on the artificial and self-chosen aspects of ethical life shows that he was still struggling with a conflict from Japanese Confucianism described by Maruyama Masao: that between the ethics of ontology—conceived of as Heaven or the Way—and the ethics of invention (*sakui*).[188] The ethics of ontology, represented by the orthodox Confucian Chu Hsi school of the Tokugawa era, portrayed norms and convention as dictated by the Way, the stratified world of humans justified as an instantiation of the hierarchical ontology of the Heaven. In contrast, the ethics of invention, represented

---

183 Ibid., 73–74.
184 Ibid., 56–57.
185 Ibid.
186 Ibid., 59.
187 Ibid., 60.
188 Maruyama, *Studies in the Intellectual History of Tokugawa Japan*, 189ff.

by the School of Ancient Studies and, later, the Kokugaku School, denied the "lawlike character of heaven" governed the nomic sphere of norms and conventions: these, instead, were created by humans. According to Winston Davis, "Katō Hiroyuki was trying to offer his evolutionary theory of ethics as a third option" beyond this dichotomy which he sees as an Eastern version of the relation between nomos and physis in Western thought. Construing the ontology of Heaven or the Way as "nature" and then linking this naturalism to that offered by modern science, Davis argues that, for Katō, "morality is not created by nature or human artifice working alone, but evolves naturally as a result of the symbiosis of natural and artificial selection. Katō tried to devise a comprehensive theory of biological, social and moral development by subordinating invention (microevolution) to nature (macroevolution)."[189]

In the pages that follow, we will see that Oka Asajirō, at least initially, developed a similar "third option," a "human-way" which he endorsed the shaping of human nature according to evolutionary law. I will argue, however, that this third option between nature and invention was not itself invented by Katō and Oka but instead borrowed from German evolutionism. The notion that morality is the active acceptance of necessity is a commonplace of the idealist tradition out of which Haeckel's evolutionism emerged and has been critiqued extensively by Karl Popper, Friedrich Hayek, and, more recently, Tzvetan Todorov as indicative of scientism, historicism, and philosophical monism.[190] Katō and Oka, as self-conscious proponents of Haeckelian monism, should be understood as having appropriated their ethical positivism—which is Popper's term for this third position[191]—from this source. As we will reveal, Oka's ethical positivism explains how he could be both a champion of enlightenment through science education and a promoter of eugenics and, ultimately, a regenerative nationalism that contributed to fascism.

Ethical positivism fit in nicely with the technocratic attitude that reformists such as Katō and Oka adopted in order to establish a metapolitical basis for the organic state. Attempting to reduce the systems of norms (nomos) to a nature defined by evolutionary science, both men, as we will see in Chap-

---

189 Davis, *The Moral and Political Naturalism of Baron Katō Hiroyuki*, 89.
190 Popper, *The Open Society and Its Enemies, Volume 1*; Popper, *The Poverty of Historicism*; Hayek, *The Counter-Revolution of Science*; Todorov, *Imperfect Garden*; Todorov, *Hope and Memory*.
191 Popper, *The Open Society and Its Enemies, Volume 1*, 71.

ter 5, tangled with reactionaries throughout their respective careers. However, the differences between the two are highly significant and point to why Oka, despite his apparently greater fidelity to rationalist evolutionism, inadvertently found greater potential rapport with the extreme measures that are usually blamed on ultranationalism. While he warned of the dire consequences of reactionary ideology, his solution to the problems with which such ideology preoccupied itself rendered his evolutionism potentially more radical than Katō's.

On the surface Katō would clearly seem closer to the reactionary position delineated by Hozumi's reactionary statism. Not only does he emphasize imperial sovereignty—identifying the emperor with the state—and devise an evolutionary history of the nation that is tribalist, but in later years he sought coexistence with the theocratic orthodoxy. For instance, he, as we will see in Chapter 6, endorsed the political uses of ancestor rites, and, more importantly, refused to question that emperor-centered historical view, pretending that evolutionary history somehow leaves off when it arrives at the appearance of ethnic nations.[192] In contrast, though he never mentions the imperial house and avoids questions of sovereignty, Oka consistently denigrates theocracy. His vision of the state as an organism is more horizontal, not including such hierarchal elements as the controlling *Denkcentrum* organ that Katō imagines. He also, as we will describe in Chapter 6, was engaged in a protracted struggle to displace "superstition" in the public school curriculum and worked to introduce evolutionary theory to the masses both through his popular writings and his efforts on the Ministry of Education's textbook committee. Finally, in an essay published during the first years of the Taisho era, Oka boldly lambasted theocratic government and warned of its fatal liabilities to the scientific and technological prowess of the nation. As scholars such as Migita would argue, Oka's credentials as an antireactionary could not be more unambiguous.

Nevertheless, this greater distance from reactionary positions did not prevent Oka's evolutionism from featuring two elements that would contribute to the radicalization of ultranationalism after the Meiji period. The first has to do with what we will call evolutionary realpolitik in Chapter 4. In contrast to the world organism that Katō imagines eventually evolving

---

192 Migita, *Tennosei to Shinkaron*, 56–57.

out of the nations that occupy the earth, Oka will leave no room for international law or the future *Weltreich*. All he will allow for are temporary expedient alliances between ethnic nations (*minzoku*) and he will depict war as the inexorable natural state between such nations—nations, which, in order to be viable, must be homogenous biological unities. Racial autarky will be the implicit goal of his geopolitics. Conforming the nation-state to the universal pattern of world historical development will not result in the realization of universal harmony but the acceptance of a perpetual total war between incommensurable races.

The second element is equally critical and involves the priority Oka places on organicism. As we have seen, Katō builds up his superorganism out of self-interested individuals: ethics emerges from the expediency of cooperative arrangements, first appearing in cells but eventually on display in individuals within groups who come to regard collective life as the best way to ensure survival and satisfy ego drives. Oka, in contrast, conceives the "ideal group" or superorganism as coming first: it is, as Haeckel explained, a higher order of organic individuality and individual persons should be properly understood as constituents that emerge from and are subordinate to the preexisting whole in precisely the same way cells develop from and support the body of a complex organism. Though he does admit that the cooperation of self-interested individuals can build up the social organism, this is mainly portrayed as a measure to repair the original natural unity of human groups. The purpose of his *shinkaron*, in fact, is to remind members of the Japanese ethnic nation of their proper place within the national organism and to encourage in them the instinctive ethical life that has always held them together with the whole.

Thus, unlike Katō, who extols egoism, Oka will depict it as a sign that a collective ethos has not been internalized and the higher individuality of the nation is disintegrating. For him egoism is anomic and therefore decadent. It is this conceit that will introduce a regenerative rationale into the sociopolitical uses of evolutionism and organic state theory. It will also render Oka's *shinkaron*, despite his defense of scientific method, potentially far more radical than Katō's political thought. Overcoming decadence by reviving the primordial social or nomic instincts of the Japanese *minzoku* will become Oka's quest. In Part II we will see that Oka will initially attempt to engender these instincts through a metapolitics much like Katō's: through education, society could be reformed to match the interdependence seen in superorganismic examples from the natural world. The nomic crisis, as we will call it, after the Russo-Japanese War, will, however, expose the shortcomings of this moderate metapolitics: not only will egoism appear to run amok in a contagion of social fevers but the reactionary attempt to curb these excesses will directly threaten the role of biological science in education, thereby undermining Oka's evolutionist program of reform. Oka's regenerative vision of national destiny, which we will describe in Part III, will represent, among other things, a more radical confrontation between organicism and the dangers of decadent egoism. For Oka the rehabilitation of ethical life and the organic unity it supports will ultimately involve the sort of extreme measures of nomic internalization that Katō was hardly capable of imagining: the use of eugenic science to reengineer the national body and thereby eradicate the kind of egoism that Katō extols.

To more fully understand how Oka's evolutionary version of reformist statism found its way to a eugenic correction of decadence, our next chapter turns to the scientific background of Oka's *shinkaron*.

CHAPTER 2

PALINGENETIC POLYPERSONS:
EVOLUTIONARY MORPHOLOGY
AND THE QUESTION OF
ORGANIC INDIVIDUALITY

Oka became only the fifth student to graduate from the zoology section at Katō Hiroyuki's Todai. Written in English, his graduation thesis of 1889 was entitled "Observations concerning Fresh Water Moss Animals (*Koke-mushi*)." Not only would its object of investigation come to serve, as we have already intimated, as the basis of the scientistic essays in *Evolution and Human Life*, but the scientific problem that the thesis explored accounts for why Oka found himself pursuing his graduate studies under Professor Rudolf Leuckart, a renowned zoologist at Leipzig University. Though Leuckart had mentored Charles Otis Whitman, the American zoologist who taught for two years at Tokyo University in the early 1880s, and Iijima Isao, one of Oka's professors during his undergraduate studies, it was without question the zoological research institute that Leuckart founded at Leipzig that lured Oka. According to Nyhart, this institute was, "between the late 1870s and the early 1890s,"[1] the largest and perhaps the most highly regarded laboratory where the question Oka addressed in his graduation thesis was investigated. This was the question of organic individuality.

As we will see, evolutionary morphology, the scientific paradigm through which organic individuals were conceived, came to serve a double function in Oka's career: it supplied him with both cutting-edge expert knowledge and a means by which to articulate a biological correlate to the

---

1   Nyhart, *Biology Takes Form*, 310.

organic statism that had already gained currency in Japan. In other words, Oka's student years in Germany qualified him to take up the statist idiom of his Todai teachers and infuse it with up-to-date insights from evolutionary biology and, ultimately, eugenics and racial hygiene. This merger of political and scientific organicism, we will come to see, became the basis of his Oka's own reformist approach and, eventually, his regenerative vision of the nation-state.

LEUCKART'S COLONIAL JELLYFISH

Oka's experience as a *ryūgakusei* (foreign study student) was an extension of the reformist statism that had come to prevail at Todai from the late 1880s, the same period the constitution and the Imperial Rescript on Education were being codified. As the last chapter alluded to, numerous figures from the university, including Kanai Noburu, Inoue Kaoru, and even Hozumi Yatsuka, spent years of foreign study in Germany beginning in this period. Not only would they retrieve cutting-edge knowledge from scientific disciplines such as *Staatswissenschaft* but they would gradually help achieve Katō's goal of integrating the university into the international research community. The choice of Germany as a destination, though partly due to the high reputation and open admissions policies of its university system, can be mainly attributed to the fact that "German political philosophy had won considerable favor with the majority of Japanese officials."[2] The trend in favor of German-based *ryūgakusei* study for students in science during the Meiji period is stark: whereas in the 1870s, 27 percent of science students had gone to Germany for their foreign studies—with 20 percent heading to Britain and 35 percent to the United States—in the 1880s the number of German-bound science students shot up to 59 percent, reaching 69 percent by the 1890s, and peaking in the 1900s at 74 percent. Meanwhile, a staggering 90 percent of students sent abroad to study medicine were selecting Germany as their destination. Summarizing about science in the Meiji period as a whole, James Bartholomew concludes that "overall two-thirds of the man-years of study were spent in Germany during the period 1869–1914."[3]

---

2 Bartholomew, *The Formation of Science in Japan*, 71.
3 Ibid.

Oka's entry into Professor Leuckart's orbit at Leipzig University was circuitous: after obtaining a loan through some of his banker relatives in Shizuoka he spent his first year in Germany at Freiburg University studying under another internationally famous zoologist, August Weismann, father of the Neo-Darwinian "germ plasma" theory which many consider the precursor to modern genetics. Oka initially chose Freiburg most likely because one of his teachers at Tokyo Imperial University, Ishikawa Chiyomatsu, had studied under Weismann (see Chapter 1). Yet despite this connection Oka complained that he did not like Weismann's teaching approach, presumably because it denied the central tenet of Lamarckism: the notion that traits acquired during an organism's lifetime were inheritable. A Lamarckian throughout his long career, Oka made use of the liberal enrollment policies at German universities to transfer to Leipzig.

In Oka's words "the three years of study in Germany were for me the happiest years of my life"[4] and he formed an especially close relationship with Professor Leuckart. Upon hearing of his teacher's death in 1898, Oka stated that Leuckart "alone is the man whom I consider to be my master."[5] Beyond personal bonds of affection, what tied Oka so closely to his elderly mentor was the seminal work Leuckart had done on organic individuality, work which had begun well before the appearance of Darwin's *Origin of Species*. During the early years of Leuckart's career, "in the 1850s, defining the individual was a source of considerable controversy in all realms of biology."[6] Leuckart and his contemporaries were particularly perplexed by the structure and function of certain aquatic organisms that displayed the curious ability to live both independently and as organlike parts of a larger living entity. In Leuckart's case he investigated a species of jellyfish called the siphonophores or, as Ernst Haeckel would later dub them, the "social medusae," in which particular jellyfish possessed "swimming bodies" and seemed to be "animated by a unified will"[7] yet also integrated into the colonial life of a larger interfused siphonophore collectivity.

Appearing in his 1851 essay "On the Polymorphism of Individuals, or the Phenomenon of the Division of Labour in Nature,"[8] Leuckart's solution

---

4   Watanabe, *The Japanese and Western Science*, 84–85.
5   Tsukuba, "Kaisetsu" [Commentary], 435.
6   Nyhart, *Biology Takes Form*, 135.
7   Di Gregori, *From Here to Eternity*, 126.
8   Nyhart, *Biology Takes Form*, 96–97; Di Gregori, *From Here to Eternity*, 418–19.

to the challenge these creatures posed to classification was to propose two types of individuality which were closely interlinked. On the one hand, the free-swimming jellyfish were physically discrete and should be conceived of as distinct individuals in the morphological sense. On the other hand, these same medusae bodies were dependent for nutrition and other essentials on the greater whole and were thus subordinated to the physiological individuality of the colony or overindividual. Structured like self-contained organisms yet functioning like organs which relied on a greater being for nourishment, the jellyfish enjoyed a dual existence, half-corporate, half-autonomous—an ambivalent double self whose position in nature Leuckart tried to clarify.

Leuckart's solution to the problem of organic individuality, which would render Leuckart "in many ways the spiritual leader of scientific zoology,"[9] also included an innovative account of how this peculiar arrangement had emerged. According to Leuckart, a temporal process of differentiation had taken place within the siphonophores such that over generations a specialization of function had appeared among the various parts of the feature. As M. Winsor explained, this process was likened by Leuckart to the division of labor within a national economy:

> Just as an organ may be drastically modified according to its function in an organism, so too, said Leuckart, entire individuals may be modified according to their role in the community to which they belong. And how are they modified? In obedience to the principle of the division of labour, answered Leuckart. As early as 1827 it had been suggested that physiological economy, like the economy of a nation, required specialization of function by the division of labour.... Now Leuckart suggested that siphonophores were communities in which the jobs of capturing prey, swallowing food, sensing the environment, and so on were divided up among individuals specialized for these functions. The phenomenon of polymorphism which results from the principle of the division of labour is not limited to the peculiar case of siphonophores, in Leuckart's view.[10]

Not only did Oka Asajirō's investigations into freshwater moss animals or *kanten kokemushi*, which we described in the introduction, closely follow

---

9   Nyhart, *Biology Takes Form*, 310.
10 Quoted in Di Gregori, *From Here to Eternity*, 419.

Leuckart's analysis of "polymorphism," but this implicit analogy between polymorphism and the nation-state became the basis of what we will call his metapolitics. However, to fully appreciate how this examination of individuality and "division of labor" was able to blend together with the idiom of the organic state, as explored in the last chapter, and eventually develop into a vision of national rejuvenation in the face of degenerate anomy, a sense of the research tradition within which Leuckart operated is required. Known as morphology, it was this tradition that, through its struggle to delineate the structures of living nature, injected organicism into biology. For morphologists natural forms came to be seen as the product of developmental patterns which were themselves initiated by underlying organic drives. As P. J. Bowler explains:

> Morphology is the science of form, the attempt to describe the structure of things and to understand the laws that govern the way a certain class of objects is structured. Much of nineteenth-century biology was still essentially descriptive and, hence, morphological in character. It involved the study of the structure of living organisms and sought to explain how the different forms were related to one another. It would be misleading to suppose that the study of form was conducted without any interest in the physiological processes that built and maintained the living body, but all too often it proved far easier to describe form than to understand function. In their efforts to go beyond mere description, the morphologists tried to understand the laws governing the construction of living bodies, but these laws were often conceived in a purely morphological sense. They were not laws of cause and effect as understood by the materialist, but patterns that were seen as limits imposed upon the diversity of natural objects. It was hoped that the bewildering variety of living forms could be unified by recognizing their underlying pattern.[11]

The underlying pattern that most fascinated morphologists was the one that embryology had revealed in the development of growing organisms. Leuckart's groundbreaking work on siphonophore individuality, in fact, comes toward the very end of morphology's early, pre-Darwinian phase—a phase referred to as idealist or transcendental morphology by historians—

---

11   Bowler, *The Non-Darwinian Revolution,* 50.

when studies in cell biology and embryology infused natural philosophy with its central organicist insight based on the pattern of growth. Examining the process of differentiation and continual integration by which embryos "evolved"—the term evolution was actually first used in this context—from single-celled zygotes to mature organisms, idealist morphologists of a romantic disposition hypothesized a generative force inherent in living nature. This developmental impetus, which contained within it a ground plan of the final end into which organic forms would be realized, was all-purpose, occurring at every echelon of living nature. That is to say, not only would it steer the growth of individual organisms to self-actualization as adult forms, but its inner plan metamorphosed into the species extant in the natural world. In the words of the English morphologist Robert Chambers it revealed "the universal gestation of nature."[12]

Perhaps most importantly, idealist morphologists noticed that, in the course of their development, embryos appeared to phase through the mature forms of all of their ancestors going back to the most primitive one-celled life forms. From this observation figures such as Johann Friedrich Meckel drew a basic conclusion that had far-ranging implications for modern philosophy: "The development of the individual organism obeys the same laws as the development of the whole animal series; that is to say, the higher animal, in its gradual evolution, essentially passes through the permanent organic stages which lie below it."[13] Called the law of parallelism or the growth analogy, this developmentalist insight was extrapolated into a conception of the entire process of evolution as unfolding like the growth of an individual organism. Indeed, in the hands of the more mystical and speculative of the romantic nature philosophers, such as Lorenz Oken (1779–1851), not only did particular organisms but species and, by extension, the totality of organic nature itself all constituted organic individuals: the generative force had actualized itself at each of these levels, differentiating into complex living wholes which manifest the unity-in-difference that exemplifies organisms.

It was from the more sober investigations of the most famous of the idealist morphologists, Goethe (1749–1832), that there emerged a mode of analy-

---

12 Ibid.
13 Coleman, *Biology in the Nineteenth Century*, 50.

sis that would help Leuckart explain how the generative force within nature achieved an organic division of labor among siphonophores. Goethe conceived of the generative force as an archetype (*Bildungstrieb* or *Urtypus*), an original vitalistic, form-creating inner plan that possessed a predisposition to metamorphose into the living forms observed in nature. Though he imagined an original archetype of organic life itself, the focus of Goethe's studies was on the "four most basic animal structures" into which this original organic archetype had metamorphosed, namely "the radiata (for instance, starfish and medusae), articulata (insects and crabs), mollusca (clams and octopuses), and vertebrata (fish and human beings)."[14] In particular, he performed studies on the phylum of vertebrates, examining the transformation of mammalian skeletons over generations. In Goethe's reckoning, the abstract pattern of bones laid out in the original vertebrata archetype metamorphosed, through interaction with external pressures of the environment, in different ways to form the various vertebrate species. Individual bones not only transformed into comparable structures but they retained "the same relative position throughout the vertebrates." In this manner, "the bones in the legs of man and steer would exhibit the same abstract, topological relationships, while differing greatly in detail."[15] Goethe called this process homology and he famously employed it to explain how "the bones of the skull were really six transformed vertebrae."[16]

Writing several decades after Goethe's death from a functionalist standpoint that sought to subordinate morphology's teleological inner drive to the physio-chemical workings of the natural world, Leuckart used his own updated version of this organicist metamorphosis to explain the development of siphonophore individuality. In his account the archetype was reconceived as a "teleo-mechanism" that, in the case of the jellyfish colony, attempted to realize the inner plan of its archetype over successive generations via chemical processes. Through interaction with the surrounding environment, the parts of the siphonophore had thus "evolved" its various specialized organs, organs which eventually became morphologically detached free-swimming jellyfish bodies that were, at the same time, physiologically dependent on the colony. As the title of his ground-breaking essay

---

14 Richards, *The Romantic Conception of Life*, 8.
15 Richards, *The Meaning of Evolution*, 35.
16 Ibid., 36.

suggests, it was this complex homological process of organic differentiation that Leuckart used to explain the division of labor—or, as his younger colleague Ernst Haeckel later summarized, "Leuckart suggested that siphonophores were communities in which the jobs of capturing prey, swallowing food, sensing the environment, and so on were divided up among individuals specialized for these functions."[17]

Working within the same organicist tradition that encompassed not only the idealist morphology of Goethe, Oken, Meckel, and Schelling, but the philosophical idealism of Hegel, Leuckart regarded this particularization of function as a process of integration, not disintegration. In adapting specialized functions individual jellyfish were evincing the unity-in-difference that characterized organic life: their self-actualization as specialized individuals ultimately served the needs and final purpose of the organic whole of which they were parts. As in Hegel's system in which ethical life—a manifestation of the underlying evolution of *Geist*—unified the diverse polity into an organic whole, in idealist morphology it was the presence of this self-actualizing engine—for Goethe the archetype, for Leuckart the teleo-mechanism—that caused natural forms to cohere as individuals even as they differentiated.

EVOLUTIONARY MORPHOLOGY

By the time Oka wrote his graduation thesis and headed off to Germany the idealist morphology that Leuckart had employed to analyze siphonophore superorganisms had undergone a decisive transformation. The impetus for this change, Darwin's *Origin of Species*, has often been described as having a revolutionary impact on nineteenth-century naturalism. Yet, as Peter J. Bowler argues, Darwinian natural selection was more a "catalyst" for the reconstitution of prior theories of nature than a completely new paradigm that was accepted by the scientific community. Darwin's theory was "just a steppingstone that helped" biologists "cross over to full acceptance of transformation"[18] in living nature. Especially for mid-nineteenth-century morphologists such as Leuckart, who had been groping to discover a way to reconcile the organicist vision of a teleologically ordered hierarchy of liv-

---

17 Quoted in Di Gregori, *From Here to Eternity*, 419.
18 Bowler, *The Non-Darwinian Revolution*, 67.

ing forms, which they had inherited from Goethe and the *Naturphilosophen*, with the mechanical laws of physics and chemistry, Darwin's notion of species transmuting into one another over time made this reconciliation possible. However, once biologists in the morphological tradition became convinced that transmutation did occur, "they turned their backs on Darwin's message and got on with the job of formulating their own theories of how the process worked."[19] Thus, idealistic developmentalism, or what we have been calling organicism, did not just simply survive Darwin. Instead, in the guise of evolutionism, it adopted "an evolutionary viewpoint within an essentially non-Darwinian framework."[20] Labeled evolutionary morphology by historians of science, it became the dominant theoretical outlook in the late nineteenth century—the organicist paradigm which Japanese such as Oka Asajirō appropriated when they traveled to Germany to study the biological sciences.

The success of this new paradigm, which represented a creative synthesis of many strains of nineteenth-century naturalism, can be attributed primarily to one man, a figure we have encountered already several times in passing: the Jena zoology professor Ernst Haeckel. In Stephan Jay Gould's estimation Haeckel was not only "the chief apostle of evolution in Germany" but was "even more influential than Darwin in convincing the world of the truth of evolution."[21] According to Robert J. Richards, "prior to the First World War, more people learned of evolutionary theory through his voluminous publications than through any other source."[22] Among the science community, the pull of Haeckel's influence can be measured by the fact that "after the publication of his *General Morphology* (*Generelle Morphologie*) in 1866, almost any German scientific writer responding to Darwin also found himself responding to Haeckel."[23] What the charismatic Haeckel accomplished was the conversion of the organicism of pre-Darwinian idealist morphology

---

19 Ibid. Despite his search for a more functional and mechanistic approach to the problem of individuality, Leuckart appears to have accepted the premise implicit in all idealist organicism—namely, that nature was a single overarching unity of life, an organism, and that a developmental impetus from within this organism caused the constituent living beings that comprised it to evolve and cohere in order to realize its final end. One of the more surprising and significant facts about the history of nineteenth-century biology is that not only did morphology (the study of form) survive the Darwinian revolution but it managed to do so with this particular speculative, quasi-metaphysical aspect largely intact.

20 Ibid., 5.

21 Gould, *Ontogeny and Phylogeny*, 77.

22 Richards, *The Tragic Sense of Life*, 2.

23 Nyhart, *Biology Takes Form*, 108.

to a materialist theory of naturalistic descent. This conversion involved accepting the developmental premises upon which the archetype theory had been based and reworking them into a principle of evolution. "Biogenetic law" is the neologism Haeckel coined for this principle. Despite its clearly non-Darwinian provenance, this law was understood as integral to most understandings of Darwinism by the end of the nineteenth century—an era that historians of science, not coincidentally, refer to as the eclipse of Darwinism due to the plethora of non- and even anti-Darwinian theories being put forth by the scientific community.

Biogenetic law is, in a sense, the granddaddy of non-Darwianian theories, mainly because, as we will see shortly, so many of the other non-Darwinian mechanisms, such as Lamarckism and orthogenesis, that continued to find scientific constituencies into the 1920s and beyond, began with biogenesis as their premise. To grasp biogenetic law and its organicist ramifications it will be instructive to distinguish its vision of evolutionary change from that implied by Darwin's selectionism. According to Bowler, natural selection represented a radical break with previous theories in that it eliminated the kind of order, purpose, and direction from living nature that we saw with idealist morphology. In Darwin's conception, transmutation occurred due to disturbances in the reproductive process. These disturbances resulted in random variations among offspring, some of which were more suited to the environment into which they had been born, others less suited. These better-suited progeny tended to be more likely to survive to maturity and therefore multiplied in greater numbers. While such descent with modification favored the "fittest," evolution itself lacked direction and purpose: it was a "haphazard, branching, and open-ended process, with no rigid trends and no goal toward which everything is striving."[24] Species came and went according to happenstance, their rise and fall at the mercy of alterations in the natural environment and the vagaries of a reproductive mechanism that Darwin did not claim to understand.

In contrast to selectionism, evolutionary morphology understood the origin and life history of species to follow a preestablished developmental trajectory. Though it readily accepted Darwin's notion that species had naturalistically transmuted from prior ancestors, Haeckel's system also pre-

---

24 Bowler, *The Non-Darwinian Revolution*, 51.

served the law of parallelism or growth analogy from idealist morphology, which portrayed species as the product of the process of archetype metamorphosis evident in the phases of embryonic growth. Haeckel's masterstroke was in synthesizing these two apparently contradictory conceptions into an account of evolution that was at once naturalistic and organicist. How he achieved this was by identifying each of the stages of embryonic growth which had led up to the fully mature organism with an actual ancestor from the evolutionary past of the species. In idealist morphology, the archetype of the phylum had metamorphosed directly through the sequence of these embryonic growth stages, with extant species each having a separate yet parallel path of development. In evolutionary morphology, though this directed pattern of growth was preserved, it unfolded genealogically: both the archetype and adult forms, seen in stages of embryonic growth, came to represent historical species that had successively transmuted into one another through a natural process culminating in contemporary species. The archetypes were now ancestors and the developmental progress of forms into present-day species was no longer conceived as a ladder but a branching family tree.

The difference between these pre- and post-Darwinian forms of morphology can perhaps best be seen in how they related living species to one another. Idealist morphology conceived of extant species from a given phylum as only related because they shared the same archetype, even if, as was often thought to be the case, their embryonic development manifested adult forms that were still living creatures. Living nature possessed unity and harmony because its multitudinous forms had separately metamorphosed from the same original generative force. Evolutionary morphology, in contrast, depicted all species from within a phylum as related through a common ancestral species from the evolutionary past. The generative force from within nature was no longer just a plan that separately metamorphosed into the various species. It was now understood as unfolding as an historical process of species transmutation. Living nature possessed unity and harmony because its multitudinous forms were part of a single family tree. It was, in other words, an organicist process in which differentiation preserved unity through adherence toward an in-built ultimate goal. In adhering to a single underlying directed pattern of growth, species evolved not from an abstract archetype, but from one another.

Despite having instigated a conversion to naturalism, Haeckel, who had been deeply influenced by the Hegelian philologist August Schleicher, was quick to emphasize this idealist provenance of evolutionary morphology. Each of the thirty chapters that comprised his *General Morphology* of 1866, a massive work which meticulously laid out his entire system of biology, began "with some passage from Goethe that represents aesthetic understanding of nature's developmental processes."[25] In his more accessible and concise follow-up, the global best-seller *The History of Creation* (1868), arguably the most influential work of evolutionary biology ever written, Haeckel went further, jointly attributing the theory of evolution to Lamarck, Darwin, and Goethe. It is, however, in the principle of evolution itself, his biogenetic law, that the developmentalist contribution of idealism is most apparent. Like many of his idealist forerunners, Haeckel restated the law of parallelism as a theory of recapitulation—hence, his famous formulation of biogenetic law as the incantation-like "ontogeny recapitulates phylogeny." What this meant was not substantially different from Meckel's law of parallelism quoted above: individual offspring in their progress from conception through to full maturity (ontogeny), replayed, in compressed form, the evolutionary stages through which all of its ancestors up until its very own parents had passed (phylogeny). Where Haeckel's recapitulationism differed from that of Meckel, Oken, and others is that, in keeping with his Darwinian conversion to a strictly materialist transmutation, it made phylogeny—the history of the species—the material cause of ontogeny—the growth of the individual. As Haeckel would explain in his *The Evolution of Man* of 1874: "Phylogenesis is the mechanical cause of ontogenesis. In other words, the development of the stem, or race, is the cause, in accordance with the physiological laws of heredity and adaptation, of all the changes which appear in a condensed form in the evolution of the foetus."[26]

This mechanical law possessed tremendous explanatory power for reconstructing the evolutionary past. With the fossil record full of yawning gaps, paleontologists in the late nineteenth century were at pains to delineate lines of descent. Armed with biogenetic law, embryology came to the rescue: ontogeny now could be understood as providing an index or map

25 Richards, *The Meaning of Evolution*, 29–30.
26 Haeckel, *The Evolution of Man*, 5. First published in German in 1874.

for phylogenetic development. In other words, where fossils happened to be lacking evolutionary morphologists could plug in the adult forms that were exhibited in embryonic development, treating them as hypothetical ancestors. Haeckel was particularly zealous in applying this technique. The popular works which he published in the decades after setting down the parameters of evolutionary morphology in his grand *General Morphology* feature myriad examples of stem-trees (*Stambaum*), which Haeckel himself illustrated, that conjectured on the genealogy of life and the pedigree of man.[27] His *History of Creation*, in particular, strove to provide a complete picture of evolution on earth, meticulously tracing in its twenty-two chapters the train of creatures from single-celled organisms up until man. His *Evolution of Man* continued this work, elaborating a full genealogy of mankind. In both cases lacunae in the paleontological records were filled in with hypothetical creatures derived from studies in human embryology: in the case of *The History of Creation* the monera and in *The Evolution of Man* the missing link.

It was in how biogenetic law described adaptation that evolutionary morphology became a facilitator of other pre-Darwinian conceptions. The most prominent of these was Lamarckism, the evolutionary mechanism from the early nineteenth century that posited that inheritable traits were acquired during the lifetime of an organism through a process of use-inheritance. Such use-inheritance was most famously employed to explain the long neck of the giraffe: attempts by successive generations of these creatures to stretch for leaves had resulted in the progressive elongation of the neck, an acquired trait that was passed along to offspring until a new species had evolved. In Haeckel's system, Lamarckism performed the primary progressive function that drove evolution forward: after recapitulation had occurred—that is, once the embryo had cycled through the adult forms of its ancestors and reached maturity—new traits would be acquired through use-inheritance as adaptations to the environment. These newly acquired traits would then become the last stage of recapitulation in the gestation of the subsequent generation. In a sense, these traits were added on to the phylogeny of the species and thus, according to biogenetic law, became part of the ontogeny of its offspring. Natural selection only came in to decide which of the acquired traits would survive in order to reproduce.

---

27 Bowler, *Evolution*, 192–93.

This account of variation is markedly different from Darwin's, which focused on random disturbances in the process of reproduction. Though Haeckel did leave a place for such variety-producing disruptions during the growth of embryo—he referred to them as cenogensis—gestation was for him primarily a conservative process that reiterated the "evolution of the tribe,"[28] which is how he often alluded to phylogeny. He sometimes applied the term palingenesis for such a purely conservative recapitulation, one that occurred without disturbances. In keeping with the sense of this term, each new offspring, each successive generation, was conceived as a regeneration, a renewal of the past, a rebirth of tribal history. In this way it can be seen how evolutionary morphology suppressed the radical, potentially nihilistic aspects of Darwin's selectionism that rendered new offspring as the product of random variations and the course of evolution as haphazard, subject to the happenstance of environmental change. Under biogenetic law evolution possessed, in contrast, an orderly inner direction, with each generation bodily inheriting its own history of organic development. Though the progressive variation-producing function of Lamarckian use-inheritance seemed to open the possibility of steering evolution in unanticipated directions, it tended, in fact, to reinforce the quasi-teleological character of transmutation. Especially where it pertained to human evolution, which is what concerns us here, Lamarckism came under the subtle pressure of palingensis: the inheritable traits that it acquired through force of habit would, within a generation, become part of the "evolution of the tribe," a continuation of its development recapitulated in the growth of offspring. Aware that it was advancing a legacy, use-inheritance was constrained—path-dependent on—by the direction and purpose of phylogeny.

As will be seen, this path-dependent Lamarckism inclined evolutionary morphologists toward a reformist outlook with a heavy emphasis on science education. The efforts of both Haeckel and Oka in this area were informed by the recognition that adding on to the genealogical legacy of the tribe would require broad understanding of evolutionary history. The mechanism of acquired traits also opened Oka, who remained an unabashed Lamarckian throughout his career, to an offshoot of biogenetic law that fell

---

28 Haeckel, *Evolution of Man*, 7.

beyond the purview of evolutionary morphology: orthogenesis, a non-Darwinian evolutionary doctrine that can be best understood in reference to his systematic presentation of organic individuality. According to orthogenesis, the ontogeny of each such individuality—whether that of an individual, a group, or an entire phylum—did not just culminate in the unity-in-difference of mature forms, but proceeded, inevitably, in a logical extension of the growth analogy, to eventual disintegration and dissolution. In short, organic individualities of every order of complexity come to the end of the life cycle: they grow old and die out. In our penultimate chapter we will discuss how Oka drew on aspects of this doctrine to identify the onset of decadence and to devise his theory of degeneration.

The Hierarchy of Organic Individuality

The preservation of direction, purpose, and meaning by evolutionary morphology is nowhere more evident than in its analysis of organic individuality—the very analysis that Oka employs in both his research into moss animals and his sociopolitical evolutionism. As we have seen, Oka's mentor Rudolf Leuckart established his reputation in the early 1850s by portraying siphonophores, a species of colonial jellyfish, as displaying two interlocking types of individuality, morphological and physiological. The division of labor that resulted in the organs of the colony developing into physiologically dependent but morphologically discrete individuals in their own right was attributed to a process of homology driven by the "teleo-mechanism" inherent in living nature. Haeckel's evolutionary morphology, a research paradigm that Leuckart subscribed to after the appearance of the *Origin of Species*, elaborated on Leuckart's analysis to devise a hierarchy of individuality that would become the foundation of Oka's evolutionism. What would make Haeckel's systemization of individuality so appealing was not just the analogy with the human nation-state that Haeckel promoted, but its organicism. A holdover from the idealist phase of morphology and its archetype theory, the organicist developmental drive would invest nature with generative potential that it lacked in Darwinian selectionism. In our next chapter it will be revealed how organicism, from the outset, goaded evolutionism beyond its reformist metapolitics and ultimately turned it into something akin to a value-positing religion.

The generative drive described by Haeckel's biogenetic law emanated from and developed into what he called "unities of life."[29] Each unity possessed an active predisposition, conceived by Haeckel in strictly material terms, to differentiate and grow. This impulse not only guided the process of differentiation—through which the potential for higher complexity built into each such life form was realized—but it ensured that the newly evolved complexity cohered as one—that its many parts remained subordinated to the living whole and its inner purpose. This was precisely the process that cell biology and embryology described in the gestation of the fetus: a developmental progression in which differentiation and specialization preserved unity through adherence to an in-built ultimate goal. As the fetus matured, it actualized the inner plan it received at conception thereby manifesting the developmental law of nature.

Haeckel's organicism consisted in taking the development undergone by this unity of life—that is, by the individual organism—and applying it to all levels of living nature. Such a derivation was implicit in the recapitulationism that he preserved from idealist morphology: "ontogeny recapitulates phylogeny" meant that the differentiation of the embryo in the course of its growth was identical to the evolutionary unfolding of the species line. For Haeckel this led to the conclusion that the species as a whole, in fact, represented an individual organism: its phylogenetic evolution was nothing but the ontogeny of the species, the growth of a living being. In other words, just as an embryo differentiated through cell-division into a mature form in which the parts cohered, so species differentiated through evolutionary change into extant life forms that, in their totality, functioned as an integrated organic individual of a higher order. Having extended the growth analogy in this manner, Haeckel then, in the spirit of his *Naturphilosophen* predecessors, took his hypothesizing one step further: since all life emerged from a single source, its evolutionary differentiation represented the growth of the most inclusive example of the unity of life. Living nature was an organism and evolution its ontogeny. Biogenetic law did not just explain evolution but the organicist structuring and self-organizing of life at every level of complexity.

How this all fit together into a genealogy of living nature can be delineated by starting from the most rudimentary form of organic individuality:

---

29 Haeckel, *The Wonders of Life*, 147ff.

the cell or "plastid" as Haeckel called it. Lynn Nyhart explains the organicist process, coupling Lamarckism and natural selection, by which this plastid initiates the evolution of not only new species but more and more complex orders of individuality:

> According to Haeckel, the form at the origin of all phyla, at the beginning of organic life, was the plastid, which also constituted the initial form present in ontogeny. Everyone agreed that primitive organic forms developed little if at all during their life cycle, but did reproduce. During their lifetimes, the initial forms would differentiate to adapt to different conditions of existence; those adaptations would be passed on through inheritance. In the process of differentiating the plastids added a stage on to their development. The new species that eventually emerged from this differentiation would have two stages to their development, one corresponding to the plastid and another to the differentiated form. These species constituted the second morphological and physiological order of individuality, in which the individuals possessed tissues and organs. As evolution continued, natural selection of favorable adaptations yielded increasing differentiation and progress. This led to the emergence of successively higher orders of individuality.[30]

As Nyhart's account suggests, Haeckel had appropriated Leuckart's analysis of morphological and physiological individuality. In fact, the research that established Haeckel's reputation among scientists in 1862 described these kinds of individuality among radiolarians, "a large class of one-celled marine organisms that secreted skeletons of silica,"[31] and he had followed this up with investigations off the coast of Italy of the same aquatic invertebrates that Leuckart had studied, the siphonophores.[32] Drawing on these studies, Haeckel's mammoth systematic work of 1866, *General Morphology*, the text which laid down the paradigm of evolutionary morphology, featured an entirely new field of study that focused on organic individuality. Called techtology, it devised "a hierarchy of six orders of morphological and physiological individuals ranging from the 'plastid' or cell to the 'corm' or colonial organisms. Each level of individual was made up of an aggregation

---

30 Nyhart, *Biology Takes Form*, 134.
31 Richards, *The Tragic Sense of Life*, 63.
32 Ibid., 180–89.

of individuals of the next lower order."[33] *General Morphology* sets down a hierarchy of organic individuality in the following fashion:

> Morphological individuality can be divided into six hierarchical categories or orders of individuals, and each of these orders appears in specific organisms as physiological individuality. For each species there is, however, a particular order that is most highly characteristic, and represents in that case its actual physiological individuality, at least by the time the organism is fully mature. The six orders of organic individuality are as follows:
>
> i.   Plastids (cytodes and cells) or "elementary organisms."
> ii.   Organs (clumps or amalgamations of cells, simple or homoplastic organs, compound or heteroplastic organs, organ-systems, organ-mechanisms).
> iii. Antimeres (counterparts or parts of a single sort). "Rays" of radial organisms, "halves" of true dipleural (bilaterally symmetrical) animals etc.
> iv.   Metameres (sequential parts or parts of a single action). "Articulated stems" of phanerogams, "segements," annuli or zonal sections of articulated animals and vertebrates, etc.
> v.   Persons (Prosopae). Shoots or buds of plants and coelenterates etc. "Individuals" in the strictest sense in the higher animals.
> vi.   Corms (clumps or colonies). Trees, shrubs etc. (compound plants). Chains of Salpae, clumps of polyps, etc.
>
> Each of these six different orders of morphological individuals is capable of occurring as an independent unit of life and of representing the physiological individual.[34]

As we will reiterate many times in the course of this book, it is on the transition from Order V (persons, or individuals as we usually understand them) to Order VI (corms or colonies, also known as overindividuals, superorganisms, and poly-persons) that scientistic attempts to apply evolutionary morphology to human affairs will focus. The organicism implicit in this type of evolutionism will be invoked to reintegrate differentiated persons back into

---

33   Nyhart, *Biology Takes Form*, 133.
34   Quoted in Di Gregori, *From Here to Eternity*, 127.

the harmony of the corm. Anomy will be identified with disintegration and Oka's regenerative vision will seek to overcome such decadence and instinctively reunite the highest organic individuality—the ethnic nation.

Before exploring the dynamic of these poly-persons in more detail, a third type of individuality which Haeckel added to Leuckart's two, must be discussed: genealogical individuality. Where morphological individuality concerned indivisibility, such that the constituent part of a whole "cannot be separated without destroying the nature or character of the whole," and physiological individuality concerned self-maintenance, such that a unity of function enables the whole to "lead its own existence completely independently,"[35] genealogical individuality was defined by life-cycle continuity, the succession of organic stages through which its original inchoate unity had differentiated while remaining integrated. Nyhart explains that there were three orders of genealogical or temporal individuals added to the six orders of listed above:

[O]ne constituted by the life cycle of the single organism, one constituted by the life span of the single species, which also had birth, maturity and senescence, and a third consisting of the life history of the phylum or tribe of species sharing a common primitive ancestor. Just as each order of morphological individual was made up of an aggregate of individuals of a lower order, so too were the genealogical individuals organized in a hierarchy such that the phylum was made up of species' life cycles, which in turn were constituted by the sum of individual life cycles. Each level of individual at once had an independent existence and constituted an aggregate of individuals of a lower order.[36]

This conception of genealogical individuality would have a significant impact on geopolitical calculations. As we will see in a subsequent chapter, the tendency of evolutionary morphologists, and most especially Haeckel, toward the speciation of human races meant not only that they were thought to emerge from separate genealogies but that they, in fact, each represented biologically distinct individuals. Each racial "unity of nature" was, in a sense, an organism whose survival in the arena of global politics required it to struggle for autarky.

---

35 Richards, *The Tragic Sense of Life*, 132.
36 Nyhart, *Biology Takes Form*, 133–34.

A passage from one of Haeckel's popular works will help convey, in more concrete terms, how the immense and intricate edifice of his hierarchy of organic individuality readily translated into a vision of the human polity. In his best-selling *The Wonders of Life*, which appeared at roughly the same time as Oka's *Lectures on Evolutionary Theory*, Haeckel simplifies the orders of organic individuality into three, with "one building upon the other—the cell, the person (or sprout), and the stem or state (cormus)."[37] Structurally and functionally—that is, "morphologically" and "physiologically"—each order constituted an indivisible and self-maintaining individuality composed of individuals from the next lower order. Thus, the cormus or superorganism was a poly-person and the individual person was a cell-state (cells, meanwhile, were constituted of inorganic processes). Temporally—that is, "genealogically"—each order of individuality was subject to its own process of life-cycle growth that was made up of the ontogeny of individuals in the next lower level. Thus, the history of the superorganism was comprised of the lives of persons who had cycled through birth, growth, maturation, senescence, and death, and, in turn, these persons were, embryonically speaking, the product of the epigenetic process of cell-division. The elegance of Haeckel's organicism comes into view if we imagine the construction of these orders of individuality unfolding from beginning to end: individual cells differentiate and integrate with other cells to form cell-states, and these higher individuals or persons cycle through the stages of their lives and integrate with other persons to comprise the highest stage of individuality, that of the superorganism or the corm.

Haeckel's frequent application of the term "state" to this highest level of organic individuality, the corm or superorganism, was deliberate and quite literal. For him the colonial life of siphonophores and the collective lives of humans were roughly equivalent. In fact he considered social existence to be just another name for organicist integration: "[T]he same fundamental laws of sociology hold good for the association throughout the entire organic world; and also for the gradual evolution of the several organs out of the tissues and cell-communities."[38] What distinguished human superorganisms from those of siphonophores was that the persons that comprised

---

37 Haeckel, *The Wonders of Life*, 148.
38 Ibid., 169.

the human corm enjoyed the freedom of physical separation. In this sense, "the formation of human societies is directly connected with the gregariousness of the nearest related mammals. The herds of apes and ungulates, the packs of wolves, the flocks of birds, often controlled by a single leader, exhibit various stages of social formation; as also the swarms of the higher articulates (insects, crustacea), especially communities of ants and termites, swarms of bees, etc."[39] In all such gregarious creatures "the social elements are not bodily connected."[40] Instead their actions were coordinated through what he called "the ideal link of common interest."[41]

While it was admitted that "it is not so easy for the imagination to grasp a human commonwealth or a colony of bees as a real 'over individual'"[42] in the same way as a siphonophore colony, Haeckel, nevertheless, considered the development achieved by way of this internalized "ideal link" to be of a much higher order. Indeed he proclaimed that the "complicated modern state, with its remarkable achievements, may be regarded as the highest stage of individual perfection which is known to us in organic nature."[43] What qualifies the state for this distinction is the uniquely complex extent of its differentiation. Whereas differentiation among siphonophores, for instance, eventually resulted in some jellyfish taking on specialized functions and acting as morphologically distinct unities of life, they were all ultimately tethered to the superorganism through physiological ties. In contrast, humans, bound only by the ideal link of common interest, were able to go through more extreme homological transformations and achieve a more complex division of labor. The state embodied the supreme "individual perfection" because its constituent individuals had been fully able to differentiate and thereby realize the latent potential of the nation or tribe of which they were members.

The "ideal link of common interest" that integrated these differentiated persons back into the individual perfection of the state was an evolutionary version of morality which Haeckel regarded as part of the process of adaptation and inheritance. The basis of such morality could be seen at the most rudimentary stage of life—in unicellular individuals, "cell individu-

---

39   Ibid.
40   Ibid.
41   Ibid.
42   Bölsche, *Haeckel*, 245–46.
43   Haeckel, *The Wonders of Life*, 150.

als," who, through habitual "association," "adapted to each other and the common environment" to form communities.[44] Through this Lamarckian mechanism, the cell individual inherited traits that bound it physiologically to the community: cell-states or multicelled organisms came into being—what Haeckel's hierarchy referred to as persons. At a later and much more complex echelon of organic development, higher up the tree of life, gregarious mammals, such as human beings, formed this physiological bond not through bodily connections but via social instincts. According to Haeckel, the Lamarckian inculcation of such social instincts, which were altruistic, was especially crucial among humans because the extreme individuation that occurred with the differentiation of human communities threatened to exacerbate to egoism. Individuals, in other words, would be tempted to act out of unalloyed selfishness, rending the social fabric. To curb this anomic tendency, morality, engendered as social instincts through altruistic use-inheritance, would be encouraged.

In the next chapter we will see that these ruminations on evolutionary morality became the jumping off point for Haeckel's confrontation with organized religion, particularly Christianity. Here, it will be enough to note that this vision of community building and ego-curbing through the internalization of ethical imperatives is not terribly different from the *Sittlichkeit* described in the last chapter. Products of the same organicist tradition of German idealism, the Hegelian organic state and the Haeckelian corm or superorganism both look to the organic process underlying life to reintegrate the differentiated plurality it had produced. In both examples untethered individualism is associated with an egoism that threatens to dismember the community. Only through the inculcation of a communitarian morality that taps the generative force driving development can this anomic egoism be sublimated to serve a higher end—the nation-state. The Haeckelian social instincts that subordinate persons to the higher individuality of the superorganism perform the same function as the Hegelian ethical life that englobes individuals so that they come to regard the interest of the state as their own. Whether intended by Haeckel or not, the supreme manifestation of organic individuality in nature, the state organism, constituted a correlate to the organic state, which occupies an equally lofty position in

44 Ibid.

Hegel's system. In short, common organicism begat a common conception of ethics founded on the integrated life of the corporate state.

JAPAN'S HAECKEL

For Oka Asajirō this correlation instilled his research activities with a political potential that he would not tap into until the Russo-Japanese War. As the last chapter discussed, Todai, where he first came to investigate moss animal superorganisms as an undergraduate, was the same institution in which organic theories of the state were being promoted to shore up the Meiji state and its monarchy of social reform. The Hegelian conception being fostered by scholars and budding bureaucrats at Todai was utilized across the ideological spectrum: not only establishment intellectuals of a reformist bent, such as Katō and Minobe Tatsukichi, but reactionaries, such as Hozumi, who began to articulate a family-state orthodoxy, developed their political philosophies on the basis of the state-science taught at the imperial university. Groomed for a reformist establishment whose role included procuring advanced knowledge from abroad in order to modernize the institutions and conventions of the new nation-state, Oka found in evolutionary morphology expert credentials and a biological equivalent of the organic state, both of which would uniquely qualify him to take up the prevailing state-science discourse and authoritatively refashion it in light of cutting-edge evolutionary theory. Though his esteem for Haeckel's contribution was not without reservation, Oka, as his *Lectures on Evolutionary Theory* illustrates, associated Darwinism with the paradigm of evolutionary morphology. It was on this basis that the centerpiece of this paradigm, the hierarchy of organic individuality, came to define the sociopolitical vision he began to articulate beginning with the outbreak of war with Russia in 1904.

A decade passed between Oka's departure from Leuckart's Leipzig University laboratory and the publication of *Lectures on Evolutionary Theory* in the early months of this war. During this time his academic career became firmly established on several fronts. For instance, within a year of his return to Japan Oka was awarded a PhD in the physical sciences from Todai and was quickly granted a two-year position at the Peer's School in Yamaguchi. In 1897 he moved on to the position that he would occupy until his retirement thirty-two years later: a professorship at the Higher Normal School in Tokyo. As its name suggests, this college was less a university and more a professional school, training its students to become future public school teachers or preparing them for placement in teacher-training colleges. It thus had close ties with the Ministry of Education, taking part "intimately in the compilation of government-authorized school textbooks" and participating in the education conferences and research investigations over which the ministry presided.[45] Because most of his students would go on to become middle school instructors, Oka was freed from having to procure positions for them. As a result, he was able to apply himself wholeheartedly to research and gained a reputation for diligence and commitment among the student body.

Tsukuba Hisaharu speculates that the intensity with which Oka pursued his studies also may have had something to do with the tragic circumstances of his personal life. Echoing the untimely deaths of his siblings and parents while he was a student in Osaka, Oka, who had married the daughter of a high-level Meiji bureaucrat in 1897, lost his first two sons prematurely to illness during his early years at the First Higher Normal School. Despite this heartbreak and other hardships, such as the sorry condition of the school's physical plant—one of his former students described the building he was assigned as a "derelict barn"—and the lack of research assistants, Oka flourished as a scholar. Some of the articles he published in the early years after securing his position at the Tokyo Higher Normal School include: "General Remarks on Arthropods," "The Classification System of Animals in Middle Education," "The Structure and Uses of Compound Eyes," and "Water Leeches," all which appeared in *Zoological Magazine*, and "Parasites of Malaria," which was printed in *Eastern Arts and Sciences Magazine* (*Toyo Gakugei Zasshi*). Eventually Oka's researches and scholarly writings were to build him an international reputation as a scientist and win for him, during his later years, membership in Japan's Imperial Academy. By 1901, at age thirty-four, he was appointed head professor of biological studies at the Tokyo Higher Normal School. Only the paucity of positions in his field available at this juncture in Japanese history seems to have prevented him from moving on to a research institution.[46]

---

45 Migita, *Tennosei to Shinkaron*, 34.
46 Tsukuba, "Kaisetsu" [Commentary], 432–33.

Though there were some grumblings by colleagues at the college concerning how Oka's research focus prevented him from providing his students with adequate guidance, any questions about his commitment to education were dispelled by his prolificacy as a textbook writer. In 1896, he began publishing, in quick succession, a series of textbooks on zoology and biology for use in middle school education and among the general populace. The eleven titles he was to put out over the course of his career include *Modern Textbook of Biology* in 1896, *Modern Textbook on Physiology* in 1898, *Modern Textbook of Zoology* in 1899, *Short Lecture on Zoology* in 1902, *Women's Science Textbook of Physiology and Hygiene* in 1905, *Women's Science Textbook of Animals* in 1906, *The Newest Textbook of Zoology* in 1906, *Elementary Textbook on Physiology and Hygiene* in 1910, *Intermediate Educational Textbook in Zoology* in 1912, *Intermediate Educational Textbook in Physiology and Hygiene* in 1912, and *An Outline of Intermediate Education in Natural History* in 1914.[47] Many of these texts were reprinted as many as thirteen times. Even if Oka had never embarked on his highly successful career as a scientific popularizer and political essayist, his impact on the perceptions of the natural world among the Japanese public in the early twentieth century would still have been enormous based on his textbook writing alone.

Oka's literary activities in the service of science education soon began to extend beyond textbooks. In 1901 he released a book entitled *Education and Natural History*,[48] and in April of the following year an article on the same subject matter, entitled "Education as Seen from Biology." Appearing in a journal called *Education and Science*, this would not only become the first of many articles that eventually came to comprise *Evolution and Human Life*, the anthology that is our focus here, but earn for Oka a position on the Ministry of Education's commission for the compilation of a nationally authorized science textbook.[49] He was by this time a member of the Ministry's committee for teacher certification and when he joined the science textbook commission in July of 1904 there were already two other faculty from the Tokyo Higher Normal School who were members. As we will discuss in a later chapter, Oka's unsuccessful struggle to promote evolutionary science as a member of this commission was one of the factors

---

47 Ibid., 456–61.
48 Migita, *Tennosei to Shinkaron*, 107.
49 Ibid., 106.

which eventually pushed him to expand his evolutionism beyond a mere reformist metapolitics.

Lectures on Evolutionary Theory, the best-selling primer that would turn Oka into a household name and help launch his career as an essayist, appeared in print six months before he became a member of the science textbook commission. Drawing on Oka's authority as a scientist and college educator and coinciding with the outbreak of war against Russia, the book employed a lively and colloquial style full of proverbs and vivid illustrations to introduce the broader Japanese public to various aspects of the theory of evolution. With most of the text divided in two broad sections on "Natural Selection" and "The Evolution of Living Things," the book provided an accessible overview of evolutionary science circa 1904, featuring individual chapters on the history of evolutionary theory, artificial selection, speciation, heredity, variation in nature, the struggle for existence, selectionism, anatomy, embryology, paleontology, ecology, classification and distribution, adaptation, "Evolutionary Theory since Darwin," and finally, "Man's Position in Nature." Though Darwin's *Origin of Species* had been first translated in 1896 and Oka himself had overseen a new and more comprehensive translation in 1905, never before had the facts of evolutionary biology been rendered so accessible to so many in Japan. The reading public was dazzled. A matron from a well-to-do family of legal scholars, for example, recorded the following in her diary shortly after Oka's work went on sale: "January 31 (1904), cloudy weather. I buy Professor Oka's work *Lectures on Evolutionary Theory* at the Senbuto bookstore. In the evening I read with great rapidity to everyone present. I read more than a hundred pages. Meshing written and spoken language it was easy to understand and greatly interesting."[50] Meanwhile, at the other end of the political spectrum, the nineteen-year-old anarchist Ōsugi Sakai also obtained a copy, which he had been "pining for unbearably" and, in a fever, quickly rifled through its pages: "Right away I began to read it. It was interesting beyond endurance. Each line was like an unknown, fantastically wondrous world that came to emerge before my eyes to the point that I was dizzy. In the end, I got through it reading from day till late into the middle of the night. Science and human life: for a long time we have been yearning to hear about these matters from scientists and at long

---

50 Ibid., 34.

last there is this good [treatment of the] topic about which, before Professor Oka, we had almost no chance to learn."[51]

Not only did the book quickly sell out in large numbers—a report in 1922 claimed that 60,000 copies had been purchased[52]—but its popularity was sustained over several decades. Between 1904 and 1940 fourteen editions of this book would appear, with revised enlargements incorporating new developments in biology appearing in 1914 (the eleventh edition) and 1925 (the thirteenth edition).[53] According to Matsunaga Toshio, "many famous writers attested to its impact"[54] and the book, along with its equally popular sequel, *Evolution and Human Life*, had such a wide impact across society that a "Darwin boom" gripped Japan toward the end of the decade. Increasingly asked to contribute featured articles to leading publications, Oka by 1909 was acknowledged in a survey of the reading public conducted by the populist magazine *Taiyō* (The Sun) as one of the leading "authorities in the world of science."[55] The full impact of *Lectures on Evolutionary Theory* in early-twentieth-century Japan is perhaps best intimated in Tsukuba Tsuneji's report that this book was the one item which returnees from Manchuria after the Second World War wished they had been able to bring back with them.[56]

As testified by Ōsgui's claim that an "unknown, fantastically wondrous world" had been unveiled to its readers, the primary appeal of *Lectures on Evolutionary Theory* seems to have been the inviting way Oka depicted natural phenomena. Though Oka did not completely shirk theoretical issues as he traversed such topics as artificial selection, adaptation, and anatomy through the main body of the text, he tended to focus on specific examples, many of which were illustrated with pictures, and all of which, it was understood, were meant to exemplify Darwinian science. It was not until one of his final chapters, "Evolutionary Theory since Darwin," that it becomes evident—at least to astute historians if not Oka's contemporaries—that his "Darwinism" had been filtered through the organicist paradigm that was Darwinian mainly in name alone—that of evolutionary morphology.

---

51 Ibid., 36.
52 Ibid., 34.
53 Ibid., 35.
54 Matsunaga, "Evolutionism in Early Twentieth Century Japan," 221.
55 Migita, *Tennosei to Shinkaron*, 35.
56 Tsukuba, "Kaisetsu" [Commentary], 430ff.

A clear indication of his morphological perspective is the long discussion concerning the mechanism driving evolutionary change which occupies a large section of this chapter. Writing in the middle of the so-called "eclipse of Darwinism," a period from the late 1880s until the First World War during which natural selection was marginalized by a variety of non-Darwinian theories of transmutation, Oka offers a three-part distinction regarding the types of evolutionary theories endorsed by his contemporaries. First are theories which regard the "cause of the evolution of organic life mainly to be outside of natural selection." Though he mentions De Vries's mutation theory, a doctrine that would latter reconcile with Darwinism to become an antecedent for the modern theory of genetics, the non-Darwinian theory Oka has in mind here is Lamarckism, or, as it was called at the time "neo-Lamarckism." Second come theories which view natural selection as the main cause, but recognize other causes as well. Finally, the third position is that "the evolution of living things is due to natural selection alone and there are no other causes to the evolution of life besides natural selection."[57] Oka explains that this position, often referred to as neo-Darwinism, is represented by the germ plasm theory of his former teacher, August Weismann, whom he had abandoned in order to study under Rudolf Leuckart.

Most of Oka's discussion centers on critiquing how Weismann's vehement rejection of Lamarckian use-inheritance misrepresents Darwinism. Oka chides that "among today's self-described 'Darwin group,' the name Darwin is used as a cover for their own theories."[58] To illustrate this distortion, a long passage devoted to Weismann methodically explains how the so-called anti-Lamarckian hard heredity of his germ plasm theory breaks with Darwinism. Quoting Weismann, Oka argues that the basis of this germ plasm theory is the notion that "newly acquired characters are not inherited by offspring."[59] In contrast, Oka emphasizes that "it is absolutely certain that Darwin thinks there are causes of the evolution of living things other than natural selection" and that Lamarckism is the most important of these causes.[60]

While Oka correctly concludes that "the theory of Darwin himself is included in the second group" outlined above, it becomes quickly apparent

---

57 Ibid., 206.
58 Ibid., 198.
59 Ibid., 214.
60 Ibid., 206.

from the other names he places in this group that the version of evolution Oka has in mind is not the random variations and haphazard branching produced by natural selection. Not only are Thomas Huxley, the morphologist, and Herbert Spencer, the Lamarckian, mentioned, but Haeckel himself is held up as an example of the "great many scholars" who combine natural selection with Lamarckism. As previously mentioned, Lamarckism provides a critical function in Haeckel's evolutionary morphology: in adapting to the environment it adds on traits after recapitulation has been completed—traits which become, in turn, the last stage of recapitulation in the succeeding generation. By endorsing a position that called for the accommodation of Lamarckism and selectionism, Oka, it is not too difficult to see given his training, was, in so many words, subscribing to a program of evolutionary morphology. He would, in fact, call himself a Lamarckian throughout his career, writing a tract defending this evolutionary mechanism as late as 1919 and suggesting its priority over natural selection. As our analysis in the coming chapters will reveal, Oka often blurred the distinction between Lamarckism and selectionism in his political essays. Though, technically speaking, he was justified in calling his position Darwinian, the paradigm through which he conceived evolution was that of evolutionary morphology and its attendant organicism.

Where Oka's subscription to the organicist program of evolutionary morphology becomes undeniable is in the centrality he accords to biogenetic law. Oka introduced biogenetic law during his chapter on embryology and referred to it as the "principle of growth in living things." After explaining how certain organs only show up during embryonic growth, how various animals resemble one another during the first stages of this growth, and how the divergence of animal types parallels the stages of individual development, Oka restates the recapitulation theory in his own words: "The growth of an individual repeats the evolutionary course of its species."[61] To illustrate how this law works, he cites the example of whales: "If there were once a period in the course of the evolution of whales into their present-day form when they had teeth, there will be also a time when teeth appear during the growth of the whale ovum into an infant." He also applies this central principle of growth to humans: "If there were once a period in the

---

61   Ibid., 122–23.

course of the evolution of humans into their present-day form when they had gill slits, there will be also a time when gill slits occur during the growth of the human ovum into a child."[62]

This second example of the gill slits alludes to an illustration that serves as the centerpiece of Oka's chapter on embryology. This is Haeckel's famous woodcut from his *Evolution of Man* comparing the ontogeny of eight vertebrate species: fish, salamanders, tortoises, chickens, hogs, cows, rabbits, and humans. The illustration shows each species at three stages of embryonic development, and it is used to explain how similarities and differences in ontogeny can be used to reconstruct genealogical relationships between such species. The appearance of gill slits on human embryos during the first stage depicted provides an important clue to these relationships and to human evolution.[63]

In Haeckel's representation, all eight vertebrates during this first stage of ontogenetic development not only possess gill slits, but appear nearly identical to one another. According to biogenetic law, this establishes that they all shared a common ancestor at some point in their evolutionary history. Conversely, the differences in embryonic form that become more and more evident in the second and third stages indicate degrees of genealogical divergence. Thus, in the second stage human embryos still resemble those of rabbits but no longer those of the other vertebrate species. This points to the fact that humans share a genealogical branch that they do not have in common with fish, salamanders, chickens, hogs, and cows. In short, because ontogeny recapitulates phylogeny, genealogical relationships between species can be inferred from disparities in embryonic growth. Oka actually goes so far as to translate this woodcut into a family tree of vertebrate species in order to make the relationship between ontogeny and phylogeny explicit—something even Haeckel himself did not bother to do in *The Evolution of Man*.

In keeping with his tendency in this text of focusing, first and foremost, on the colorful facts of evolutionary science, it is not until later in the book, in his chapter on "Evolutionary Theory since Darwin," that Oka draws on this presentation to equate biogenetic law with evolution itself. As he states in the subsection entitled "Facts Become More and More Certain": "Consid-

---

62 Ibid., 123.
63 Ibid., 118–19.

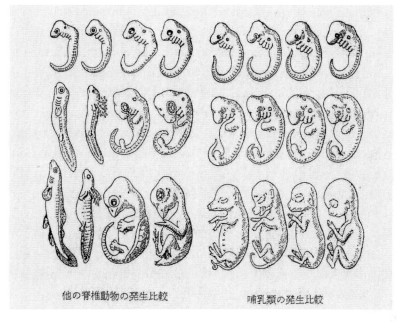

他の脊椎動物の発生比較　　　哺乳類の発生比較

Figure 3. Comparison of Ontogeny. "A Comparison of the Ontogeny of
Nonmammalian Vertebrates [Left Side]. A Comparison of the Ontogeny of
Mammals [Right Side]."

Source: Oka, *Shinkaron kōwa*, 109.

ering, in light of this [biogenetic] law, the biological facts which have come to
be discovered since Darwin and up until today, it seems sufficiently certain
that each species of living thing has diverged and descended from a common
ancestor in a tree of life." Biogenetic law provides such confirmation for evolution according to the method already discussed: it allows biologists to map
the stages of embryological development back onto the history of the species.
As Oka explains it: "when the anatomy and growth of a single animal comes
to be clarified we are able to discover some characters of ancestors which certainly existed. As a consequence, we can estimate, on this basis, something
about the path such an animal has passed through in its line of descent."[64]

This method of phylogenetic reconstruction, with its implicit subscription to the developmental vision of Haeckel's system, actually undergirds
the presentation of evolution throughout Oka's text. For instance, the cluster of chapters under the heading of "The Evolution of Living Things," which

---

64 Ibid., 203.

deals with subjects ranging from anatomy and paleontology to embryology, ecology, and the sciences of classification and distribution, implicitly accept morphological parallelism as inherent to evolution. In the other main section, "Natural Selection," though this conceit is less apparent, Oka's presentation there suggests the orderly, hierarchical, and directed transmutation of morphology, not the accidental, potentially willy-nilly changes implied by natural selection. He is able to achieve this by first introducing the phenomenon of evolution to his readers through the example of artificial selection. The pattern of directed change seen in the selection carried out by animal breeders becomes a model for selection occurring in nature.

It should not be assumed that because Oka subscribed to Haeckel's system that he also shared his dogmatism.[65] Like Darwin, Oka tended to be more cautious and doctrinally ecumenical in his outlook. As the years passed he came to incorporate the widest variety of scientific approaches in the various primers he produced for the reading public, including doctrines that flatly contradicted his own Lamarckism. This openness also injected a healthy skepticism into his presentation, even toward biogenetic law. Though, as the title of the subsection suggested, "facts" were becoming "more and more certain" due in part to this law, Oka ultimately regarded the period in which he was writing as one in which theory had not caught up with the wealth of data suddenly available. As he saw it, phylogenetic reconstructions of the past, for instance, were makeshift approximations that awaited further refinement in the future. Such approximations are not mere guesswork, but rather, according to Oka, reflections of scientific reality: "Because these estimates rest on very certain grounds, it is probably that they are taken as true." In Oka's view, "more truthlike estimations are not at all possible in today's circumstances" and they have been of immense help since Darwin in "clarifying the branches of the evolutionary tree" and "the genealogical tables of individual animal species." In "gathering together the facts of embryology" and synthesizing them into an account of the evolutionary past, biogenetic law is something which, in short, "must of course not be doubted."[66]

This qualified skepticism also extended to Haeckel himself. Oka extols Haeckel as a "leading figure" in the development of modern science for his

---

65 James Pusey, writing about Haeckel's influence on the Chinese writer Lu Xun, refers to him as "Darwin's Doberman." See Pusey, *Lu Xun and Evolution*, 37.

66 Tsukuba, "Kaisetsu" [Commentary], 430ff.

discovery of "an all-inclusive law of nature out of the miscellaneous, disparate facts gathered together by embryology" and to "express it as a single principle."[67] However, he also voices misgivings about the facile manner in which Haeckel himself has applied this biogenetic law to construct evolutionary phylogenies. In a section on Haeckel and Huxley, which appears in his chapter on "Evolutionary Theory since Darwin," Oka writes: "When reading Haeckel there is a feeling that the border between conjecture and known certainties based on research is not clear. Thus, it is said that there is a danger of misunderstanding for general readers, and among biologists there are many who express disapproval."[68]

In this spirit Oka levels criticisms at two of the popular books that made Haeckel famous, *The History of Creation* (1868) and *The Evolution of Man* (1874). The former is, according to him, "a book which describes a situation in which everything we see today between heaven and earth does not draw on the power of a godlike being outside of nature, but instead gradually achieves completion by the power of nature."[69] Yet at the same time he admits that the "greater part" of the book "is, of course, conjecture." In his view, Haeckel "makes up for the lack of factual evidence with beautiful inferences," that "when reading this book it seems as if the facts of heaven and earth have perhaps already been interpreted completely."[70] Similar charges are directed in *The Evolution of Man*, which, in attempting to delineate systematically the twenty-two evolutionary stages preceding man, speculates freely about extinct species based on the evidence of embryology. In Oka's words: "Though it clearly describes the history of mankind, beginning with an explanation of the course of human evolution from its starting point as a simple organism without any structure which gradually evolved finally into today's complex human beings, it too is, of course, mostly conjecture and there are not a few points in the book that are not exactly correct. If one were to criticize it succinctly, one would say the book is too clear. With today's incomplete knowledge, it is hardly the case that we can already clearly explain the course of human evolution from beginning to end."[71]

---

67 Ibid., 204.
68 Ibid., 210.
69 Ibid.
70 Ibid.
71 Ibid.

Oka is concerned that this speculative approach has caught on and it has become popular for biologists to make "public hypothetical theories concerning the path of animal evolution" so that "even among university dissertations there are hardly any that do not refer to hypothetical genealogical tables of the evolution of animals."[72] The danger here is that once these hypothetical speculations are disproven, the public might come to doubt the theory of evolution itself. Nevertheless, he regards Haeckel's conjectures as tolerable because Haeckel is aware of what he is doing. Thus, the conjectures in *The History of Creation* "are absolutely different from conjectures thought to be empty due to the fact that they are based only on the knowledge of biology we are aware of today. They must be thought of as being more or less close to the truth."[73] Likewise, in *The Evolution of Man*, Haeckel "is just concretely articulating conjectures deduced from the facts of presently known human embryology, and, indeed, making public something to be thought of as 'missing the mark but not far off.'"[74]

As Oka's use of this well-known Japanese proverb, "Missing the mark but not far off," insinuates, approximation is for him not just a necessary evil due to the incompleteness of science, but part of the method of popularization. In Haeckel's case, Oka says he "likes *The History of Creation* and *The Evolution of Man*" because "these two books he wrote are both easy to understand" and "those who want to do research into evolution should try to read them once."[75] To Oka's mind, Haeckel has realized that "in writing popularly about evolution and causing it to spread among the general public, it is not quite sufficient to do things in a careful way such that one only publishes biologically sound facts." Attempting to be too exact may reveal ambiguities in present knowledge and thereby breed doubt among laymen and prospective scientists. In order to promote evolutionary science effectively, it is better to "add some speculation and concretely render the conditions of the evolution of life."[76] In a sense, *Evolution and Human Life*, with its focus on the concrete renderings of biological phenomena, represents an example of this very method.

---

72 Ibid., 204.
73 Ibid., 210.
74 Ibid., 211.
75 Ibid.
76 Ibid., 210.

Along with efforts at popularization, Oka also seems to have wanted to emulate the scientific leadership provided in Germany. In his view countries that "lack figures comparable to Haeckel and Huxley," who can make evolution concrete for nonscientists, are forced to translate these authors. The result is that "the spread of the theory of evolution seems to have been somewhat slow" in these nations.[77] From all that has been said above about *Lectures on Evolutionary Theory* and Oka's attitude toward Haeckel, it is clear that he intended that he himself should occupy this role for Japan—a country which, like France, lacked its own popularizers and had fallen behind in evolutionary science. It even might not be going too far to suggest that Oka regarded himself as Japan's answer to Haeckel: a highly respected scientist in his own right who sought to make the theory of evolution, especially as described by evolutionary morphologists, palatable to the nation at large. Oka's text, *Lectures on Evolutionary Theory*, appears to be a conscious attempt to provide the Japanese people with what Haeckel provided the Germans in *History of Creation, The Evolution of Man* and other works: an accessible yet highly sophisticated account of evolutionary science.

As we will see in the coming chapters, Oka's effort at popularization will extend beyond explications that "concretely render" the latest in evolutionary theory by "adding some speculation." Just as Darwin, after his *Origin of Species* laid out an account of the natural world, waited until the *Descent of Man* to address human evolution, so did Oka, in the wake of *Lectures on Evolutionary Theory*, begin to focus consistently on human beings only in the companion piece that is the subject of this study, *Evolution and Human Life*. Evolutionary morphology and, most especially, the organicism that animated it from within came to play a far more explicit role in this follow-up book. While in *Lectures on Evolutionary Theory* Haeckel's program subtly shaped the presentation of "Darwinian" *shinkaron*—its principle of growth, biogenetic law, verifying evolution itself—in *Evolution and Human Life* the hierarchy of organic individuality which is the centerpiece of evolutionary morphology defines Oka's biopolitical vision. In particular, the pinnacle of this hierarchy, the corm or superorganism, comes to be Oka's model for human polities. The organicism passed down from the morphological tradition will figure centrally in Oka's efforts, and not just because

---

77 Ibid., 211.

it allowed him, as we have already suggested, to gesture toward an implicit comparison between the superorganism and the organic theory of the state. Just as importantly, the developmental or growth dimension of organicism, the formative disposition of inchoate forms to differentiate and reintegrate in realizing themselves, will challenge Oka to see the nation-state not as a static structure, but a palingenetic poly-person, a superorganism that cycles through distinct life stages like any organism.

Before turning to the essays that comprise *Evolution and Human Life* it will be necessary to explore how this formative or generative disposition serves to transform what it meant to "apply" evolution to human affairs. We will see that Oka's initial straightforward assumption, that science education should reform institutions, gradually gives way to another stance which regards nature as the source of both human institutions and the values that inform them. Drawing on the organicism handed down from the morphological tradition, this generative approach will enable evolutionary science not only to compete with religion but to remake human beings. Founded on organicism, what we will call Oka's generative scientism will form the basis of his contributions to eugenics, degeneration theory, and even ultranationalist ideology.

CHAPTER 3

GENERATIVE SCIENTISM: ORGANICISM BEYOND REFORM

Lectures of Evolutionary Theory, Oka Asajirō's best-selling primer of 1904, concludes with a telling assertion: "If the theory of evolution gradually spreads, the arrival of the day when the words 'Humans are a kind of animal, and are descended together from apes' appear on the pages of elementary school readers cannot be far off."[1] Migita Hiroki, in his recent *Tennosei to Shinkaron* (The emperor system and evolutionary theory), rightly contends that this statement speaks to the reformist quest to enlighten the general public that motivated Oka's work as a research scientist, classroom instructor, education bureaucrat, and evolutionary activist. By disseminating information about evolution throughout the nation, a work such as *Lectures on Evolutionary Theory* would facilitate the introduction of a biologically correct view of "man's place in nature"—as Oka, quoting Huxley, entitled one of the subsections of his book—to every level of the educational system. Knowledge of the common ancestry of human beings and other living creatures would liberate the *minzoku* (ethnic nation) from the superstitions that reigned over it.

In Migita's view, the common ancestry argument was a means not only of suggesting that human norms and conventions should be grounded in nature but of indirectly critiquing the emperor system, *tennosei*. Citing the testimony of various figures on the political left, such as Ōsugi Sakae, Sakai Toshihiko, and Kōtoku Shusui,[2] who were inspired by Oka's book at a young

---

1   Migita, *Tennosei to Shinkaron*, 108–9.
2   Ibid., 35–36.

age, Migita tries to explain how reading *Lectures on Evolutionary Theory* and the works that followed it constituted acts of subversion—its portrayal of humans as descended from primates having the effect of undermining the supposed divine origins of both the emperor and his extended family, the Yamato race. In Migita's narrative Oka's enemies are not limited to the reactionary state ideologues who held a creationist view of the imperial line and sought to inculcate their brand of Shinto fundamentalism among the masses. They were also the reformist establishment that was willing to countenance state Shinto, at least for a time, as an "exoteric" truth necessary for unifying the nation, while they themselves, by virtue of their university education, understood the harsher underlying reality needed for effective governing—the "esoteric" truths of evolutionary science. According to Migita, Oka, in keeping with the materialist left-wingers he helped to inspire, struggled throughout his career against these adversaries, seeking to render the esoteric truth of evolutionism exoteric.[3]

Though Migita is correct to portray Oka as a reformer who sought to enlighten the public through evolutionary science, he was no subversive. As we will argue in later chapters, Oka was just as dismayed with the anarchists and socialists who picked up evolutionism as he was with the reactionaries and fellow reformists who resisted its wide dissemination. His position was not that of a revolutionary but a reformer, in line with the technocratic scholar-officials that Todai was producing. In his view evolution should describe the conditions for a viable polity, not overthrow that polity. As he stated very clearly, and Emperor Hirohito himself reiterated, ideology and evolutionary science must be aligned. What Oka was delineating in the sociopolitical essays that followed up *Lectures on Evolutionary Theory* can be thought of as a metapolitics: the laws of evolutionary necessity that political structures and ideological concepts had to take into account if the nation-state was to survive and thrive.

However, where Migita's analysis runs most into trouble is in his unquestioning stance toward the scientism behind Oka's metapolitics. By scientism I mean the assumption that the norms, conventions, and laws—the nomos—constructed by humans should be definitively reduced to the natural ontology made transparent by modern science. Scientism presumes a

---

3   Ibid., 60–62.

nomos-to-nature direction of fit,[4] and Migita's narrative, in accepting that the Japanese nation-state would inevitably modernize along scientific lines, enunciates a central ramification of this scientism: the ineluctable progress of scientific knowledge and methodology. To underline this point, his book, in fact, concludes with a discussion of a postwar photograph of Hirohito seated in his study between busts of Lincoln and Darwin. Appearing in a text entitled "Emperor" which the Occupation authorities approved in 1946, this photo, in Migita's estimation, represented the inevitable triumph of science in general and evolutionary theory in particular over the superstitions of the emperor system and its creationist account of human origins: "An historical moment in which the long fight for supremacy between evolutionary theory and the emperor-centered historical view has tentatively concluded with the 'victory' of evolutionary theory."[5]

Yet, as the rest of this study will examine, Oka, though he began with a similarly sanguine disposition toward modernizing science, soon came to understand that unintended consequences accompanied modernization and the march of progress. In particular, he became cognizant of the fact that the subjective freedom that enabled the masses to learn the truths of evolutionary science might also allow them to distort, misapply, or even reject this same science. These individuals could also decide to utterly disregard the communitarian concerns that implicitly inspired metapolitics and invest themselves exclusively in the wants and desires of the private sphere. The appearance of such potentially subversive "egoists" was, in fact, identical to the disruptive future developments that Itō and the other oligarchs had feared when they devised the Meiji political order. Suddenly aware that they were free to construct their own nomos in the marketplace of modern life, the self-aware individuals that emerged in the mid-1900s might chose egoism over ethics and thereby prevent the higher self of the human collective from ever emerging.

---

4   My explanation plays off of John Searle's discussion of direction of fit. See Searle, *Intentionality*.

5   Migita, *Tennosei to Shinkaron*, 234. Migita's scientism seems to follow from the Marxist framework he adopts in evaluating state Shinto. The term *tennosei* (emperor system) from the title of his book imagines Meiji orthodoxy as an all-enveloping "feudal" ideology and, therefore, utterly incommensurable with science and, by extension, universal progress. Migita makes Oka the hero of his text because he misconstrues Oka's scientism for his own. Oka's developmentalism and his disdain for superstition blind Migita—as it did for many on the left during the Meiji and Taisho eras—to his aspiration to regenerate traditional nomic cohesion in a modernist fashion by drawing on the palingenetic qualities of organicist evolutionism.

This is a problem that Oka came to confront over the course of his early career, and in this chapter we will discuss how the scientism he drew upon widened its purview to counter such anomic responses to the modern setting. It will be argued that the scientism connected with evolutionary theory expanded from a reformist doctrine that sought to modernize extant institutions into a generative doctrine that aimed to harness the laws of development to create human beings who would satisfy the value-laden requirements of evolutionary necessity. The initial section of the chapter explains how scientism achieved this expansion by drawing on the historicist vision implicit in the organicism of evolutionary morphology. Where the reformist approach to scientism focused on the structural and functional aspects of organicism, the interdependence of parts, the expanded version brought into play the generative drive, the "principle of growth" that not only caused differentiating life forms to cohere into wholes but directed their evolution. This engagement with the temporal, epigenetic process of growth—as exhibited in embryology and cell biology—will enable evolutionism to go beyond reform and present naturalistic development as the creator of values in place of religion. Not just the structure and internal functions of the superorganism but its evolution will become transparent "without residue"[6] and the scientist will be a position to raise it up, develop its parts, cultivate its growth, and determine its health.

The second section will discuss Haeckel's career as an example of this expansion of scientism from a more modest reformist stance, to a generative doctrine that tried to vie with and ultimately supplant organized religion—and which, in the process, established the framework for eugenics and race-hygiene. Finally, in a third section, Oka's early essays on ethics and eugenics will be explored as examples of how the organicism of evolutionary morphology eased him toward a "generative" stance even at a time when his metapolitics were manifestly reformist in their outlook. The coexistence of these stances is key to understanding how Oka's evolutionism came to both genuinely enlighten the masses, promoting science education and disseminating Darwinism in Japan to an unprecedented degree, and contribute to the scientistic framework of eugenics and, much later, totalitarianism. As the epilogue will argue, it is within the organicist framework of genera-

---

6   Todorov, *Hope and Memory*, 19.

tive scientism that *shinkaron* and so-called *tennosei* will approach an accommodation that is much more intimate than the uneasy and segregated coexistence that Migita describes.

SCIENTISMS—REFORMIST AND GENERATIVE

Generative scientism can best be explicated in reference to the account of scientism provided in two of Tzvetan Todorov's works, *Hope and Memory* and *Imperfect Garden*. Todorov explains that "scientism as a doctrine starts from the hypothesis that the real world is an entirely coherent structure. It follows that the world is transparent, that it can be known entirely and without residue by the human mind. The task of acquiring such knowledge is delegated to the requisite praxis, called science. No fragment of the material or spiritual world, of the animate or inanimate domain, can ultimately resist the grasp of science.[7]

Why the "coherent structure" of the "real world" cannot elude science is due to determinism—"the inexorable linking of causes and effects."[8] Functioning within a universe of homogeneous matter, this "causality is not only omnipresent, it is also the same everywhere: scientism is a universalism."[9] Such universalism does not imply, however, uniformity of conditions, for though "the laws (of nature or history) are everywhere the same, the facts they govern are not."[10] Thus, "races are different, as are historical epochs but all are strictly obedient to the forces that determine them and provoke equally predictable consequences."[11]

These all-determining causal forces are what can be "thoroughly known"[12] without remainder by the human mind. According to scientism, "modern science is the royal road to this knowledge."[13] Such knowledge, however, though it is of a deterministic nature is actually "opposed to the passive acceptance of the world as it is."[14] As Todorov makes clear: "if human science can indeed unravel all the secrets of nature, if it can identify the causes of

---

7   Ibid., 19–20.
8   Todorov, *Imperfect Garden*, 22.
9   Ibid.
10 Ibid.
11 Ibid.
12 Ibid.
13 Ibid.
14 Ibid.

all facts and all beings, then it should be possible to modify the processes involved and to steer them in a more desirable direction. Science is a tool of knowledge, but it also underpins techne, a tool for changing the world."[15] Implied in scientific knowledge then is technology which "allows the manufacture of improved existing conditions."[16] "Not satisfied with describing what exists but searching for the mechanism that produced it, scientism can envisage that another reality, better adapted to our needs, might emerge from the same laws…. He who has penetrated the secret of plants can produce new ones, more fertile and nourishing; he who has understood natural selection can institute artificial selection."[17]

The totalistic conceit at the heart of scientism—"everything is determined, everything is knowable, everything can be improved"[18]—raises a basic question: what are the values that decide how the world, which has been made utterly transparent by science, will be transformed? As Todorov poses the problem: "when we speak of the production of something new, we are also speaking of an ideal that stands behind our production. What is a *better* vegetable or animal species, how do we judge one country is *superior* to another, by what criteria do we decide that a certain political regime would be *preferable* to the one that already exists?"[19] Scientism's reply is straightforward: "values follow from the nature of things, they are an effect of the natural and historical laws that govern the world, so again, it is up to science to make those values known to us. Scientism, in effect, involves basing an ethics and a politics on what is believed to be the results of science. In other words, science, or what is perceived as such, ceases to be simple knowledge of the existing world and becomes a generator of values, similar to religion; it can therefore direct political and moral action."[20] Everything, in other words, is submitted to "the rule of necessity,"[21] including values. What is particularly remarkable is that the "nature of the transformation," the imposing of these inexorable laws on the constructed reality of human institutions, "doesn't even deserve mentioning, because it is the ineluctable prod-

---

15 Ibid., 20.
16 Ibid., 22.
17 Ibid.
18 Ibid., 25.
19 Ibid., 22.
20 Ibid., 22–23.
21 Todorov, *Hope and Memory*, 84.

uct of knowledge."[22] As Todorov asserts, the "ends of humankind and of the world become a secondary effect, an automatic byproduct of the search for knowledge—so automatic, in fact, that followers of the cult of science often don't bother to formulate them."[23]

Todorov emphasizes two interrelated consequences that follow from the value-generating natural ontology rendered transparent by science. The first involves defining freedom and, by extension, the artificial, nomic constructions of human willpower, as extrapolations of this ontology. "The only freedom is that of knowledge"[24]—by which Todorov means that the will is truly free solely when it is exercised in adherence to the rule-governed mechanisms of nature. "Freedom, formerly reduced to zero, is here reborn; but it can exist only thanks to the mediation of science."[25] Todorov reasons:

> [T]he cult of science dissolves the contradiction between determinism and free will by introducing a third term, that of "scientific" knowledge. If the world is entirely knowable, if historical materialism does indeed show us the real laws of all societies, and if biology reveals the truth of all living things, then we who possess this knowledge not only have the power to explain existing forms of society and of life, but we also have the power to transform them in the direction we choose. That is how techne, which lies in the domain of the will, can claim to have the authority of science, which in itself seeks only to lay bare what is determined.[26]

As this passage implies, technological engineering, as conceived by scientism, extends beyond tools and other useful artifacts to the entirety of human norms, conventions, and laws. "Having discovered the objective laws of the real, the partisans of this doctrine decide that they can enlist these laws to run the world as they think best."[27] This paradox of absolute freedom to shape and determine nomoi through absolute submission to nature culminates, almost inevitably, according to Todorov, in a eugenic approach to humanity itself: "There is no contradiction here between an entirely determined universe, which rules out freedom of action, and the free will of the

---

22 Ibid., 20–21.
23 Ibid., 20.
24 Todorov, *Imperfect Garden*, 4–5.
25 Ibid., 22.
26 Todorov, *Hope and Memory*, 40.
27 Todorov, *Imperfect Garden*, 23.

scientist-technician, which presupposes freedom. On the contrary: if the transparency of the real includes the human world, then there is nothing to stop us from imagining how to create 'new man,' a human species without the blemishes of the original strain. The logic of livestock breeding ought to work for humankind as well."[28]

The second consequence of scientism concerns the "new man" devised by this channeling of inexorable laws of nature: his existence dissolves utterly into the life of the collective. Todorov explains how this inevitability follows from the "free" submission of human willpower to forces of nature:

> [S]cientism does not eliminate the will but decides that since the results of science are valid for everyone, this will must be something shared, not individual. In practice, the individual must submit to the collectivity, which "knows" better than he does. The autonomy of the will is maintained, but it is the will of the group, not the person. The followers of scientism act as if there were a continuity between the constraints that man endures at the hands of nature and those that society inflicts on him, effacing the boundary between two kinds of freedom: freedom that is opposed to necessity and freedom that resists constraint. Postulating the absence of the one, they conclude the desirable absence (for the individual) of the other.[29]

Believing that "truth is one" the scientistic technicians, the breeders of the new man who harness the group will in the name of necessity, conclude that "pluralism becomes an irrelevant concept."[30] Such scientism, "by evacuating all subjectivity from its vision, takes no account of the contingency of individual wills."[31]Collectivistic technocrats act for the "benefit of nature, humanity, a certain society, not the individuals being addressed."[32] In the end, "nature, the world, and humanity give orders; individuals submit to them."[33]

For Todorov totalitarianism represents a primary political manifestation of this collectivist commandeering of "implacable laws."[34] "A state founded on scientistic principles may veer toward totalitarianism: if one masters the

---

28 Todorov, *Hope and Memory*, 20.
29 Todorov, *Imperfect Garden*, 23.
30 Ibid.
31 Todorov, *Hope and Memory*, 26.
32 Todorov, *Imperfect Garden*, 23.
33 Todorov, *Hope and Memory*, 26.
34 Todorov, *Imperfect Garden*, 227.

whole range of biological and historical processes, one can dispense with consulting the will of individuals."[35] In this sense "the rulers of the countries in which these [totalitarian] regimes prospered believed, or encouraged the belief, that the evolution of the world obeyed strict laws of a social or biological nature. But far from viewing this as a reason for passive resignation, they judged that, with truth on their side, they could pursue their goal with even more assurance. Everything is necessary, of course, but one has the freedom to accelerate necessity in order to follow the direction of history or the direction of life."[36] Seeing that "the world is entirely homogeneous, entirely determined, entirely knowable, on the one hand; but on the other, [that] man is an infinitely malleable material," what Todorov calls "utopian scientism" united "systematic determinism" and "boundless voluntarism"[37] to impose a monism on human life. "The monism of totalitarian regimes comes from the same axiom as the cult of science. Because there is only one rational way of grasping the entire universe, there is no reason to maintain artificial distinctions such as those between different social groups, between the different spheres of individual life (public and private), or between different opinions. Truth is one, and so should the human world be."[38] It is this monism, with its fixation on total social cohesion and complete uniformity of ends, which resulted in "brutal consequences" during the twentieth century: "since class enemies are destined (by the laws of history revealed by science) to disappear, one can eliminate them with impunity. Since inferior races are both harmful and fated to perish in the struggle for survival, according to the laws of evolution established by science, the extermination of these races is a benefit to humanity, a way of giving destiny a hand."[39]

Todorov also recognizes a milder, gentler variant of scientism which appears in apparently nonauthoritarian settings such as Western democracies. Still sharing the belief that political and moral "ends flow automatically from the processes described by science"[40] but not quite seeing themselves as a hand of destiny, the technicians or experts who promote science in these so-

---

35 Ibid., 32.
36 Ibid., 23–24.
37 Ibid.
38 Todorov, *Hope and Memory*, 22.
39 Todorov, *Imperfect Garden*, 24.
40 Ibid., 25.

cieties look to "intervene in numerous aspects of public life"[41] while leaving society itself intact. "Economists, sociologists, and psychologists observe society and individuals, and believe they can identify the laws governing their behavior, the direction of their evolution; politicians and moralists (the 'intellectuals') then urge the population to conform to these laws. The expert replaces the sage as purveyor of final aims, and a thing becomes good simply because it is frequent."[42] Todorov, citing Victor Goldschmidt, goes so far as to identify these experts as comprising a "technocratic collective"[43] that sees itself, and not autonomous subjects, as the exclusive locus of free will. However, it is clear that he regards these scientistic technocrats not as totalistic transformers of the human world but as invasive reformers who are satisfied, at least initially, with adopting a gradualist approach to human improvement.

Throughout his discussion Todorov is quick to reiterate that scientism is not itself scientific. "Science," he claims, "in itself seeks only to lay bare what is determined,"[44] while scientism is "a perversion of determinism" making it "absolute,"[45] thereby conferring on so-called science unlimited authority to impose itself on human affairs. This is in keeping with other critiques of scientism. The classic statement is offered by Hayek who viewed it as preoccupied "not with the general spirit of disinterested inquiry but with slavish imitation of the method and language of science."[46] In an analysis which we will see is highly relevant to Oka's case, Hayek describes how "the sciences had in their beginning to fight their way in the world where most concepts had been formed from our relations to other men and in interpreting their actions."[47] According to Hayek, "the momentum gained in that struggle" carried "science beyond the mark."[48] The resulting product, scientism, is "decidedly unscientific in the true sense of the word, since it involves a mechanical and uncritical application of habits of thought to fields different from those in which they have been formed."[49] Richard Olsen stream-

---

41 Ibid.
42 Ibid.
43 Ibid.
44 Todorov, *Hope and Memory*, 40.
45 Todorov, *Imperfect Garden*, 228.
46 Hayek, *The Counter-Revolution of Science*, 25.
47 Ibid., 27.
48 Ibid.
49 Ibid., 25.

lines this definition somewhat, employing the term scientism "to indicate the transfer of ideas, practices, attitudes, and methodologies from the context of the study of the natural world (which was assumed to be independent of human needs and expectations) into the study of humans and their social institutions."[50]

Where Todorov's approach to scientism differs is that he is as interested in the prescriptive potential of science as in its descriptive and methodological power. The interpretation of the world by science does not just provide a method to analyze sociopolitical institutions, but values that shape and guide their transformation. The suggestion is that the laws and the specific examples described by natural science should be understood as determining the contours and ultimate ends of human norms, conventions, and laws. The reality made transparent through science offers normative exemplars that come equipped with techniques for their implementation in human affairs. Beginning from genuine empirical science, scientism comes to promote technologically loaded prescriptions for human improvement that are more like religion than science.

This use of normative exemplars from the natural world is especially evident in scientistic evolutionism which involves extrapolations from biological phenomena. As we have already indicated, Oka's evolutionism makes this extrapolating move, deriving nomic prescriptions from zoological specimens: moss animals embodied for him "how life in human societies should be."[51] In order to fully unpack Oka's evolutionism, an account of scientism is needed that fully explores the manner in which evolutionary morphology offered, on the one hand, models for human improvement and, on the other, values, purpose, and ultimate ends that replaced religion and envisioned the creation of a new humanity. The nonexclusive, overlapping relationship between the two varieties of scientism we will delineate here—reformist and generative—follows from the organicism that, as we saw in the last chapter, infused evolutionary morphology and its hierarchy of organic individuality. Evolutionists working from this paradigm, such as Haeckel and Oka, used the historicist principle within this organicism to expand their scientism from a program to reform nomoi, to one that sought

50 Olsen, *Science and Scientism in Nineteenth-Century Europe*, 1.
51 Oda, "Oka Asajirō Sensei no Ōmokage," 121.

to generate them. In Oka's case, this generative potential served as an antidote to the anomy that was thought to come with the allegedly degenerative pluralism of late Meiji modernity.

Reformist scientism corresponds roughly with the scientism Todorov ascribes to democratic and other nonauthoritarian regimes. The project this scientism set for itself is one of modernization: nomoi will be corrected to approximate the ontology described by natural science—they will be reformed to fit this "nature." However, though science promises to make this natural ontology utterly transparent, thus opening the way to perfecting improvements, reformist scientism works within the constraints of the values and ultimate ends posited by the particular existing nomos. While the practitioners of this scientism may hope that the ends they recognize in nature may one day remake the norms and conventions of human society—that normative laws will collapse into natural laws—they acknowledge that nomoi are human constructions and their strategy is to seek piecemeal, progressive changes within the parameters of the status quo. Accordingly, a central aspect of their program is educational: the subjective freedom intrinsic to modernity allows individuals to reject traditional ontologies and subscribe to the nature depicted by modern science. This new knowledge of natural necessity will enable an educated society to participate in the construction of a modern nomos based on science. In the case of evolutionism this would mean customs, ethics, and forms of government were all rendered modern in the specific sense of being evolutionarily correct.

The reformist establishment described in Chapter 1 endorsed this variant of scientism. The normative law laid down in the Meiji Constitution established constraints within which reform based on modern science could be enacted. The imperial house and the familialist or tribalist conception of society posited values and ends within whose horizon of meaning the modernizing Todai intelligentsia functioned. Though an Haeckelian such as Katō Hiroyuki may have hoped one day to convert such normative laws to naturalism, his approach was one of gradualist, piecemeal reform. His evolutionism—and, as we will see shortly, that of Oka—can be thought of as a form of metapolitics: it sought to describe the evolutionary preconditions on the basis of which the nomos of the Japanese nation-state must adhere if it wished to survive and prosper. In a sense, the modern knowledge imported through the imperial universities had this reformist, metapolitical intent: the gradualist fitting of the makeshift and malleable Meiji normative laws to the natural laws of modern science.

Organicism contributed decisively to this reformist scientism but it constituted what we can call a soft or atemporal organicism. That is to say, its main focus was not on development but structure and function. It especially stressed the interdependence of parts and the priority of wholes over these parts. Thus, a reformed nomos was one which would mimic this holism, its internal interdependence and intimate interfusion of its constituent parts. In Chapter 1 we saw this at work in the appropriation of Hegelian state science and Katō's development of a correlate to the organic state based on evolutionary science. The intent of Katō, the Todai founder, and others involved, in one way or another, in the state-science project was to use the examples of interdependence and holism—often identified with the division of labor—found in nature to educate the nation to an evolutionary ethos that would reinforce the ultimate ends established by the Meiji state. The atemporal functions and structure of the superorganism would gradually convert the similarly organicist tribalism of the family-state into a modern, evolutionarily correct political order. As we will argue in later chapters, Oka's organicism initially adhered to this same basic approach: it was a metapolitics that sought to undergird and eventually fully modernize existing arrangements.

Generative scientism goes beyond this reformism by identifying organicism with the principle of growth. In this fuller, more consistent organicism, functional-structural interdependence becomes an aspect of the dynamic process of organic development whereby inchoate unities differentiate and reintegrate into fully elaborated, coordinated wholes. Living nature, to which this form of scientism attributes ontological status, is understood in temporal terms: at every level it undergoes growth in the same way an organism does, unfolding like an embryo through stages of development toward full maturity. Grasping the inexorable causal laws that underlie this epigenetic unfolding, the practitioner of scientism is empowered: just as Todorov suggests, the real is made utterly transparent and with this transparency the scientistic technocrat attunes his will with the laws of nature and engineers' improvements.

As with reformist scientism, these improvements are carried out in the nomic sphere, the realm of normative laws. However, the difference in generative scientism is that nomoi no longer simply mimic nature, but are completely generated by it. Norms, conventions, and laws are, in their totality, literal outgrowths of natural ontology. Human constructions and indeed humanity itself are generated by the processes of evolutionary necessity. Most critically of all, the trajectory of this growth process determines values and ultimate ends. Nomoi gain purpose and meaning automatically from nature: not only human institutions but humans themselves acquire worth and significance to the extent that they positively further the implicit direction of the evolutionary growth process. The temporal realization of organicist unity-in-difference, particularly at the societal level, comes to serve as the ultimate measure of human value. Controlling and cultivating the development of human life via the transparency afforded by the laws of evolutionary necessity define an augmented role for technocrats, most of whom began as moderate reformers.

The unannounced radicalism of this generative scientism—reducing normative laws to natural laws of growth—derives from its historicism. As proposed by Hayek and Popper, historicism describes an all-encompassing and purposive vision of human reality premised upon a holism identical to the integrated unities of life assumed by the organic principles of growth. Rejecting "methodological individualism," historicism makes social wholes the main object of scientific enquiry and proceeds to delineate laws of development which these wholes display. The radical aspect of historicism follows from the manner in which knowledge of these historical laws allows for predictions concerning the future course of development. This knowledge enables historicists to serve not only as seers and prophets who prognosticate the future but as activist technocrats who can "accelerate necessity," manufacturing social wholes with the complete and consistent knowledge supplied by historical laws. Like Todorov, Hayek and Popper implicate this methodology in totalitarianism: in such regimes individuals are fashioned from the inside out with the aid of science to ensure the "political hygiene"[52] of the utopian organic collectives, the social wholes governed by historically oriented biological laws. Adopting a "vivisection morality"[53] that follows "every thought down to its final consequences and act[s] accordingly," this

---

52 Popper, *The Open Society and Its Enemies, Volume 1,* 107.
53 Koestler, *Darkness at Noon,* 160.

utopian scientism takes upon itself, in Arthur Koestler's words, "the whole weight of responsibility for the superindividual life to come."[54]

Yet historicist prophesy not only offers a methodology by which to justify and implement total control over social wholes. By reducing nomoi to a natural or ontological process of development, it also appropriates the value-positing, nomos-anchoring function traditionally reserved for religion. As Peter L. Berger explains, religion preserves the fragile contrivances of human norms and conventions by attributing ontological status to them: normative laws are no longer properly understood as man-made but as extensions of cosmic processes. Along with an illusion of ineluctability this "cosmization"[55] imparts ultimate values to nomoi: the cultural world becomes a "sacred canopy" that precludes the terror of anomy in a universe otherwise bereft of inherent meaning. The historicism of generative scientism performs a cosmicizing "world-maintenance" function analogous to that of religion. The law of growth that governs its organicist ontology grants nomoi not only natural status but meaning and purpose by situating them within a grand cosmic process of evolution. That is to say, the direction and intimated final ends of evolutionary development confer meaning in the same manner that the cosmic or heavenly order of religion does. Participation in the furtherance of this cosmic organic growth process delineated by evolutionary science establishes the worth of all living entities. In short, the particular organism acquires value to the extent that it positively contributes to the evolution of a higher individuality—a social whole or the "superindividual life to come"—of which it is a constituent part.

Religious-like value-creation, complete technological control of developmental processes, and an assumed ideal of collective health—all of these elements of generative scientism come together in eugenics. As Todorov suggested, the "logic of livestock breeding" seems an automatic byproduct of the propensity to discover ultimate, nomos-generating values in the transparency of the real. The founders of the eugenics and race-hygiene movement explicitly drew this connection between the sacralization of health and a mastery of the inexorable laws of nature. As Francis Galton explained to the sociological society at London University in 1904: "[Eugen-

---

54 Ibid., 100.
55 Berger, *The Sacred Canopy*, 24–25.

ics] must be introduced into the national consciousness like a new religion. It has, indeed, strong claims to become an orthodox religious tenet of the future, for eugenics cooperate with the workings of nature by securing that humanity shall be represented by the fittest races."[56] It is this religious emphasis that perhaps most distinguishes generative scientism from its education-focused reformist sibling: not only are the normative laws now engineered by science treated as unquestioned tenets of scientific faith but the technique of cooperating with the "workings of nature" tempts the technocratic upholders of this faith to transcend their reformist stance, which involved educational construction of norms and conventions, and to entertain the possibility of manufacturing humans who embody their religious ideal. In particular, the social wholes—whether conceived as societies, nations, races, or other biological groups—that are subject to the laws of organic growth must be cultivated, through knowledge of these very laws, to develop and integrate in a healthy manner in order to achieve the organism-like unity-in-difference that was their implicit end. The primary danger to this healthy integration is the various parts of the social organism that have differentiated and become specialized in the course of growth—individuals. Thus, maintaining collective health—the ultimate value of generative scientism—meant, essentially, using knowledge of the communitarian commandments of organic development to breed individuals that instinctively live out these commandments, subsuming themselves automatically to the integrated superindividuality of national life.

Because they reduce individual persons to the cells of the social whole, superorganisms are the ideal actualization of this scientistic faith based on evolutionary morphology. However, as often as not, the ideal they represented was invoked in the negative: instead of directly extolling the evolution of progressively higher and more inclusively holistic stages of individuality through the process of differentiation and integration, generative scientism frequently resorted to bemoaning dysgenic phenomena that impeded or diverged from the realization of such organic health. Especially with the spread of evolutionary science across the Europeanized world toward the fin-de-siècle, theories of degeneration began to appear, providing a necessary precursor to the eugenics movement. According to Roger Griffin,

---

56 Quoted in Griffin, *Modernism and Fascism*, 148.

the "dramatic rise to prominence in early-twentieth-century history" of eugenics is, in fact, largely attributable "not to disinterested scientific curiosity or even human idealism, but to the prospect it offered of purging society of its degeneracy through an unprecedented alliance between modern science and the power of the modern state."[57] Such degeneration manifested itself as a decline in physical and spiritual health: "Moral decadence, chronic diseases like tuberculosis, venereal diseases and alcoholism, crime and deviant social behavior—which included merely having two children or less—were diagnosed as symptoms of hereditary degeneration."[58] Thus, "social problems could be treated as diseases in a malfunctioning social organism."[59] Why these symptoms of decline called for drastic measures by the technocratic overseers that ministered to collective hygiene was because it was individuals who were the carriers of social disease. These cells of the "cell-state" were degenerate in that they obstructed the development of the social organism into a higher, more fully elaborated unity. The well-being of future generations, which constituted an ultimate value in generative scientism, was put in danger by such unhealthy cells—with the criterion for what is unhealthy now extended to any uncooperative part of the social organism that prevented nomic integration.

It is in this sense that individualism itself could come to be understood as potentially pathological and, in the normative sphere, a source of anomy. As the coming pages will illustrate, the envisioned absorption of nomos into nature often led the practitioners of generative scientism to regard sociocultural phenomena as natural events that required technological or biomedical correctives. The perceived threat to norms and conventions that came with the emergence of modern individualism falls into this category: the very subjective freedom that, ironically, allowed members of society to question received ontologies and employ the scientific method also empowered them to comprehend the malleability and, indeed, the artificiality of nomoi—even those constructed on natural "facts." The difficulty in getting such subjectively awakened and, often, self-interested individuals to accept natural science as the new generative source of norms and conventions—a scientistic religion of national health—posed a challenge to those who as-

---

57 Ibid.
58 Weindling, *Health, Race and German Politics*, 9.
59 Ibid., 19.

pired to engineer the superorganism. In many cases this could inspire, as we just suggested, initiatives to circumvent education and directly implant collective values into humans through the eugenic breeding of appropriate social instincts.

The final section of this study will argue that Oka Asajirō began to make overtures of just this sort when the allegedly decadent individualism in the period after the Russo-Japanese War seemed to have worsened beyond educational remedy. Dreading both the anomy brought on by the new pluralistic consumer culture and reactionary proposals to combat this anomy with state Shintoism, Oka's theory of decadence invokes an historicist law of cosmic or, more precisely, evolutionary development that would simultaneously generate nomos in the way religion does and inform eugenic programs for national rejuvenation. Though Oka never abandoned his modernizing, reformist stance as educating the nation about evolutionism (*shinkaron*), his generative scientism surmised that the egoism of contemporaries had become so decadently overdeveloped that supplementary, extraeducational measures would be required to restore national health. The new humans that constitute the cells of the regenerated national superorganism would come to occupy their proper station in the collective division of labor not through educational understanding but through instinct. Rejecting the degeneracy of the present, Oka, as we will see, employs the organicist principle of growth at the heart of scientistic evolutionism to suggest a future alternate modernity for the nation, one in which wayward individuals have been reconstituted as products of evolutionary growth—and norms and conventions come to emanate from this same generative ontology.

Generative scientism, as we have described it, constitutes an example of what Roger Griffin calls programmatic modernism. As we saw in the introduction, programmatic modernism rebels against the decadent, dissolute, anomic present by advancing a comprehensive transformative vision that will help rejuvenate community and establish a credible, alternate account of ultimate reality. According to Griffin, programmatic modernism realizes such visions through programs that will "transform not just art but humankind itself, or at least a chosen segment of it."[60] The vision which generative scientism draws upon is, as we have seen, the hard organicism based on the

---

60   Griffin, *Modernism and Fascism*, 116.

principle of growth in nature which focuses not only on interdependency but the temporal process of development through which inchoate unities differentiate and reintegrate into fully elaborated wholes. This evolutionism encompasses the human cultural world of normative laws and thereby overcomes the anomy of decadent contemporary modernity. Though generative scientism never gives up on inculcating this vision through education, its ultimate program for transforming humankind involves eugenic techniques. The organicist laws of biology promise to provide the full transparency of the real and thereby make possible this total transformation, one which encompasses human nomos and human "nature" together. Thus, the programmatic modernism of generative scientism amounts to engineering future human superorganisms as healthy alternatives to the decadent, anomic modernity of the present.

What finally distinguishes generative scientism from its reformist brethren is this rejection of contemporary modernity. While both scientisms sought to reduce nomos to nature, and both, being based on evolutionism, found in organicism a model for this reductionism, reformist scientism placed implicit trust in modern individuals and their subjective freedom. Through education in the atemporal truths of organicism on display in nature, these differentiated unities of life would consent to integrate themselves back into the collective existence of society. In this manner nomoi that had been established by traditional or extrascientific means could be gradually modernized from within: their norms and conventions adjusted to the natural ontology through piecemeal reform. In contrast, generative scientism has come to understand that the conditions of modernity which make science possible also undermine the possibility of remaking nomoi on a scientific basis. In particular, the awakening of subjective freedom is seen as hindering organicist integration and threatening permanent anomy. This decadence, which results from individuals devising their own willy-nilly plans and projects based on their own private cogitations on ultimate reality, can only be overcome by turning organic nature into a generative source of nomoi akin to religion. Invoking the temporal aspect of organicism, a new horizon of meaning is established for existence by placing all phenomena of living nature, including human societies, within a process of evolutionary growth whose direction of development defines ultimate value. Nomoi are rejuvenated and humans themselves regenerated once this new cosmic order of differentiation and reintegration into higher unities of life is instantiated. Superorganisms and the individuals that comprise them overcome anomy and rediscover health, value, and transcendent purpose by aligning themselves with this historical law of evolutionary growth. Finally, the same scientific method that prognosticates the future can be employed to engineer instincts and produce healthy humans congenitally immune to anomy.

Contrary to what might be expected, such starkly contrasting stances toward modernity do not render these scientisms mutually exclusive. In fact, as we will see in the case of Oka, they often coexist side by side. This may be attributed, at least in part, to the convoluted maneuver involved in transferring "positive science" and evolutionary biology in particular into a "source of transcendence"[61] that could cosmicize nomoi. As Migita indicates in the opening chapters of *Tennosei to Shinkaron*, the materialist ontology of evolutionism had the same impact in Japan as it did in the West: undermining traditional cosmologies that undergirded normative laws and opening the possibility of "disenchantment of the world" or "advent of nihilism" along with the encouragement of subjective freedom. For evolutionists such as Oka the impetus to move from a reformist to a generative mode of scientism came from conditions which evolutionism, paradoxically, helped usher in. The modernity which generative scientism sought to overcome was the same one that the modernizing science helped foster. This paradox was hidden from generative scientism due to the tremendous effort involved in battling reactionary forces that responded to this same anomic modernity by dogmatically defending traditional cosmologies in the face of science. Fighting superstition in the name of rationalism, modernity, and science, proponents of scientism were often blind to how their own proposals to counter this threat and ground nomos in an ontological substrate often came closer to revelation than science.

Thus, we will see Oka endorsing the spirit of science in education while, at the same time, developing a theory of decadence that treats evolutionism as a value-creating, organicist cosmology that can eugenically remake human life. In the last section of this study, it will be argued that it is this programmatic modernist aspect of generative scientism that provoked a response from Shinto ultranationalists which would result in the transforma-

---

61   Ibid., 148.

tion of its orthodoxy into a radical, proto-totalitarian doctrine. The historicist organicism of generative scientism will be seen to constitute nothing less than the "scientistic foundations"[62] for this and other Japanese ideologies in the twentieth century.

ONTOGENY OF THE NATION-STATE: HAECKEL'S SCIENTISMS

The distinction ventured here between reformist and generative varieties of scientism is particularly evident in the career of the founder of evolutionary morphology, Ernst Haeckel. In this section we will show how the frustrations that Haeckel experienced in reforming the normative sphere according to the ontology of evolutionary science goaded him to radicalize his evolutionism into a monist religion. Constituting a prime example of programmatic modernism, it is this scientistic faith that would prove integral to later historicist, palingenetic ideologies, such as fascism, that looked to the processes of organicist development for values and techniques by which to remake social wholes in the manner of a gardener or animal breeder.

The social whole that Haeckel hoped to reform with the "organicist Darwinism" of his evolutionary morphology was the nation-state. As Di Gregorio explains, the historical circumstances surrounding the German wars of unification and the establishment of the Second Reich shaped Haeckel's scientism: "Haeckel could not avoid thinking of the concept of Nation, given the changes his own country were undergoing at the time. The concept of Nation had to be reconsidered in light of the new science, or better, in light of the scientific reform Haeckel felt he was helping shape. There was almost a messianic quality in the absolute duty he felt he had to spread the new creed. The aspect of *reform*, on which he insisted all his life, is vitally important in order to understand Haeckel's actions and conceptions."[63]

Reconsidering "the concept of the nation ... in light of the new science" meant, from the very beginning of Haeckel's academic career, understanding it as an organic individual. As early as 1860, within a year of the publication of the *Origin of Species*, he was writing to a friend about "our common German nation" in terms of a "healthy embryo which is capable of

---

62 Ibid., 184.
63 Di Gregori, *From Here to Eternity*, 125.

evolution."[64] As discussed in the previous chapter, Haeckel's *General Mor-phology* (1866)—which not only established the scientific paradigm of evo-lutionary morphology but was published the same year as the Austro-Prus-sian War—envisioned a hierarchy of organic individuality, the top echelon of which consisted of "corms, clumps or colonies,"[65] or what we would re-fer to today as superorganisms. Haeckel's explicit and literal identification of the nation-state with superorganisms, their inner workings and external relations, continued right up until his final major popular work, *Eternity*, in which he observed that "The biologic [sic] relation of the cells to the tissues and organs' of lower organisms is the same as that which exists among the higher animals between the individuals and the community of which they are component parts. Each cell, though autonomous, is subordinated to the body as a whole; in the same way in the societies of bees, ants and termites, in the vertebrate herds and the human state, each individual is subordinate to the social body of which he is a member."[66] Situated at the top of the or-ganizational hierarchy of living nature, "civilization and the life of nations" were not only "governed by the same laws as prevail throughout nature and organic life,"[67] but nation-states represented "the culmination of the evolu-tion of life from simple to complex organisms."[68]

This "corporatist biology"[69] as Paul Weindling has called it, was not sim-ply a matter of applying biology to the normative realm of politics, society, and morals, as Haeckel claimed he was doing.[70] Instead, much as laissez-faire liberalism in mid-nineteenth-century England influenced Darwin's selectionism, Haeckel's later "synthesis of evolution and cell biology"[71] in-corporated statist conceptualizations into his evolutionary morphology, re-flecting "the integrating needs of Wilhelmine imperialism."[72] Thus, Haeckel "developed the concept of an animal economy in such a way that it could be reapplied in a biological form to social problems"[73] and "emphasized how

64   Gasman, *The Scientific Origins of National Socialism*, 3.
65   Di Gregori, *From Here to Eternity*, 127.
66   Gasman, *The Scientific Origins of National Socialism*, 83.
67   Weindling, *Health, Race and German Politics*, 34.
68   Ibid., 30.
69   Ibid., 45.
70   Gasman, *The Scientific Origins of National Socialism*, 91.
71   Weindling, *Health, Race and German Politics*, 27.
72   Ibid., 47.
73   Ibid., 41.

the organs formed from tissues were like state departments and institutions: rule by a central government was comparable to the power of the brain as nerve center."[74] Most significantly, in evolutionary morphology "there was a concern to establish elemental categories such as the cell, the individual or the family in a way that would not lead to atomistic disintegration but would reinforce organic unity."[75] Haeckel's frequent reference to the nation-state as a *Gesamtperson* or collective individual signifies perhaps the culmination of his successful efforts to vividly articulate a "biological nationalism" by employing "organicist terminology"[76] in descriptions of living nature. According to Gasman, "the Germans, Haeckel and his followers contended, must either accept a new philosophy based on evolution and science and unite with the forces of nature, or cease, through weakness and deterioration, to exist as a nation."[77] The statist rendering of biology in Haeckel's hierarchy of organic individuality facilitated not only the formulation of this new philosophy, what Haeckel called "monism," but also efforts to reform the nation as an organicist superorganism. In this manner, understanding the nation as a *Gesamtperson* became intrinsic to reforming that nation on the basis of evolutionary necessity.

Having in his best-selling *The History of Creation* made his grand system of organic individuality available to a global public, Haeckel was particularly enthusiastic for the founding of the German Reich in 1871 which he "glorified" as "highly evolved."[78] The "organicist vision of a reformed society through applying biology,"[79] which he continued to offer up in his popular writings during the early decades of the regime, was intended to serve as a modernizing metapolitics: it would deploy cutting-edge science to transcend internal divisions and act "as an ideology of social integration."[80] According to Weindling, Haeckel was particularly eager to avoid

pinning his evolutionary world view to a specific political party. He reacted strongly against bourgeois commercialism of the "railway fever" and con-

---

74 Ibid., 44.
75 Ibid., 30–31.
76 Ibid.
77 Gasman, *The Scientific Origins of National Socialism*, 31.
78 Weindling, *Health, Race and German Politics*, 43.
79 Ibid., 47–48.
80 Ibid.

demned socialist materialism. He endeavored to establish biology as a popular and participatory science, and as providing objective standards beyond the
limitations of all parties whether liberal, socialist or conservative. Science was
thus a surrogate for civic values and party political activism. His distinctive
position is intelligible within the context of Wilhelmine intellectual imperialism; as critical of the repressive old regime, and yet concerned to develop revitalized forms of national power.... Biology was to take a leading role in social
and psychological affairs. The expectation was that it would be emancipatory
and objective, dissipating superstition and patriarchal prejudice.[81]

This metapolitical "popular and participatory science" was to be inculcated by making "evolutionary theory ... the basis of education in the newly
united nation."[82] Haeckel hoped that "in the school of the future nature will
be the chief object of study; a man shall learn a correct view of the world he
lives in; he will not be made to stand outside and opposed to nature."[83] Instilling a "correct view" of the natural world through the educational system and his popular writings was especially critical for Haeckel, given the
role that evolutionary morphology ascribed to Lamarckism in rounding out
the process of growth: through the mechanism of use-inheritance habitual
actions would add new traits on to the mature organism and these would
be passed along to its offspring. Haeckel's reasoning vis-à-vis education was
that if individuals were taught about their proper subordinate station within
the social whole from which they had differentiated, then they would forgo
egoism and adopt other-directed habits that identified self-interest with the
welfare of the organic nation state. These "altruistic" habits, as Haeckel, after
Darwin and Huxley, referred to them, would engender acquired traits that,
when inherited by subsequent generations, internalized a predisposition for
gregariousness. Eventually social instincts would evolve and on their basis
duty and national allegiance could be cultivated. In this manner educational
enlightenment sought to ground normative laws in the organicist natural ontology delineated by evolutionary biology: first by getting the population to
subscribe to biologically correct moral-political habits and then by permanently ingraining these integrating naturalistic norms as instincts. The ca-

---

81 Ibid., 47.
82 Ibid., 43.
83 Quoted in Gasman, *The Scientific Origins of National Socialism*, 38.

pacity to question tradition that the scientific revolutions of the previous centuries had bestowed would enable properly educated humans to ground norms, conventions, and laws in a natural ontology, one that would eventually, via Lamarckism, permanently transform humanity itself.

Haeckel not only looked to "central state direction"[84] to fit nomos to nature and keep the differentiated nation integrated, but he singled out the founder of the new Reich, Otto von Bismarck, as the agent of this scientistic reform. Famously, in 1892, two years after the chancellor had been ousted from office, Haeckel and other members of the Jena academic community extended an invitation for him visit to the university. During the former chancellor's July appearance in the Jena market square,[85] Haeckel addressed the gathered crowd and grandiosely conferred on "Prince Otto von Bismarck [the] Honorary Doctor of Phylogeny—the first and greatest Doctor of Phylogeny."[86] The basis for "this new honorary title," Haeckel explained, was Bismarck's role as "the creative genius of modern German history" and "the deeply perceptive observer and anthropologist of mankind, the far-seeing historical investigator and ethnologist, the practical creator of history.'"[87] Alluding to the publication of his own masterwork, *General Morphology*, during the war with Austria, Haeckel directly associated the beginning of the new Reich with the establishment of evolutionism: "While the booming guns at the Battle of Koniggratz in 1866 announced the demise of the old Federal German Diet and the beginning of a new splendid period in the history of the German Reich, here in Jena the history of the phylum [*Stammesgeschichte* or phylogeny] was born."[88]

In spite of the clever parallelism that Haeckel drew between the ontogeny of the Reich and the birth and development of evolutionary theory under his own scientific leadership, the years of Bismarckian rule did not always facilitate the growth of a reforming evolutionism. In fact, during the very decades of the 1870s and 1880s in which Haeckel began to disseminate his system in both its popular and academic manifestations, instruction in biology and evolutionary theory met with stiff resistance across Germany. As Weindling explains:

---

84   Weindling, *Health, Race and German Politics*, 42.
85   Richards, *The Tragic Sense of Life*, 357–59.
86   Gasman, *The Scientific Origins of National Socialism*, 18–19.
87   Ibid., 18.
88   Ibid.

Soon after unification ... restrictions were imposed on the teaching of biology in schools. In 1876 a school teacher, Hermann Müller, was censored for having taught the evolutionary popularization by Carus Sterne, stating the chemical origins of life from carbon. Haeckel reacted with a campaign for reinstating the teaching of biology in schools, leading a series of ferocious debates at the *Naturforscher Versammlungen* in 1877, 1882 and 1886. At the height of the campaign, in February and March 1878, he toured Germany and Austria holding popular lectures on the cell soul and the monistic unity of man and nature. In 1879 a debate on the teaching of Darwinism in schools in the Prussian House of Representatives resulted in the banning of the teaching of evolution in schools. In 1882 an education order excluded natural history teaching from higher classes in schools.... The authorities suspected biology of subversive materialism and as aiding the spread of socialism. Biology was a casualty of the anti-socialist laws.[89]

Why this hedging on the question of evolutionary education did not stand in the way of Haeckel's hyperbolic bestowal of the honorary doctorate in phylogeny on Bismarck can be explained by the chancellor's response to an even more crucial issue: national integration. For Haeckel this was the essential question. When he extolled the "German nation as among the highest evolved of social organisms,"[90] he meant the differentiation and specialization in form and function that had led to an unprecedented division of labor. While such individuation increased the power and capacity of the nation-state by diversifying its attributes, the resulting progressive differentiation could also threaten to become a fatal, centrifugal process. Whether in a siphonophore superorganism, an ant colony, a beehive or a pluralistic civil society, polymorphism and the division of labor might result in dissolution, with each cell of the cell-state dysgenically breaking off and going its own way. Bismarck's centripetally oriented "social technologies of integration"[91] responded to this danger by countering the impediments to a healthy, national cohesion, such as socialism. Though the antisocialist laws contributed to the restriction of evolutionary theory from schools because it was thought to encourage materialism, Haeckel endorsed Bismarck's illiberal measures, believing that "Darwinism stood for order, differentia-

89   Weindling, *Health, Race and German Politics*, 43.
90   Ibid., 42.
91   Ibid., 16.

tion, and specialization in contrast to egalitarian socialism"[92] and its fixation on divisive class conflict. Likewise, at the other end of the political
spectrum, Haeckel approved of Bismarck's attempts to curb free-market
excesses. He strongly believed that the "civic individualist tenets of liberal
economic theory, derided as vulgar Manchestertum,"[93] had been discredited by the economic upheavals of the 1870s. The protectionism and inter-
ventionism of the Bismarck regime were necessary to establish a healthy
national collectivism and rein in the "doctrinaire individualism"[94] of laissez-faire economics.

What ultimately won over Haeckel, however, was Bismarck's vigorous, albeit ill-fated, campaign against the greatest threat to national cohesion and the acceptance of evolutionism: conservative Christianity and, in
particular, the Catholic Church. According to Weindling, Haeckel and his
colleagues were powerfully inspired by "the conviction that every original
fact—each discovery of a species of microscopic plankton or observation
on the contortions of embryos—was a nail in the coffin of Christianity as
an archaic superstition."[95] In Bismarck's Kulturkampf, which took aim at
the Catholic Center Party and featured an aggressive program of discrimination against the influence of the church on civil institutions, Haeckel,
in particular, seems to have recognized a Germany that was evolving into
a "progressive, civilized and educated society"[96] immune from debilitating
superstition. As he was fond of reiterating in his popular writings the pa-
pacy's retrogressive influence was particularly glaring at the onset of the
war, which led to the creation of the Reich: just five days into the fighting
with France in 1870 the "militant head of the church" claimed "infallibil-
ity for himself and all his predecessors in the papal chair,"[97] an act—along
with the proclamation of immaculate conception in 1854 and the condem-
nation of modern civilization in 1864—which Haeckel depicted as a "*guerre
a l'outrance* against independent science."[98] For Bismarck's efforts to struggle against this ultramontane reaction Haeckel hailed him as "the great

92 Ibid., 43.
93 Ibid., 46.
94 Ibid., 15.
95 Ibid., 40–41.
96 Ibid., 43.
97 Haeckel, *The Riddle of the Universe*, 324.
98 Ibid., 323.

hero, not only of the national unity, but also of the rational emancipation of Germany."[99]

Yet Haeckel's passion for the Kulturkampf and his conviction that "religion is generally played out,"[100] did not mean he endorsed the immediate and wholesale overthrow of all things Christian. Integral to what we are calling his reformist scientism is Haeckel's surprising affirmation of the central normative principle of Christianity: "Do unto others as you would that they should do unto you."[101] In his view, this Golden Rule, which he believed was endorsed by all major religions, was an expression of the natural law of association, the sociological principle that held throughout organic nature and was responsible for the coordination and integration into higher unities of life of constituent parts which had individuated in the cycle of growth. Not only cells within an individual organism but the "persons" that comprise superorganismic groups cohere according to this rule of association. Among humans association required balancing the egoism of persons against their altruism toward fellow members of the group and, by extension to the collective interest of the group as a whole: "[B]oth these concurrent impulses are natural laws, of equal importance and necessity for the preservation of the family and the society; egoism secures the self-preservation of the individual, altruism that of the species which is made up of the chain of perishable individuals."[102]

Though Haeckel insisted repeatedly that egoism and altruism were to be counterbalanced, one against the other, it was evident that he regarded the latter to be the basis of ethics and organic unity: "If a man," Haeckel wrote, "desires to have the advantages of living in an organized community, he has to consult not only his own fortune, but also that of the society, and of the 'neighbours' who form the society." He had to comprehend his responsibility to the broader community. "He must realize that its prosperity is his own prosperity, and that it cannot suffer without his own injury." Haeckel sought to remind the Germans that "this fundamental law of society is so simple and so inevitable that one cannot understand how it can be contradicted in theory or in practice; yet that is done today, and has

99 Ibid., 335.
100 Ibid., 331.
101 Ibid., 350–51.
102 Ibid., 351.

been done for thousands of years."[103] Echoing Hegel's *Sittlichkeit*, which we discussed in the first chapter, Haeckel claimed that only a "highly developed moral sense" truly recognized the "value of the state": the state was a higher unity in which the lower unity of the moral individual came to identify its own "welfare, true happiness and satisfaction."[104] Any doubts about the relative importance of such "altruism" over egoism were erased during the Great War, when Haeckel urged ethical youth to battle by arguing: "If his ethical development is high enough for him to have achieved the proper balance between egoism and altruism, he will also be mindful of his social duty to the state and will gladly offer up his life for the preservation of the fatherland.... [Soldiers will] sacrifice even their family happiness to the higher interests of their country."[105]

Haeckel's conclusion that "the old Golden Rule of morals" should become the "norm within the state" and "guide the conduct of the different social classes to each other"[106] epitomizes his reformist scientism. Altruism among human beings was a manifestation of natural laws in the normative sphere: the sociological law of association, the integrating principle by which internally differentiated unities of life cohere into full-fledged individualities at every echelon of the natural world. For Haeckel the Golden Rule represented a soft, atemporal organicism that recognized interdependence and properly identified the existence and welfare of constituent parts with the continued survival of the whole. Accordingly, the Christian nomos was to be scientistically reformed, not overthrown: "[I]n spite of its errors and defects, the Christian religion (in its primitive and purer form) has so high and ethical value, and has entered so deeply in the most important social and political movements of civilized history for the last fifteen hundred years, that we must now appeal as much as possible to its existing institutions in the establishment of our monistic religion. We do not seek a mighty *revolution*, but a rational *reformation*, of our religious life."[107]

The agent of this reform was the kind of rational, metapolitical entity that Haeckel thought he recognized at times in Bismarck's Reich: poised above the fray of divisive parties, subversive ideologies and egotistical strivers that

---

103 Gasman, *The Scientific Origins of National Socialism*, 45.
104 Ibid., 44.
105 Ibid., 131.
106 Ibid., 83.
107 Haeckel, *The Riddle of the Universe*, 336.

threatened to pull the nation asunder, the state would gradually modernize the nation by enforcing scientifically grounded policy measures and making educational appeals to the population. Such modernizing metapolitics would begin its work within the values set down by the existing nomos. While ultramontane extremism that denied modern science had to be rooted out, traditional norms, conventions, and laws, which emanated from original Christianity and the Protestant Reformation, were to be carefully rationalized to reflect the natural ontology set down by evolutionary science. Above all, the organicism implicit in the altruistic Golden Rule had to be refashioned to fit the real organicism of living nature. In short, Haeckel's reformist scientism posited that "the Christian system must give way to the monistic."[108]

It was largely out of fears the "monistic" system grounded in evolutionary morphology would not achieve normative status that a more radical, temporal organicism began to emerge in Haeckel's scientism. While never explicitly rejecting reformism, this generative scientism did not derive ultimate values from the existing nomos but from the evolution of life. The epigenetic growth process that characterized living nature at every level of complexity came to be treated as an evolving cosmological order whose progressive trajectory would establish ultimate values. A system of norms, conventions, and laws would be generated by this developmentalist ontology—and the cultural world inhabited by humans would acquire meaning and purpose in accordance with the actualization of growth. With nomoi conceived as direct outgrowths of determinate nature, the role for humans was confined to cultivating institutions that expressed the laws governing natural processes. By the 1890s, Haeckel, as we have already seen, was referring to this radical scientism as a monistic religion. Even though he continued to enunciate his moderate reformist stance, which sought to convert the organicist elements of received religion to naturalism, this attempt to present evolutionary morphology as a religion in its own right—an ontological source of norms and values—would supply a younger generation with a template for programmatic modernist activism. As we will see, not only the eugenics and racial hygiene movements but the accompanying declinism that called for an alternate modern mode of existence would make use of the generative framework at the basis of this secular religion.

---

108 Gasman, *The Scientific Origins of National Socialism*, 64.

Haeckel cosmicized his monism into a religion by emphasizing the temporal aspect of organicism when describing the lives of nations and civilizations. In contrast to the soft organicism of his reformism, which merely focused on the interdependence and implied holism of the Golden Rule as a basis for biological nationalism, this hard organicism stressed the law of growth (biogenesis) that governed the cosmic, historical process out of which human superorganisms evolved. In his *The Wonders of Life* of 1905, a globally circulated book which clarified many of the issues enunciated in his blockbuster, *The Riddle of the Universe*, from five years earlier, Haeckel makes it clear that this superorganismic growth is an epigenetic unfolding through developmental stages—an actualization of unity-in-difference in the manner of an embryo progressing to maturity:

> The history of civilization teaches us that its gradual evolution is bound up with three different processes: (1) Association of individuals in a community; (2) division of labor (ergonomy) among the social elements, and a consequent differentiation of structure (polymorphism); (3) centralization or integration of the unified whole, or rigid organization of the community. The same fundamental laws of sociology hold good for the association throughout the entire organic world; and also for the gradual evolution of the several organs out of the tissues and cell-communities. The formation of human societies is directly connected with the gregariousness of the nearest related mammals. The herds of apes and ungulates, the packs of wolves, the flocks of birds, often controlled by a single leader, exhibit various stages of social formation; as also the swarms of the higher articulates (insects, crustacea), especially communities of ants and termites, swarms of bees, etc. These organized communities of free individuals are distinguished from the stationary colonies of the lower animals chiefly by the circumstance that the social elements are not bodily connected, but held together by the ideal link of common interest.[109]

Haeckel's depiction of the evolution of nations, civilizations, and species in terms of such ontogeny—the growth of an organic individual—follows from his biogenetic law. As we saw in the last chapter, biogenetic law was based on the concept of parallelism that had survived from idealist mor-

---

109 Haeckel, *The Wonders of Life*, 169.

phology: "ontogeny recapitulates phylogeny" and does so, in part, because both echelons of organic individuality, the embryo and the phylum (a genealogical individual), cycle through parallel life stages as they develop from inchoate unities, into differentiated polymorphic entities and before finally reintegrating into complex wholes that displayed a mature unity-in-difference—a holistic, higher individuality. Haeckel attempted to verify this law by illustrating the history of its ancestors (phylogeny) repeated during the epigenetic growth of the individual organism—a palingenetic process that, as we will see later on, also had great political significance for programs to rejuvenate the nation. However, for our purposes here what is important is that the treatment of unities of life at the apex of the organic hierarchy as superindividuals with their own ontogenetic life cycles committed monism to an historicist vision of the nation-state. In particular, the foreseeable developmental stages of differentiation out of an inchoate unity and reintegration into full and mature organic complexity came to serve as an historical law by which the growth of the nation could be predicated, controlled, and, perhaps most importantly, assigned value. Whether a nation was seen as "valuable" or not was determined by how successfully it had achieved the unity-in-difference of epigenetic development—that is, by adherence to a standard of healthy growth. Conceptualized as intrinsic to evolution, a universal process of organic development, such health took on a cosmic value akin to that laid down by a religion.

Haeckel's discussion of the "Value of Life" in his *The Wonders of Life* delineated how his scientism came to generate ultimate values that had the potential to not only reform but supplant received religious belief. The "value" that Haeckel has in mind when considering the lives of particular organic individualities is their worth to the "outer world."[110] In his view, "it is just as true of the species as of the individual that it lives for itself, and looks above all to self-maintenance."[111] For the individual organism this makes its own life "the first aim and standard of value."[112] Haeckel, however, contrasts this "subjective estimate of life" with an objective evaluation grounded in natural ontology:

---

110 Ibid., 410.
111 Ibid., 387.
112 Ibid., 410.

This objective value increases as the organism develops and presses into the general stream of life. The chief of these relations are those that come of the division of labor among individuals and their association in higher groups. This is equally true of the cell-states which we call tissues and persons, of the higher stocks of plants and animals, and of the herds and communities of the higher animals and men. The more these develop by progressive division of labor and the greater the mutual need of the differentiated individuals, so much the higher rises the objective value of the life of the latter for the whole, and so much the lower sinks the subjective value of the individual. Hence arises a constant struggle between the interests of individuals who follow their special life-aim and those of the state, for which they have no value except as parts of the whole.[113]

Though Haeckel reiterates in this context that "the chief task of the modern state is to bring about a natural harmony between the social and the personal estimate of human life" and that the best way to achieve this harmony is through "reform of education, the administration of justice and the social organization,"[114] his chief focus is on the powers that such nation-states will need to develop in order to healthily maintain themselves and survive. In fact, a "might is right" form of ethical positivism had been implicit in Haeckel's monism since *The History of Creation*, where he stated that "[a]s a rule, for organic life the utmost violence justly triumphs."[115] In *The Wonders of Life* he not only makes the acquisition of powers and capacities that will strengthen the most elaborate organism in nature, the state, a prerequisite for healthy self-maintenance, but he depicts the development of such powers as part of an historical process driven by the epigenetic law of growth. The life of a nation-state or civilization becomes more objectively valuable to the degree it has advanced and empowered itself by differentiating and specializing. Actualization of unity-in-difference, augmentation of power, and sheer survival success together come to define a standard of health generated from within the evolutionary processes of nature that can be used as an historical measure of ultimate value.

Haeckel employs this measure to describe the history of human civilization as a grand ontogenetic process that establishes the superior value of

---

113 Ibid.
114 Ibid.
115 Asajirō Oka, "Jindō no Shōtai" [The true character of humanity: the human-way], in *Shinka to Jinsei* [Evolution and human life] (Tokyo: Yūseidō Shuppan, 1968), 64.

nation-states founded on monism. Borrowing from Alexander Sutherland's *The Origin and Growth of the Moral Instinct* (1898), he sets down successive stages of "civilization and mental development"[116] represented by four classes of humans: savages, barbarians (or semisavages), civilized races, and cultivated races. Elaborating substages of development within each of these four primary stages, his account can be best understood as a global unfolding of epigenetic differentiation and reintegration, with specific peoples and races evincing greater or lesser levels of mental complexity and social organization. Thus, savage tribes exhibit a nearly undifferentiated form of life that Haeckel repeatedly asserts is inferior in its organization to certain "herds of mammals (apes, gregarious carnivore, and ungulates) and the flocks of social birds (hens, geese, ducks)."[117] Living in "families or scattered small groups"[118] which, even at the most advanced "higher savage" stage, never exceed 500 members and display only the very rudiments of social organization, these savages have little mental capacity as evidenced by their crude implements, primitive clothing, and lack of permanent housing. Represented by the contemporary "races" such as the Veddahs, Ainu, Tasmanians, American Indians, Hottentots and Negroes of Australia and Africa, this inchoate humanity was, in Haeckel's estimation, like "our own ancestors ... ten thousand or more years ago."[119] For the most primitive of these hunters and gatherers, "the value of the life ... is like that of the anthropoid apes, or very little higher."[120]

The value of life only begins to increase with the "slight division of labor"[121] among the first agriculturalists whom Haeckel dubs "barbarians or semisavages." Residing first in agricultural villages of up to 5,000 persons and later in towns ten times that size, these barbarians, by the time they evolve into "higher semisavages," not only evince specialized labor functions but other indicators of growing mental and organizational complexity such as stone dwellings, advanced metalwork, hereditary distinctions of rank, and the beginnings of writing and the arts. The "civilized races" which succeed these barbarians usher in a truly sophisticated differentiation with their "ad-

---

116 Haeckel, *The Wonders of Life*, 392.
117 Ibid., 419.
118 Ibid., 392.
119 Ibid., 393.
120 Ibid.
121 Ibid., 394.

vanced division of labor and improvement of instruments,"[122] creating the conditions for a complex, bureaucratic polity. As Haeckel explains: "The increasing specialization brings about a great elaboration of individual functions, and at the same time a great strengthening of the whole body politic, as there is complete mutual dependence. The citizens see that they must submit to the laws of the state."[123] By the time humans have evolved into "higher civilized races" they are living in cities of "ten millions or more" with stone houses and paved streets, using science to navigate the seas and fight wars, distributing books, and enjoying the fruits of a "highly centralized state" which features courts, a system of codified laws, and "numbers of government officials" of "settled rank."[124] Typified by the "Romans of the empire, and the Italians, French, English, and Germans of the fifteenth century,"[125] these most advanced examples of "civilized races" also include, significantly, contemporary Chinese and Japanese.

The culmination of this global epigenetic process, the full realization of unity-in-difference for human beings, is found in the "cultivated races."[126] Haeckel reserves this stage of historical development for the modern West: the European nations of the sixteenth to eighteenth century are categorized as "lower cultured races" representing the "full growth of mental life" in the age of exploration, scientific discovery, and religious reformation, while the Europe and North America of Haeckel's own nineteenth century qualify as "middle cultured races" for their starling advances in science, industrialization, and political participation. Referring to his contemporary era as the "century of science,"[127] Haeckel identifies the achievements of these middle cultured races with modern life itself. For him modern advances in the "personal and the social value of life"[128] are stark and undeniable, and he hammers this point home by contrasting the superior differentiation and integration of the "social body" of the modern nation-state over the primitive existence of the lowly savage in all "fields of vital activity."[129] As examples he points to the "self-maintenance" that the modern state provides through

---

122 Ibid., 396.
123 Ibid.
124 Ibid., 397.
125 Ibid.
126 Ibid.
127 Ibid., 399.
128 Ibid., 401.
129 Ibid.

medicine, hygiene, and nutrition; the capacity for "complex sensations" that are made available by education and technological aids such as the microscope and telescope; and vast improvements in locomotion that have come with the new "invaluable means of rapid and convenient travelling."[130] Haeckel sees the latter making an especially crucial contribution to the higher individuality of the nation-state: "This progress in the means of transit is not less valuable socially than personally. If we conceive the state as a unified organism of the higher order, the development of its means of transit corresponds in many ways to that of the circulation of the blood in the vertebrate frame."[131] Haeckel even finds benefits to superorganismic integration in the reproductive practices of modern humans: unlike their savage counterparts who regarded women "merely as an object of lust,"[132] civilized men of the present have refined sexual love and opened the possibility for "pure marriage[s]" that can not only serve as "the most solid foundation of the state" but promote "the balance of egoism and altruism," the "ethical golden rule"[133] that coordinates individuals within the national collectivity.

Of all "these brilliant triumphs of modern civilization"—which, again, Haeckel believes have "only been made possible by the various forces cooperating in a vast division of labor, and by the great nations utilizing their resources zealously for the attainment of the common end"[134]—none is more important than the sophisticated mental life of civilized men—what he calls their "higher psychic activity."[135] According to Haeckel, "never, in the whole of history, has true science risen to such an astounding height as it has at the beginning of the twentieth century. Never before did the human mind penetrate so deeply into the darkest mysteries of nature, never did it rise so high to a sense of the unity of nature and make such practical use of knowledge."[136] In his estimation, these developments, which he directly links to the "construction of the monistic and realistic philosophy,"[137] have brought about "a higher development of the whole mind of a modern community."[138] Em-

130 Ibid., 404.
131 Ibid., 405.
132 Ibid., 402.
133 Ibid., 403.
134 Ibid., 408.
135 Ibid., 407.
136 Ibid., 408.
137 Ibid., 399.
138 Ibid., 408.

bodied in its individuated yet integrated social organization, this collective mind represents a vast increase in the value of life and in the capacity of the nation-state to act.

Yet it is also in precisely this area that Haeckel identifies serious obstacles to the final evolution of "middle cultured races" of the present into "higher cultured races." His fears that the political realization of the "perfect state" of the future, in which the epigenetic process of growth has finally resulted in a completely harmonious "rational balance between egoism and altruism,"[139] is being stalled and thwarted by forces within society that are discouraging the individuated parts of the nation from "altruistically" reintegrating into its collective life. Haeckel's invocation of evolutionary necessity as a value-generating historical process as well as his increasingly rhapsodic promotion of his monism as a religion appear to have been triggered by the sense that after the removal of Bismarck these forces were on the ascendant. In 1892, the same year as the former chancellor's visit to Jena, Haeckel found himself once again having to campaign for the unrestrained teaching of biology and evolution in school, an experience which prompted "the fiery statement of philosophy of monism"[140] in his *Monism as Connecting Religion and Science: The Confession of Faith of a Man of Science*. The pages of his *The Riddle of the Universe* and *The Wonders of Life*, to which we have just been referring, bristle with attacks on the resurgent Center Party and ultramontane Catholicism which he perceived to be the primary threat to his integrative monist ethic. However, his anxiety also extended to the market economy which was enabling an unregulated egoism by turning individuals into fashion apes. He also insinuates that internal conflict could potentially be fomented by "uneducated sections of the community" who, in contrast to the more valuable educated members, "wander far below in the valley, treading their monotonous and weary way in a more or less stupid condition."[141]

Thus Haeckel's generative scientism was largely a response to the socialist, capitalist, and, above all, conservative Christian forces that he worried would prevent normative *Kultur* from attaining the highest stage of cultivation and realizing a "perfect" organic polity in line with evolutionary science. What Haeckel confronted in his frustrated attempts to disseminate his or-

---

139 Ibid., 400.
140 Weindling, *Health, Race and German Politics*, 45.
141 Haeckel, *The Wonders of Life*, 409.

ganicist Darwinism were the liabilities inherent in appealing to modern subjects through a program of mere reform: reforming nomos implied that the new nomos being put forth was something that individuals had to decide to endorse—it was something they had to understand and embrace. Despite his continued advocacy of education as the leading edge of national transformation, Haeckel, in the end, did not believe dissent from the sociopolitical truths of monism was an option: the superorganismic state was an outgrowth of all-determining nature, and the only choice involved was internalizing evolutionary necessity or perishing. By describing the emergence of this state as a direct product of the development of the cosmological order, Haeckel was attempting to establish that the values and conventions of his monistic nomos were ineluctable—coextensive with a nonnegotiable natural ontology. More than the vitalistic unity of *Geist* and matter, which Haeckel appropriated from Goethe and natural philosophy and which is usually pointed to explain his monism, it is this ontological embedding of human institutions within this universal process of epigenetic growth that renders his monism a religion. Such cosmicization did not represent an abandonment of reform but rather an attempt to make the dire necessity of evolutionary science apparent to a fickle public bedeviled by superstitions. Haeckel's fierce battles with implacable opponents, especially on the Christian right, served to paper over any contradictions between the reformist and generative stances and to make his dogmatism appear rational.

Along with the resurgence of these opponents to monist philosophy, the pessimistic atmosphere of the 1890s also contributed to Haeckel's generative scientism. Rumors of degeneration were rife among the European intelligentsia and Haeckel's emphasis on nations and civilizations increasing their value by fully completing the epigenetic process of growth should be understood as offering an alternative vision of healthy development. In *The Wonders of Life* he specifically mentions Max Nordau who had warned, the very same year in which *Monism as Connecting Religion and Science* appeared, that "in our days there have arisen in more highly developed minds vague qualms of a Dusk of Nations, in which all suns and all stars are gradually waning, and mankind with all its institutions and creations is perishing in the midst of a dying world."[142] Though Haeckel acknowledged "the darker

---

142 Quoted in Marius Turda, *Modernism and Eugenics* (New York: Palgrave Macmillan, 2010), 25.

sides of modern life" which "have been laid bare by Max Nordau," he himself never abandoned, as we have just seen, his "hope and confidence" in the "luminous features of modern civilization."[143] He still believed what others were calling decadence could be corrected "if reason is permitted to have its way in practical life."[144]

It was rather Haeckel's younger colleagues, deeply influenced by his generative scientistic *Lebensanschauung*, who came to identify modern civilization with decadence and sought to forge an alternate version of modern life through the techniques of eugenics and racial hygiene. Not only did Haeckel's generative vision of epigenetic civilizational growth provide a template for this movement, but from the beginnings his writings had specifically entertained the possibility of applying artificial selection to the national body. In his *History of Creation*, fifteen years before Galton started using the term *eugenics*,[145] Haeckel marveled at the "special law" that the ancient Spartans had implemented by which "all newly born children were subject to careful examination or selection" and those deemed "weak, sickly, or affected with any bodily infirmity were killed.... Only the perfectly healthy and strong children were allowed to live and they alone afterwards propagated the race."[146] In other sections of the book he went on to wonder whether "artificial medical selection" was not permitting "heredity diseases" to linger at the expense of "succeeding generations."[147] Even more chillingly, Haeckel called for capital punishment for "incorrigible and degraded criminals," reasoning that it is a "benefit to the better portions of mankind; the same benefit is done by destroying luxuriant weeds, for the prosperity of a well-cultivated garden."[148] This gardener approach to humankind which, we will see in a moment, Roger Griffin regards as indicative of scientistic programmatic modernism, remained a feature of Haeckel's monism right through to the twentieth century, reappearing in his *The Wonders of Life* nearly forty years later: "We are not bound ... under all circumstances to maintain and prolong life, even when it becomes utterly useless.... Hundreds of thousands of incurables—lunatics, lepers, people

---

143 Haeckel, *The Wonders of Life*, 400–401.
144 Ibid., 400.
145 Turda, *Modernism and Eugenics*, 19–20.
146 Quoted in Gasman, *The Scientific Origins of National Socialism*, 91.
147 Ibid., 95.
148 Ibid., 96.

with cancer, etc.—are artificially kept alive … without the slightest profit to themselves or the general body."[149]

Despite this overriding concern with the "general body" and future generations in his generative scientism, Haeckel's optimistic appraisal of modernity meant he still looked to the transformative Lamarckian potential of education to address social problems. A generation removed from mid-century German liberalism, the "dissident young doctors and intellectuals"[150] under Haeckel's influence who founded the racial hygiene movement were less restrained and more consistent in bringing the ontological claims of evolutionism to bear on every aspect of national life in the name of a healthy organic cohesion. Among the major figures who, beginning from the generative vision of Haeckel's monism, sought to cure the ethnic nation of its degenerative contagion can be counted the physician Wilhelm Schallmayer, who published the first eugenics text in Germany[151] and famously won the Krupp Prize, which Haeckel administered[152]; Alfred Ploetz who authored the seminal text on racial hygiene in 1895[153] and, twelve years later, established the International Society for Racial Hygiene; Gerhard Hauptman, who, with Ploetz, "established a League to Reinvigorate the Race as early as 1879"[154]; and Ludwig Plate, who succeeded Haeckel in his chair at the University of Jena.[155] Perhaps the most vivid representation of what monism could mean in the political realm can be found in the writings of Dr. Johannes Unold. A central figure in Haeckel's Monist Alliance,[156] Unold shared the master's disdain for the clerical influence on the nation, but he leveled his most biting criticism at mass society: "[A] people is not an aggregate, a sand-pile of loose equal granules, but is an organic unity."[157] Writing in 1907, he blamed these pathologically atomized and dissolute conditions on "exaggerated and self-seeking individualism" which "tended to ignore … connections with the community."[158] Absorbed exclusively with their own

149 Ibid., 95.
150 Weindling, Health, Race and German Politics, 19.
151 Turda, Modernism and Eugenics, 25–26.
152 Weikart, From Darwin to Hitler, 15; Popper, The Open Society and Its Enemies, Volume 2, 61.
153 Griffin, Modernism and Fascism, 149.
154 Turda, Modernism and Eugenics, 29.
155 Weikart, From Darwin to Hitler, 15.
156 Ibid., 66.
157 Quoted in Gasman, The Scientific Origins of National Socialism, 42.
158 Ibid., 47–48.

self-interest, these unregulated individuals had fallen under the sway of corrosive political ideologies and divisive mass movements, the most notorious of which was anarchism. As Unold explained: "[T]he egotistical pretensions among more or less degenerate individuals has reached its climax in the criminal madness of anarchism."[159] To counter egoism, monism endeavored to "cultivate an 'insight' into the mutual dependence of the individual and the community."[160] In particular, individuals must be made to understand that they live at "the disposal of the species"[161] and that in nature "thousands, indeed, millions of cells and individuals are sacrificed"[162] for the sake of the organic collective in which they are embedded. As we will see in later chapters, Oka Asajirō, writing at precisely the same time in Japan, would reach nearly identical conclusions based on roughly similar premises.

Paul Weindling portrays the use of eugenics and racial hygiene by these doctors and intellectuals as a form of "technocratic antipolitics": wary of the divisiveness of conservative, liberal, and socialist political factions and profoundly alarmed by the "consequences of industrialism in terms of poverty, disease, and homelessness," these promoters of eugenics and "organicist welfare schemes" sought "collectivist (but not socialist) solutions to social problems" believing that "politics could be replaced by scientific planning and administration."[163] Yet it would perhaps be more accurate to say that their particular metapolitics entailed a totalistic program that extended far beyond mere reform, comprehensively applying to "everyday life" the "categories of hereditary biology."[164] Ultimately, it meant replacing the constructed nomos of the extant nation-state with one comprehensively determined by the developmental cosmic order described by evolutionary science. In Weindling's terms, "eugenics represented a process of substitution of biological values where hitherto the categories of political economy and civil society had predominated."[165] Taking the organicist paradigm of Haeckel's secular religion to its logical extreme, eugenics proposed employing the "transparency of the real" afforded by epigenetic processes to hy-

159 Ibid.
160 Ibid.
161 Ibid.
162 Ibid., 49.
163 Weindling, *Health, Race and German Politics*, 20–21.
164 Ibid.
165 Ibid.

gienically reconstitute the body of the nation and its constituent cells. The health of future generations became the pretext for "accelerating necessity" and invasively rejuvenating the collective life of the people.

It is because of this emphasis on rejuvenation in the name of an alternative healthy modern mode of future existence that Roger Griffin identifies Haeckel, his Monistic Alliance, and the closely related eugenic and racial hygiene movements as the "outstanding example of the scientistic currents of social modernism"[166] in the critical period from the 1880s to the end of the Great War. Griffin's portrayal of this rejuvenation as a "palingenetic" move is especially appropriate when considering those who were attempting to implement the paradigm of evolutionary morphology in the nomic realm of human affairs: palingenesis is not only, as we saw in the last chapter, the critical feature in the recapitulation process described by biogenetic law, but it, in effect, imagines a replay of the epigenetic growth process that infuses all of living nature—a restart of the life that every echelon of individuality, from the cell up to the superorganism, experiences. Modernist regeneration is nothing but a call for a new beginning of the process of differentiation and reintegration, one that will unfold without the pathologies that weaken the body of the organism and prevent its final instinctual realization of unity-in-difference. For Haeckel, as we have seen, this "perfect state" was one in which altruism and egoism were in supreme, nation-affirming harmony. Dysgenic forces, especially ultramontane Catholicism, stood in the way of realizing this palingenetically renewed future but Haeckel believed that the redoubling of monism by construing it as a cosmic truth akin to religion would enable the cultivated races of the twentieth century to actualize a healthy organic unity. Meanwhile, a younger cohort, much less restrained by the traditional nomos and waging an all-out war on decadence, entertained more radical programs that involved the possibility of remaking the human fabric of the nation in order to attain organic unity.

Griffin associates this type of scientism with fascist regimes, which he refers to, after Zygmunt Bauman, as "gardening states."[167] Not only "the extensively planned, controlled and engineered society of Fascism" but "the Nazi vision of a national community culturally and eugenically purged of

---

166 Griffin, *Modernism and Fascism*, 147.
167 Ibid., 183.

all symptoms of deviancy and degeneracy" represent rebellions against "the decay of a supposedly organic nation" that sought to "'cultivate' and 'breed' healthy human beings"[168] and with the bodily instantiation of these hygienic values to overcome the horror of anomy. Griffin is careful to stress, however, that the "scientistic foundations," which we have been calling generative scientism, were laid in the nineteenth century and thus came to be "nurtured by elements within the scientific, academic, political, and cultural elites of early twentieth century 'liberal' democracies as well."[169] In the case of Oka these same scientistic foundations would, as in fascist and democratic states of the same era, come to conjoin "the modernist image of society as a defective, decaying organism to be revitalized through draconian social and political measures of improvement" with the "growing power of the modernized state."[170] As we will see, the Japanese version of generative scientism, as articulated by Oka, would be both constrained and encouraged by the pressures experienced by the Japanese state, resulting in an accommodation with fascism—not to speak of other ideologies—less forthright but perhaps equally influential.

OKA'S POTENT HOLISM: ETHICS FROM ECOLOGY

The overriding constraint on Oka's scientism was one not experienced by Haeckel: he was forbidden to challenge the cosmic legitimation of the reigning nomos. The official orthodoxy of the imperial line could not be publically questioned. This fact imposed unique conditions on Oka: all of his scientistic musings had to be overtly in the reformist mode. As with Haeckel, this entailed identifying connections between the underlying organicist ontology described by evolutionary theory and features of the nomic realm. Unlike Haeckel, though, Oka could only indirectly hint at these parallels— he could not address them forthrightly. Nevertheless, Oka set out to do the next best thing in his early writings, portraying a modernizing metapolitics whose organicism would not undermine orthodoxy—and might even reinforce it. It was only, as in the case of Haeckel, when the orthodoxy went on the offensive that Oka began to develop the generative vision that had been

---

168 Ibid., 183–84.
169 Ibid.
170 Ibid.

implicit in his evolutionism from the beginning. This generative scientism found expression in his theory of decadence. We will argue that though the cosmic vision implicit in this theory could never be overtly stated, its formula for national regeneration would have a surprising impact on the development of the orthodoxy, challenging it to become futural and organicist in the manner of developmental biology. In the conclusion we will even intimate that this orthodoxy would eventually struggle to arrive at a satisfactory synthesis with this scientism, one that wedded the emperor-centered historical view to the generative vision of evolutionism.

As what we have just laid down would suggest, Oka, like Haeckel, entertained both reformist and generative stances at once, the atemporal organicism of interdependence driving his reformism, the temporal organicism of epigenetic growth shaping his generative vision with its expansive cosmic overtures. An early essay will serve to explain how both of these coexisted from the start of his career as a popular writer attempting to influence the normative disposition of the nation. Entitled "Good and Evil in the Animal World," it appeared in December 1902, eight years after Oka's return from Leuckart's Leipzig laboratory. As the previous chapter recounted, these eight years had been extraordinarily productive for Oka on a variety of fronts. As a scholar and researcher, he had continued to publish articles in international science journals such as the *Journal of Natural History*. As a textbook writer he began to churn out titles such as *Modern Textbook of Physiology*, *Modern Textbook of Zoology*, and *Education and Natural History*. As a classroom educator he had secured a position at the Tokyo Higher Normal School. This professorship, which he held until 1929, led to a simultaneous appointment as an education bureaucrat in the Ministry of Education.[171]

All of these activities should be understood as part of the "reformist statist" enlightening project of Todai graduates who had gone abroad to bring modernizing knowledge back with them to Japan. For Oka, disseminating an up-to-date understanding of biology through the educational system, the government bureaucracy, and, eventually, society at large would help reform the nation-state without undermining its emperor-based German constitutional order. "Good and Evil in the Animal World" was written in pre-

---

171 Tsukuba, "Kaisetsu" [Commentary], 430–55.

cisely this spirit: normative notions of good and evil would not be discarded but instead properly grounded in biology. According to Oka "we must at all costs seek the foundations of ethics in ecology."[172] As he explained using language and a style of analysis familiar to us from Haeckel's writings—the term "ecology" was in fact coined by Haeckel himself[173]—from this same period: "If the habits of various types of animals are investigated through ecology, the shifting phases of these customs are clarified during the move from lower animals gradually up to higher animals, the connection between individual life and group life is sought out and we finally ascend up to the human level, then perhaps the firm foundations of ethics will be determined here for the first time."[174]

Despite this aspiration to finally ground human ethics in biology "for the first time," Oka carefully avoids discussing human beings in this early essay. Instead his focus is on the ethical life of primates and on defining what he calls the "ape-way." Not only does the device of the ape-way allow Oka to leave it to his readers to make their own inferences concerning the reform of human norms and conventions, but it facilitates the emergence of more radical insights in his evolutionism, particularly those we identified above as typifying generative scientism. When Oka finally gets around to directly grounding human ethics in biology with his "human-way," these value-generating aspects will start to call into question his reformist stance and point the way to the programmatic modernism of his later career.

As Oka depicts it, the "good and evil" of the ape-way is necessitated by the transitional state which primates occupy between two levels of organic individuality, neither of which should be described in moral terms. At the lower level, corresponding to what Haeckel called persons, Oka identifies lone individuals whose conduct merely advances their own survival. Pointing to the example of solitary wolves, Oka claims "With such an animal, the result of each action touches upon its individual self alone. Even if it succeeds, the advantage does not extend to others. Even if it fails, others are not inconvenienced. When it is strong, it prospers. When it is weak, it perishes. It neither receives favors from, nor becomes entangled with anyone."[175] In such cir-

---

172 Oka, "Seibutsukai ni okeru Zen to Aku" [Good and evil in the animal world], 54.

173 Richards, *The Tragic Sense of Life*, 4.

174 Oka, "Seibutsukai ni okeru Zen to Aku" [Good and evil in the animal world], 54.

175 Ibid., 46.

cumstances "the designations good and evil" are "utterly lost."[176] Similarly, at the higher level, Oka considers "animals which have attained the consummate group life—such as ants and bees."[177] That the "consummate group" is Oka's term for the higher individuality represented by Haeckelian "corms" or superorganisms becomes explicit in how he portrays them:

> Each group operates as if were an individual possessing a single will. Each of the individuals that make up these groups is like a developing cell in the body of the group: functioning merely at the behest of the group's will. To put it another way: for these animals the spirit of each individual transcends the boundaries of the private self—including the ego—which places importance only on individual welfare. It reaches the region of the higher self where the goal is to maintain the prosperity of the entire group. Studying ants and bees busily searching for and gathering food all day and taking care of larvae, it is evident that everything they do is only for the use of the group to which they belong, and not even one thing directly benefits the individual self.[178]

Morality does not apply to "ants and bees" and other consummate groups because they are "merely confined to doing as a single group what other animals, which lead solitary lives, do as a single individual. Such deeds cannot be criticized using the terms good and evil."[179]

For Oka, primates are like ants and bees in that they spend "their entire lives gathering together in large numbers."[180] However, where they differ is that they have not attained the "region of the higher self": individuals within the group have not integrated into a more complex unity—they remain differentiated egoists who only reside in groups so long as doing so satisfies their self-interested survival needs. Morality arises to transcend this individuated isolation of the lone ego—and it only makes sense as a facilitator of organic cohesion: "distinguishing the actions of individuals as good and evil and then criticizing them can only be done in cases when the will of the group and the desires of the individual mutually contradict among animals which lead their lives in groups."[181]

---

176 Ibid.
177 Ibid., 47.
178 Ibid.
179 Ibid.
180 Ibid., 48.
181 Ibid., 53.

As Oka portrays it in this seminal essay, morality begins as expediency and ends up, through Lamarckian use-inheritance, as social instinct. Although they are inclined to "passionately take hold of the desire to obtain advantages for themselves alone no matter how it affects others,"[182] individuals come to understand that maintaining the group and looking after its members is the best way to realize their own self-interest. Eventually, "individuals within such groups are able to narrow the gap between the desires of the self, that is, selfishness (*Egoismus*), and the requirements of the group, that is, altruism (*Altruismus*). At certain times they willingly fall in with the demands of the group, handing over all gains to the group as a whole. At other times they are weak-willed, falling prey to their desires and causing the entire group great trouble."[183] According to Oka it is at this point that "good and evil are differentiated from one another."[184] As he explains, "when the results of an individual's actions confer advantages to the whole group, comrades in charge of distributing benefits praise these results, calling them good (*Bonum*). And of course when the results of individual actions damage the whole group, comrades who share in sustaining these damages blame these results, calling them evil (*Malum*)."[185]

It is among large and semipermanent primate groups that altruistic habits promoting social cohesion translate into instincts:

the unconscious habit of each individual to act to a degree for the benefit of the whole group is left over as an instinct because it remains an unaltered fact that, no matter how big the group becomes, if each individual fails to control his desires and comply with group demands, the existence of the group cannot be preserved. Without knowing the reason why, individuals come to present an outward appearance as if they are merely doing good for goodness sake. When we read the report of scholars who travel to tropical regions to investigate the habits of apes, it is often mentioned that when an ape fights and sustains a wound, other apes provide care and comfort by aiding and protecting him and bringing him food to eat and water to swallow. Moreover, when a parent dies leaving behind a child, right away another ape takes over the nurturing duties, raising this adopted child with the same affection

---

182 Ibid., 49.
183 Ibid.
184 Ibid.
185 Ibid., 49–50.

as it shows the one to which it gave birth. Thinking of these acts alone it seems that for apes there may even be something like an ape-way (*Simianitas*) based on the spirit of philanthropy (*Philopithecia*).[186]

Even though Oka associates this "ape-way" not only with philanthropy but duty and conscience, he, following Haeckel's monistic *The Riddle of the Universe*, makes a point of distinguishing it from Kant's dualist based "*Kategorischer Imperativ*."[187] Instead these altruistic instincts, which directing conduct from "deep inside the heart," function at the behest of a "collective will [*Volitio cormi*]" that treats each individual "like a marionette acting in obedience of its strings: without knowing the reason each individual seems to conduct himself in accordance with the demands of the group."[188] The ape-way is nothing but an integrating device to ensure group survival: when the needs of the group alter, "the criterion for the terms good and evil also vary according to the time."[189] It is, therefore, "completely meaningless to take only certain acts apart from the life of the group and criticize them as good or evil."[190] Deeds count as moral to the extent they serve the preservation of the group.

The purpose of this situational grounding of ethics in ecology is not to point out the arbitrariness of morality but to intimate the preconditions for a normative order conducive to group survival. This is, in fact, the first articulation of what, in the next section, we will call Oka's metapolitics. Rather than offer ideological prescriptions in the name of evolutionary theory, as so many others in Japan had done, Oka sought to delineate the biological basis for all prospective normative visions. The implicit aim was to reform the current norms and conventions, including the prevailing orthodoxy, so that they conformed with these preconditions—that is, with evolutionary necessity. As we will see in the second section of this study, Oka's emphasis on external threats in the formulation of the "ape-way" would become a more and more pronounced feature of his reformist scientism. With the war against Tsarist Russia and particularly its increasingly anomic aftermath, Oka rebranded the ape-way as the soft organicism of what he called the human-way, an instinc-

---

186 Ibid., 50. The terms *"Kategorischer Imperativ"* and *"Volitio cormi"* are written using the original Latin alphabet in Oka's text.
187 Ibid., 51.
188 Ibid.
189 Ibid., 53.
190 Ibid.

tive ethic of interdependence that ensured the national solidarity necessary to combat external threats amid the anarchic ecology of the new imperialism.

At the opening of this chapter we suggested that Migita was wrong to characterize Oka as a subversive who believed *shinkaron* and the orthodoxy of so-called *tennosei* were absolutely incompatible. The reformist stance we have set down here implied, in contrast, that the system of norms—in this case, exemplified by good and evil—could be redefined to align with the ontology delineated by evolutionary biology. Good and evil, for instance, could be reconceptualized according to the soft organicism made available by the hierarchy of organic individuality. However, we also suggested that problems inherent in making individuals cohere into "higher unities" could result in the emergence of a more aggressive organicism, one which stressed epigenetic reintegration and tended to regard ultimate values as generated by the process of growth itself.

In Oka's case, the sense of dissolution did not come until after the conflict with Russia when the wartime national consensus was revealed to be chimerical. However, the first intimations of his generative scientism and its embrace of healthy growth as an ultimate value that potentially transcends the laws of the existing nomos could already be felt as early as 1902. In "Good and Evil in the Animal World," this generative outlook is particularly evident in how Oka depicts the internal life of his "consummate groups." Like those from his generation who were promoting eugenics and racial hygiene in Europe at this very moment, Oka portrayed the continued healthy growth of such collective bodies as an ultimate good—and individual persons as expendable. The connection he wishes his readers to draw with human institutions is quite unambiguous: "Studying ants and bees busily searching for and gathering food all day and taking care of larvae, it is evident that everything they do is only for the use of the group to which they belong, and not even one thing directly benefits the individual self. Furthermore, the individual that has already become useless to the group is killed without mercy and disposed of by the gathered members of the group. Never are they lent assistance merely because they are ants or bees: on the basis of these labels alone one does not deserve respect in one's capacity as an ant—nor is one accorded value due to one's rights as a bee."[191]

---

191 Ibid., 47.

This disavowal of the inherent rights of individuals leads Oka to suggest eugenic-like measures to preserve the health and integrity of the group. For instance, he marvels at how the individual drone within the superorganismic beehive, "once his reproductive function is used up" is "directly killed off and ejected from the group, just like a used-up baby tooth is expelled from a child's body."[192] Similarly, he accounted for the evolution of duty and conscience in the animal world by explaining how among flocks of birds the thieves who steel from other's nests to build their own are ritually eliminated through exemplary executions: "upon detecting these deeds, the birds from the surrounding area all gather together there. After surrounding the defendant and noisily caw-cawing for a short while at him, a punishment committee is selected and this offending bird is pecked to death."[193] Oka says this behavior is "not an exceedingly strange occurrence"[194] and that he has actually observed it himself on the grounds of Ochanomizu Shrine in central Tokyo. In his view, such punishments not only ingrain a conscience—which he defines as "merely the individual's fear of sanctions from the group"[195]—but are essential for maintaining the "order of bird society."[196] In short, among such instinctually united groups, "each individual possesses value only as a single element belonging to the group. Splitting off from the group it cannot be said to have any special individual value merely as an individual alone."[197]

While these examples pertain to consummate groups, Oka's presentation "ape-way" and, by extension, human morality imply that the organic cohesion displayed by these superorganisms was to be regarded as normative. To a degree greater than even Haeckel's monism, Oka's human-way will construe the balancing of egoism and altruism as an ethic of subordination of individuals to the social whole. Though like Haeckel he will attach value to the individuated organisms that emerge within the group for the specialized powers they contribute, he will regard them as not only expendable but, ultimately, a potential threat to the collective body. Making its appearance in the later essays of *Evolution and Human Life*, Oka's generative scientism

192 Ibid.
193 Ibid., 51.
194 Ibid.
195 Ibid., 52.
196 Ibid., 51.
197 Ibid., 47.

will attribute the late Meiji anomic crisis following the Hibiya Riot of 1905 to the untethered egoism of the industrializing, laissez-faire urban world. As we will see, Oka, by 1910, will be synthesizing a theory of degeneration with public proposals for racial hygiene and a critique of superstitions influence on society. Together, these will offer a vision of an organically reintegrated modern life submitted as an alternative to the decadent, anomic, and individualistic present.

Along with remedying ills of dysgenic individualism, Oka's project of resituating collectivist norms and conventions within the organicist ontology of epigenetic development will have a profound effect on the central unmentionable superstition of the Meiji constitutional order. As I shall argue in the conclusion, Oka's generative scientism will goad what Migita refers to as *tennosei* and what we will call, after Skya, Shinto ultranationalism to begin to adapt itself to evolutionism in future decades. In a sense, the reformist quest of civilization and enlightenment will be realized by grounding the makeshift myths of "*tennosei*" in modern science—the goals of reformist scientism are only achieved through the appearance of a more radical, "generative, and modernist cosmology." As the coming section will reveal, this coexistence of reformist and generative scientism in Oka's writings date from the beginning of his career as a public figure when the conflict in Manchuria inspired him to articulate a metapolitical vision of ethnic nations perpetually at war.

PART II

Metapolitics

In his recent *War of the World*, Niall Ferguson speculated on the consequences of "apparently nonpolitical ideas and assumptions that nevertheless had violent implications"[1] in the early twentieth century. The great clash of ideologies in the decades leading up to and encompassing the Russian Revolution, the rise of fascism, and the two world wars masked, he suggests, the subtle yet pervasive influence of conceptual systems not overtly political such as those promoted by science and religion. In particular, his book argues that biological ideas had an especially catalytic effect, disseminating "the hereditary principle in theories of racial difference."[2] Writing from a Dawkinsian perspective, Ferguson intimates that the notion of speciation among *Homo sapiens*, which had become widespread by the early twentieth century thanks to the rise of biology and evolutionary science, helped trigger what appears to be an innate human predisposition to favor those we perceive to be like ourselves—and to do so even in the absence of actual racial differences. Along with economic volatility and the decline of multicultural empires that had facilitated ethnic harmony, the resulting "race meme" was partly responsible for the tendency to treat other men like aliens or subhumans—a tendency which, in part, explains the unprecedented levels of violence seen in what Ferguson calls "the fifty year war" that began with Japan's clash with Russia in 1904.

What Ferguson has not adequately appreciated is the extent to which those most responsible for spreading these biological conceptions of hu-

---

1   Ferguson, *The War of the World*, xxxvii.
2   Ibid., xli.

mankind often deliberately attempted to wield influence in this indirect, seemingly disengaged manner. In large measure their success in the political realm can be attributed to not having overtly participated in ideological discourse. Instead, they sought to shape all discussions about morality, society, religion, and politics—the full spectrum of normative laws—by setting down naturalistic ontological preconditions. In the case of nation-states this meant identifying national viability with adherence to evolutionary necessity. Only those nations that modernized in a manner that fit nomos to nature would survive and prosper.

In the last chapter, we saw that Ernest Haeckel adopted such a metapolitical stance. However, he and those who came to advance his paradigm— and do so with less deference to tradition than he displayed—ultimately found themselves articulating a vision that, by its generative implications, suggested superseding mere reform. Paul Weindling calls such a stance the "technocratic antipolitics" of this younger cohort and for him it formed the background for accommodation with later ideologies. Disturbed by the turbulence of party politics and the vicissitudes of the economy, this newly minted bureaucratic and professional class attempted to construct "a scientific basis for administration and for an ideology of social cohesion."[3] For Weindling the eugenics movement had its basis in this ideal of a healthy "social integration," the combination of "apolitical" and "national commitments" enabling German biology and medicine to assume "social tasks of national reconstruction."[4] By the turn of the twentieth century, this movement, citing dangers of degeneration to the social organism, began to call for the "state and professions" to take on "unlimited powers to eradicate disease and improve the health of future generations."[5] It was this metapolitically authoritative and scientistic stance, and not any initial tenuous links "with *völkisch* racism and extreme nationalist groupings," that established the basis for a later "process of adaptation and appropriation on both sides"[6] between eugenics and National Socialism.

In this part we will illustrate how Oka exhibits a similar metapolitical tendency. As we will argue, his evolutionism, despite his clear preference for

3   Weindling, *Health, Race and German Politics*, 10.
4   Ibid.
5   Ibid., 7.
6   Ibid., 10.

statism and against superstition, did not stake out overt ideological commitments but instead described the preconditions for any polity that strove for evolutionary viability. In keeping with the reformist ethos of technocratic expertise learned at Todai, Oka accepted the nomic dimensions of the Meiji order with the understanding that its norms, conventions, and legal constructs would be gradually rationalized by science. Its nomos would be fashioned to fit the organicism described by evolutionary morphology. Oka may have had his own ideological preferences, but adherence to these metapolitical preconditions was fundamental. Yet, as with his European colleagues, such a reformist scientism ultimately proved to be inadequate. As a result, a more aggressive, value-generating scientism emerged from its organicist basis.

What distinguishes Oka's metapolitics from the ideology of health and social cohesion that Weindling describes in Germany is the acute sense of national peril that Oka believed Japan was under due to imperialism in East Asia. Oka's homecoming from Germany, in fact, coincided almost exactly with the Sino-Japanese War (1894–95). Breaking out shortly after a promise to lift humiliating unequal treaties, this quick, stunning victory culminated with the beginning of Japan's modern empire as set down by the terms of the Treaty of Shimonoseki. While this unequal treaty accorded the new empire territorial gains in Taiwan and the Pescadores, a hefty indemnity from the defeated Qing, access to Chinese ports, and a preponderant say in Korean politics, three of the European powers, Germany, France, and Russia, intervened in the settlement and self-servingly overturned the provisions that would have handed strategically vital south Manchuria over to Japan. Announcing that it needed to be done in the name of peace in East Asia, the powers got Japan to deliver Liaodong and the area up to Muken to Tsarist Russia, which was feverishly constructing a railroad eastward across Siberia and needed the warm-water harbor at Port Arthur to establish a naval presence in the Pacific.

The Japanese, who had hoped modern civilizing efforts alone would establish that they had exited from a backward Asia, drew a sobering conclusion from this humiliation: "Say what you will," wrote the journalist Tokutomi Sohō, "[I]t happened because we weren't strong enough. What it came down to was that sincerity and justice didn't amount to a thing if you weren't strong enough."[7] For Oka, who, as we have seen, was busy establishing him-

---

7   Gordon, *A Modern History of Japan*, 119.

self as a biological researcher, college instructor, textbook writer, and education bureaucrat, a realpolitik sensibility also came to inform his reformist scientism in the decade following the victory over China. With its central conceit that the interaction of groups is the same as that between "individual animals that lead independent lives: the superior wins, the inferior loses—the strong prosper, the weak perish," his "Good and Evil in the Animal World" offered a preliminary sample of this realpolitik thinking. However, it was the outbreak of a second war in the so-called "Man-Kan" region (Manchuria and Korea), this time against a European power in February 1904, which inspired Oka to turn the organicism of evolutionary morphology's hierarchy of individuality into a geopolitical vision of perpetual war and racial autarky. Seizing on the notion of *kyokoku itchi* (national unity), Oka, as Chapter 4 will reveal, depicted Japan as the biological correlate of the organic state: a racial superorganism beset by other racial superorganisms in an anarchic arena of ongoing international struggle.

As will become evident, Oka's initial wartime essay, "War and Peace," was intended to dispel humanitarian and pacifist ideals being disseminated by the anarchist-led peace movement. While *kyokoku itchi* denied such internal divisions, the aftermath of the war revealed the pervasiveness of dissent and an ominous erosion of the consensus of self-sacrifice that had held throughout the extraordinary decades of Meiji development. In response to this anomy, which found its most alarming expression in the Hibiya Riot of 1905, the late Meiji government embarked on what Rotem Kowner has called "a widespread campaign of re-indoctrination."[8] In the third section of this study we will see that the government efforts to preserve national unity in the name of the "emperor-centered historical view" amounted to an activist program of "state Shinto"—as scholars have generally referred to it[9]—a fundamentalist movement initiated by reactionary statists which occupied the same oppositional role in Oka's career as ultramontane Catholicism did in Haeckel's. In the early postwar period, however, reindoctrination manifested itself in an upsurge in commentary from public moralists lamenting the loss of solidarity and warning of dire consequences ahead. Oka did not hesitate to join this chorus of voices and his version of ethical

---

8 Kowner, "The War as a Turning Point in Modern Japanese History," 30.
9 For an intriguing alternative, see the discussion of the "Shinto secular" in Josephson, *The Invention of Religion in Japan.*

life, "the human-way," which was codified in the months immediately after the Hibiya Riot, represents perhaps the clearest formulation of his metapolitics. As will be explored in Chapter 5, the centerpiece of Oka's reconceptualization of the "ape-way" in human terms as a human-way is its anti-individualism. Clearly cognizant of the criticisms other commentators were leveling at self-interested social elements in the postwar years, Oka's essay attempted to distinguish his evolutionism from egoistic social Darwinism by evoking the higher self of the group as the proper nexus of evolutionary struggle. His scientistic vision of interdependence and holism would serve as the biological reality underlying calls for family-like solidarity. The unstated purpose of this metapolitics was for orthodox moralism to reform itself according to the modernizing truths of modern science.

As the final section of this study will argue, however, this moderate reformist scientism that sought to ground nationalism and public morals in the biological ontology of evolutionism also contained the seeds of a more radical generative program, one that would look not to society but the processes of natural development to determine the source of ultimate value. In the last chapter we explained how the eugenics movement enshrined such values and in this section we will see that Oka, while the fighting in Manchuria was still in progress, took it upon himself to introduce notions of eugenics and racial hygiene to the Japanese biomedical community. Like his other essays before and after the war, his lecture "Evolutionary Theory and Hygiene" cautiously attempts to undergird the accepted nomos, assuring the doctors in attendance of his address that what he was proposing did not undermine medical ethics or the Hippocratic oath. Yet, we will see that Oka's evolutionism, when it comes to resituating the racialist realpolitik of the human-way within a developmental cosmology, would not only intimate a new table of values based on ideals of health but invite the orthodoxy to transform itself into a palingenetic vision of national regeneration.

CHAPTER 4

WORLD WAR ZERO

During the early months of the Russo-Japanese war a controversial pamphlet by Leo Tolstoy appeared in Japan. Entitled "Bethink Yourselves!" [Doumaites!] and translated by the anarchist activists Kōtoku Shusui and Sakai Toshihiko, Tolstoy's emotional essay, despite being "unpublishable in Russia" due to its "anti-war content,"[1] was carried "in its lengthy entirety in *Heimin Shimbun* and the *Tokyo Asahi*." *Heimin Shimbun* (The commoner's news), was actually a short-lived anarchist publication, and it was reported that the special issue that featured "Bethink Yourselves!" "immediately sold out its print run of 8000."[2] According to David Wells, Tolstoy's ardent humanitarian plea, which was published around the world in 1904, was

> in effect, a sermon on two Biblical texts: "The time is fulfilled and the kingdom of God is at hand. Bethink yourselves and believe the Gospel" (Mark 1:15) and "And if you do not bethink yourselves you will all perish" (Luke 13:5). Tolstoy makes an impassioned statement against war in general and the present war in particular, denouncing it as contrary to the teaching of both Christ and Buddha. He recommends that those who are called up should refuse to bear arms, and holds up as examples several individuals who have adopted this course of action.[3]

In this chapter we will describe how Oka Asajirō's metapolitics first came to be articulated in response to not only Tolstoy's pacifist argument but a general humanitarian outlook that he worried would undermine the nation's

---

1   Wells, "The Russo-Japanese War in Russian Literature," 123.
2   Wilson, "The Russo-Japanese War and Japan," 174.
3   Wells, "The Russo-Japanese War in Russian Literature," 123.

ability to survive imperialist encirclement. First in his groundbreaking essay "War and Peace," which indirectly answered Tolstoy at the start of the war in the pages of the student magazine *Seinenkai* (Youth world), and later in his "Mankind's Struggle for Existence," which was featured in the leading intellectual journal of the day, *Chūō Kōron* (The central review), at the war's conclusion, Oka contributed a starkly contrasting vision of evolutionary realpolitik, one in which total war between nations is perpetual and racial autarky is the unstated aim of a biologically grounded approach to foreign affairs. Inspired that the spontaneous mobilization on the home front and the mass sacrifices in Manchuria confirmed government slogans about *Kyokoku itchi* (National unity), Oka capitalized on the emergency circumstances of the war to insert the higher individuality described by the evolutionary morphology of Leuckart and Haeckel as an ontological substrate for the humanly constructed nation-state. Metapolitically conceived as a superorganism, the *minzoku* (ethnic nation) would not only succeed in the endless and inevitable "war in peace" between races and nations but avoid a false humanitarianism which would fatally compromise national self-interest. At the close of the chapter we will explore whether Oka's *shinkaron* legitimized a new racialist line of thinking based on evolutionary science in Japan.

Humanitarian Perils

What must have certainly provoked Oka was not just the aggressive pacifism of Tolstoy's pamphlet but the manner in which its humanitarianism almost seemed to mimic the altruism endorsed by Haeckel's monism. As the last chapter explained, Haeckel's reformist scientism portrayed the altruism of traditional religion as an unconscious correlate to the soft organicism of interdependence found in nature. Both of Haeckel's best-sellers from the fin-de-siècle, *The Riddle of the Universe* (1899) and *The Wonders of Life* (1904), repeatedly invoked the Golden Rule of the New Testament as a universal principle promoting social cohesion and, whether intentionally or not, Tolstoy made "do unto others" the centerpiece of his argument, presenting it as not just "the law of all religions,"[4] but "the law of life."[5] Like Haeckel

---

4 Tolstoi, *Bethink Yourselves!*, 46.
5 Ibid., 37.

and, as we will see, Oka, Tolstoy regarded the moral insight contained in the Golden Rule as affording "rational guidance for human activity"[6] and a means of reconciling each human being with his or her destiny as an "organic being" in a "universe infinite in time and space."[7]

For Tolstoy, however, this "incontestable principle"[8] was not, as it was with monism, a group-specific device to reconcile altruism and egoism and thereby ensure the integration necessary for collective survival. Rather it represented a universalist manifestation of the will of God in the affairs of mankind. After clearing away the dogma, ritual, and superstition of a corrupt, pseudo-Christianity, Tolstoy believed the lone option available left to humanity was to become "the servant of God, because for man there is one way of being free—by uniting his will with the will of God."[9] It is this unity with God's will that cosmizes nomoi, for it "establishes the relation of man to All, to God, and, therefore, gives a general higher direction to all human activity."[10] The binding demand that "we should love our neighbor and serve him," a principle with which Tolstoy believes "it is impossible to disagree,"[11] becomes "the whole of practical religions"[12]—a universal religious law "more or less consciously" recognized "not in the Christian world alone, but in the Buddhistic, Mahomedan, Confucian, and Brahminic worlds"[13] as well.

Tolstoy attributed "the evil from which men of our time are suffering"[14] to the absence of this "law of all religions" in people's lives. Without religion men can no longer be lifted to a "higher plane of reason"[15] and they thereby descend to "the plane of animals and even lower than them."[16] For Tolstoy, wars are a prime indicator of this fall from grace because they call forth "the lowest animal passions" and "deprave and brutalize men."[17] The senseless conflict over imperial spoils between Russia and Japan is the ultimate testament to the feral state to which humans have been reduced:

---

6   Ibid., 20.
7   Ibid., 17–18.
8   Ibid., 23.
9   Ibid., 21.
10 Ibid., 20.
11 Ibid., 26.
12 Ibid., 24.
13 Ibid., 46.
14 Ibid., 20.
15 Ibid., 7.
16 Ibid., 20.
17 Ibid., 3.

Men who are separated from each other by thousands of miles, hundreds of thousands of such men (on the one hand—Buddhists, whose law forbids the killing, not only of men but of animals; on the other hand—Christians, professing the law of brotherhood and love) like wild beasts on land and on sea are seeking out each other, in order to kill, torture, and mutilate each other in the most cruel way. What can this be? Is it a dream or a reality?[18]

If Tolstoy's equating the animal side of humans with immorality failed to offend Oka's sensibilities, what he had to say about the contribution of scientists in rendering men "more and more degenerate and morally depraved"[19] certainly did. According to Tolstoy, "those who enjoy the greatest authority, so-called scientists," had committed "the coarse error that religion is a temporary and outgrown step in the development of mankind and that men can live without religion."[20] Their influence was especially pernicious because they "inculcate this error to those of the masses who are beginning to be educated."[21] It is this lack of ethical ground that leads scientists to wrongheadedly guide human "efforts to discoveries and improvements principally in the sphere of technical knowledge." As a result, "men of our time have developed in themselves enormous power over the forces of nature; but not having any guidance for the rational adaptation of this power, they naturally have used it for the satisfaction of their lowest and most animal propensities."[22]

In Tolstoy's view, "what they call science cannot replace religion." He believed earnestly that "a religion which answers to the demands of our time does exist and is known to all men." It is the role of "educated men—the leaders of the masses" to "understand that religion is necessary" and "that without religion men cannot live a good life."[23] Thus, scientists and others "who regard themselves as enlightened should cease to think and to inculcate to other generations that religion is atavism, the survival of a past wild state, and that for the good life of men the spreading of education is sufficient."[24]

---

18   Ibid., 1.
19   Ibid., 14.
20   Ibid., 22–23.
21   Ibid.
22   Ibid., 20.
23   Ibid., 31.
24   Ibid., 24.

Instead of befuddling the populace with "complicated, confused and unnecessary theories,"[25] "men of science should understand that the principle of the brotherhood of all men and the rule of not doing unto others what one does not wish for oneself is not one casual idea out of a multitude of human theories which can be subordinated to any other considerations, but is an incontestable principle, standing higher than the rest, and flowing from the changeless relation of man to that which is eternal."[26]

Perhaps most insufferable of all for a young scientist who regarded it as his special calling to inculcate evolutionary theory among the populace of a developing nation, was Tolstoy's insistence on the priority of the individual and his conscience. Tolstoy enjoined his readership, both Russian and Japanese, to understand that "all those personal, social, and even universal human aims which I may place before myself and which are placed before me by men are all insignificant, owing to the shortness of my life as well as to the infiniteness of the life of the universe."[27] Each individual should subordinate him or herself to the "higher aim for the attainment of which I am sent into the world"[28] and ground his existence in this religious commitment, not social or political roles. "Before I am Emperor, soldier, minister, or journalist," Tolstoy proclaimed, "I am a man." As a man "my destiny, my vocation, is of being a workman of God, of fulfilling His work."[29]

For secular supporters of the war effort the danger here was not Tolstoy's religious message per se but the manner in which he assigned special value to the individual and his conscience. Tolstoy's pacifism sloughs aside political obligations, concluding that "the work of my life has nothing in common with recognition of the rights of the Chinese, Japanese, or Russians to Port Arthur. The work of my life consists in fulfilling the will of Him who sent me into this life."[30] A non-Christian or secularist who accepted this ethical reasoning without its religious implications could find much to agree with in Tolstoy's insight that the tremendous sacrifices being exacted by the war were both immoral and unnecessary. Indeed, the most moving passages from his pamphlet detail what the unfolding slaughter meant for individu-

---

25 Ibid.
26 Ibid., 23.
27 Ibid., 17–18.
28 Ibid.
29 Ibid.
30 Ibid., 25.

als. An example is Tolstoy's recounting of an incident from the beginning stages of the war which seemed to have inspired the rapid publication of his pamphlet: the sinking of the Russian battleship *Petropavlovsk* in early April 1904. This event was widely reported in the international press due to the death of the ship's captain, Vice Admiral Stepan Makarov, who was not only a hero of the Russo-Turkish War of 1877–78, but an internationally renowned scientist and inventor. Makarov had been handed his command in order to inspire the Russian navy to take the initiative and it was upon returning from an engagement with the Japanese off of Port Arthur that the *Petropavlovsk* hit a mine and sank, taking the admiral down with it. Tolstoy did not lament the admiral's death so much as the loss of the 652 sailors who perished under his command. He described them as unwitting victims who had been tricked into throwing away their precious individual lives for a specious cause: "[T]hose unfortunate men drawn from all parts of Russia, who, by the help of religious fraud, and under fear of punishment, have been torn from an honest, reasonable, useful, laborious family life, driven to the other end of the world, placed on a cruel, senseless machine for slaughter, and torn to bits, drowned along with this stupid machine in a distant sea."[31]

Yet perhaps the most powerful and lasting image from Tolstoy's pamphlet was the one that excoriated the sort of biological corporatism that zoologists with Oka's training were trying to promote. His example of the super-individual life fittingly alludes to the plagues of the Old Testament: "When crawling locusts cross rivers, it happens that the lower layers are drowned until the bodies of the drowned formed a bridge over which the upper ranks can pass. In the same way are the Russian people being disposed of. Thus the first lower layer is already beginning to drown, indicating the way to other thousands, who will all likewise perish."[32] Though from his Biblical framework he prefers locusts to bees, ants, or social medusa, Tolstoy is unmistakably repudiating the eugenic reasoning of contemporary theories of the nation as a corm or superorganism which we discussed at length in the last chapter. For Tolstoy the mass sacrifice of individuals to the collective body is not only unnecessary but repugnant. His choice of image also turned out to be sadly prescient: the long siege on Port Arthur that began in summer

---

31 Ibid., 32.
32 Ibid., 34–35.

1904 and lasted until the following year would see an unprecedented squandering of expendable lives in the "human bullet" charges by the Japanese infantry on Russian artillery positions.

Oka began to warn of the dangers of Tolstoy's humanitarian individualism even before the Japanese translation of "Bethink Yourselves!" was published in June 1904. Evidently responding to press reports of Tolstoy's pacifist activism, Oka's essay "War and Peace" appeared in April in *Seinenkai* and was directed at youth that were in jeopardy of being "infected by Tolstoy and his kind" who "disdain the progress of civilization" and contemptuously call it the "civilization of masters."[33] Who Oka certainly had in mind were the socialists and anarchists at the forefront of Japan's small but highly vocal antiwar movement. In the year leading up to the conflict these activists had espoused an "anti-imperialist, anti-militarist and pro-socialist editorial position" in the pages of the "defiantly individualist broadsheet"[34] *Yorodzu Chōhō*. Though the prowar lobby, led by politically connected Todai professors, tipped public opinion in favor of war by late 1903[35] and the newspaper itself, under government pressure, abruptly switched to a prowar stance, the leaders of the peace movement—in particular Kōtoku, Sakai and Uchimura—"set up a new publishing firm, Heiminsha (Company of Commoners) and started publishing the first Japanese socialist weekly newspaper, *Heimin Shimbun*, on 23 October 1903.[36] It was in the pages of *Heimin Shimbun* that "Bethink Yourselves!" appeared in June 1904.

In a subsequent chapter we will see that, much to Oka's consternation, Heiminsha would later attempt to appropriate his *shinkaron*, publishing inexpensive overviews of Oka's *Lectures on Evolutionary Theory* in order to promote socialist materialism as the alternative to the orthodoxy of the Shintoist family-state. However, in the context of the Russo-Japanese War, the company was fully focused on opposing the conflict from the vantage point of Tolstoy's humanitarianism. As an article from the 4 September 1904 edition, entitled "The Ground of Antimilitarism," explained: "[T]he logic of those who oppose the war is very simple. They do not make any important

---

33 Asajirō Oka, "Sensō to Heiwa" [War and peace], in *Shinka to Jinsei* [Evolution and human life] (Tokyo: Yūseidō Shuppan, 1968), 94.

34 Shimazu, *Japanese Society at War*, 34.

35 Ibid., 32–33.

36 Ibid., 35.

distinction between individual morality and national morality."[37] Adroitly coupling this internationalist humanitarianism with a defense of individual freedom from an "oppressive state attempting to intervene in daily life," Heiminsha socialism, despite the relatively small readership of its newspaper, found broad appeal for a nation weary of the sacrifices of war and imperial competition. According to Shimazu, the antiwar movement was not only "a unique social feature of the 1904–5 war, never hitherto or henceforth repeated" but revealed a diverse and pluralistic "society in conflict with itself"[38]—a society ambivalent toward imperial projects and possessing a "critical social conscience."[39] In contrast to the "monolithic" wartime society imagined by most scholars, Shimazu portrays a variegated civil order in which individual initiative often outpaced the state, even in the area of nationalism. Later we will argue that the war and its aftermath represent the emergence of subjective freedom. The appeal of the humanitarianism espoused by Tolstoy and Heiminsha is that it allowed a society of newly awakened individualists to anticipate an order in which their plans and projects were not tethered to the collective needs of the national community. And, perhaps even more significantly, it exposed such a community for what it was and was not: something constructed by human artifice, the product of self-interested constituencies, not the necessary and inevitable manifestation of an all-determining ontological essence.

To counter pluralism and the "cacophony of voices"[40] it entailed, the government and the war-frenzied mainstream media promoted a vision of Japan as "an idealized society united in patriotic sacrifice."[41] This idealization was encapsulated in the wartime time slogan *Kyokoku itchi* (National unity), a notion which intimated that "the state and the nation were united as one to face the national calamity of war against Russia."[42] Orchestrated in part by commercial interests that collaborated with government ministries, an atmosphere of war-fervor gripped the nation, seeming to verify that a spontaneous organic fusion between the Japanese state and its highly patriotic society had taken place. Flags and patriotic symbols festooned trams,

---

37 Ibid., 37.
38 Ibid., 21.
39 Ibid., 42.
40 Ibid., 19.
41 Ibid., 40.
42 Ibid., 19.

streets, and other public spaces; triumphal arches to welcome home the troops sprang up in cities and towns; and pictorial magazines saturated the public consciousness with images of the war. Not only did publically displayed *nishiki-e* prints and photographs provide up-to-date documentation of the unfolding conflict but magic lantern shows and panoramic models of the Manchurian battlefront quickly emerged as forms of mass entertainment. Tokyo's cinemas, of which there were already twenty-four by 1903, fascinated rapt audiences with reenactments of the fighting. If confirmation were needed that this outpouring of patriotic expression was a grassroots phenomenon, one only had to point to the "lantern parades" that were extemporaneously organized across the country. Named after the internally lit, illustrated paper lanterns that their participants carried, the first of these celebratory nighttime processions was initiated by Keio University students at the outbreak of war and involved 2,500 people circumambulating central Tokyo. Later parades, which were held across the country, grew exponentially in size, with the largest, occurring in March 1905 to celebrate the Battle of Mukden, attracting a crowd of 212,800. Though, as Shimazu makes clear, the authorities came to wonder whether the patriotism of these parades was not merely a pretext for "public (and expensive) outbursts of popular energy"[43]—even going so far as to ban them for a time in 1904 out of, as we will see, a well-founded fear that crowds were transforming into an uncontrollable force of popular radicalism—the usual interpretation has been that they represented "a sign of the well-being of the *kokumin*, symbolic of the strength of popular patriotism."[44] Together, the parades and the media frenzy surrounding them helped to confirm for many the truth of the primary ideological trope of the war—*Kyokoku itchi* (National unity).

Oka, as we will see in a moment, seized on this semiofficial discourse. The crux of what we are calling his metapolitics begins with his identification of wartime national unity with the higher individuality described by evolutionary morphology: to achieve evolutionary viability Japanese nationalism only needed to recalibrate itself to the interdependence displayed by superorganisms. Oka certainly found further encouragement along these lines by the manner in which the Japanese state projected "its self-image as a

---

43   Ibid., 44.
44   Ibid., 46.

'civilized state (*bunmeikoku*)' fighting on behalf of 'civilization'"[45]—an emphasis which, for Oka, must have suggested Haeckel's conception of evolutionary history as the epigenetic development of civilization. Yet unlike Haeckel's biopolitics, in which the functionally differentiated and nomically reintegrated civilized nations ultimately eliminated less evolved "unities of life," Japan's wartime *bunmeiron* was enunciated on a humanitarian basis. To Oka's consternation, the authorities, many of whom shared Oka's cosmopolitan background, moderated and regulated wartime rhetoric and conduct out of "the desire to be included into the elite corps of great powers."[46] Toning down warmongering and censoring dehumanized representations of the enemy, the war was presented as a conflict "fought between 'civilized states [*bunmei koku*]'" with "'civilization [*bunmei*]'" coming "to symbolize the wartime conduct of the Japanese state and its *kokumin*."[47] Such logic went so far as to deny any separation between nationalism and humanitarianism: "[H]umanitarianism was one aspect of nationalism; in other words, one could only be a good humanitarian if one were a good patriot because love for one's country was fundamental to all proper human conduct, including love for others."[48]

Designed to win the sympathy of the West and demonstrate that Japan deserved to "join the ranks of the 'first-rate' powers" [*ittōkoku*],[49] this humanitarian "moral diplomacy"[50] was put on display in the Japanese treatment of Russian prisoners of war. The First Hague Conference of 1899, under its Convention on the Laws of War on Land, had stipulated that POWs "should be treated in a manner analogous to that of the troops of the Detaining Power."[51] Accordingly the Ministry of the Army made sure that "international lawyers were dispatched to every division within Japan's Manchurian Army"[52] and issued a statement to the international community to clarify that "wars are based on political relations between states and the objective is to decrease the fighting capability of the enemy country.... As a result, one should not possess animosity toward the people of the enemy

---

45 Ibid., 157.
46 Ibid., 15.
47 Ibid.
48 Ibid., 176.
49 Ibid., 167–68.
50 Ibid., 15.
51 Ibid., 168.
52 Ibid.

country."[53] Recognizing "a categorical distinction between the enemy state and its people on humanitarian grounds," the nearly 72,000 Russian POWs were understood to be "honored guests"[54] who were afforded comfortable accommodations in twenty-eight camps across Japan. At Matsuyama on Shikoku, the largest of these camps actually attempted to integrate prisoners into the local community, organizing excursions and leisure activities for them which included bicycling, tennis, photography, dancing, playing music, keeping pets, and performing plays.[55] Some local businesses regarded the camps as a commercial boom, treating the prisoners as "accidental tourists,"[56] and there were even stories of budding romances between local women and the Russian captives that emerged from the war.[57] The highly patriotic Japanese Red Cross, which had grown to 900,000 members by 1903, also played a significant role in demonstrating "to the world" Japan's "humanitarian mission."[58] One wounded Russian POW testified to the international press that "without exaggeration and without overestimation" the nurses of the Japanese Red Cross "are our angels and our consolation,"[59] a quasi-religious sentiment that was echoed by a Japanese magazine cover from the war that depicted the Japanese nurse as a Madonna-like figure overseeing Russian wounded.[60] Some camp wardens even worried that "excessively kind"[61] ministrations were leading the Russians to fall in love with the nurses.

EVOLUTIONARY REALPOLITIK

The success of this moral diplomacy found confirmation in the Fourth Hague Convention, which was held in 1907. According to Shimazu, Japan's humane conduct toward Russian combatants served as the convention's

---

53 Ibid., 168–69.
54 Ibid.
55 Ibid., 185–86.
56 Ibid., 190–95.
57 Ibid., 184–85.
58 Ibid., 173. For a firsthand account of the Japanese Red Cross during the war itself, see Ariga, *The Japanese Red Cross and the Russo-Japanese War.* For a discussion of international admiration for the Japanese nurses serving in the Red Cross, see Takahashi, *The Development of the Japanese Nursing Profession,* 77–110.
59 Ibid., 171.
60 Ibid.
61 Ibid.

new standard for treatment of POWs and the wounded that came into effect during the First World War. Yet despite this widespread recognition of the nation's civilized humanitarianism, the postwar experience also confirmed warnings from minority voices within the prowar punditry who, in opposition to *bunmeiron* position, had argued that Japan would never be accepted as an equal by the West. For this minority, the war with Russia was a racial conflict. The "racial discourse" (*jinshuron*) they promoted was typified by Narukawa Sei who, just one month into the war, in the first issue of *Chūō Kōron* (The central review), announced, "Now the era of race war has arrived. The war between Russia and Japan ... is the first step in the rivalry between the Aryan race and the yellow races."[62] In general, the *jinshuron* perspective

> positioned Japan uncompromisingly as a yellow race in the East, against the white European West. This group perceived Russia as symbolically representative of the West, and Japan as its antithesis in the East. No matter what amount of acculturation or assimilation took place, differences between Japan and the West remained unbridgeable; and moreover, it was desirable that they remained unbridgeable. Fundamentally, it desired to define Japan not on Western terms but on its own terms as an Asian state, as symbolically defined on the basis of race. Ultimately, the racial argument portrayed the war on the basic axis of Japan versus the West.[63]

While the *jinshuron* viewpoint remained unfashionable during the war itself, it gained in popularity and acceptance in the war's aftermath "as the Japanese gradually began to feel the brunt of Western racism, in spite of their all-out effort to integrate with the West."[64] By 1908 the populist magazine *Taiyō* had come out with a special issue entitled "The Clash of the Yellow and the White Race." The introduction to this issue traced all conflict in the world to "survival of the racial stock and self-survival" and one of its featured articles argues that harmonization with the West is highly undesirable because of the inevitability of war between the races.[65]

---

62 Ibid., 166.
63 Ibid., 165–66.
64 Ibid., 166.
65 Ibid. The quote is from the introductory essay of the 15 February 1908 edition of *Taiyō*. See "Rinji Zōkan: Ōhaku jinshu shōtotsu," introductory page. The same edition features articles which, as we will see, resonate with Oka's racial geopolitics. For instance, "The Trend of the Future" makes race "the basis of world

Oka's *shinkaron* (evolutionism) has much in common with this *jinshuron* perspective, and, in fact, his writings most likely had a direct influence on this postwar special issue of *Taiyō* with its emphasis on "racial stock" and race survival.[66] However, his evolutionism, while it emphatically rejects wartime humanitarianism—whether espoused in the name of pacifism or the name of nationalism—also clearly rejects the disavowal of modern Western science implicit in the *jinshuron* position. Shimazu depicts both *jinshuron* and *bunmeiron* as reflections of *aija-shugi* (Asianism) and *Datsu-A* ("Escape Asia") respectively, discourses which had been dominant in the late nineteenth century. In her view, "both these discourses were about Japan's 'metaphorical' distance from Asia (implying in the main China): 'Escape Asia' sought to distance Japan from Asia, and bring it into the bosom of the West; whilst, 'Asianism' sought to bring Japan closer to Asia, but with a caveat—with Japan as the leader of Asia."[67] One sense in which we are using the term "metapolitics" in this section is to indicate how Oka's *shinkaron* is crafted to describe a position more fundamental than either of these two alternatives, one that would fit them to the ontology of organic nature while discarding their scientifically incorrect excesses. For Oka one's proximity to Asia or the West was not the point. Grounding one's position in modern science—which happened to have been developed in the West—in order to maximize the prospects for Japan—which happened to be located in the East—was what was important. Thus a *jinshuron* that rejected science because it was Western was as misguided as a *bunmeiron* that indiscriminately embraced all Western ideas—especially humanitarianism—and denied the significance of Japan's geographical position in Asia. In short, Oka's *shinkaron* aspired to be a *jinshuron*, but one based on the scientific *bunmeiron* described by modern biology. Both positions could be salvaged by preserving the scientifically accurate aspects of their position and rejecting the rest.

Yet perhaps the best way to understand Oka's *shinkaron* is not primarily as a reaction to the positions we have just described but as his own uniquely

---

struggle" and envisions a collision between the white and Mongol races. Similarly, "The State of Antagonism between White and Yellow Peoples" connects the "yellow peril" in the Pacific with the "white peril" in China. Finally, "The White Peril and Corruption" [the characters for white and yellow are used here] focuses on the "white peril" in China, the importance of race exclusion, and the inevitability of racial conflict. The extent to which Oka may have directly influenced the unnamed authors of these articles is a topic I hope to take up in a future essay.

66 Ibid., 165–66.
67 Ibid., 159–60.

innovative solution to Japan's situation as conceptualized through the organicism of evolutionary morphology. As we suggested at the opening of Part I, organicism appealed to the Meiji elites because of the realpolitik logic that tends to steer modern Japan's international conduct. According to Kenneth Pyle, the combination of anarchy, weak central authority, and intense interstate competition during its protracted feudal period—which culminated in the all-out war of all against all during the Sengoku era— prepared Japan for the similarly structured modern international system under the new imperialism. As it was for the rival ministates of the Sengoku era, successful realization of state interest became the be-all and end-all of the Meiji state. Slogans of the Meiji era, such as "Rich nation, strong army" [*Fukoku kyōhei*] and "Civilization and enlightenment" [*Bunmei kaika*] implicitly acknowledge this realpolitik impetus. Though Pyle describes sophisticated patterns of realist response which include pragmatism, adaptation, emulation, a concern for rank and honor, and the quest of autonomy and regional hegemony, what the Japanese fundamentally brought to the international order was a keen sense that survival depends on mastering sources of power. By painstakingly attending to and pragmatically accommodating these sources of power, especially as they manifested themselves in great impersonal forces and trends of historical development, a state could, after a period of apprenticeship, venture power-maximizing innovations and eventually achieve prestige and autonomy within the international system.

As we argued in Chapter 1, the organic theory of the state was appropriated by the oligarchs in the 1880s as a practical measure in the spirit of Japanese realpolitik: it promised to provide access to the sources of modern development while maintaining the nomic unity needed to meet external challenges. By the 1890s, with the establishment of Todai as an imperial university and with droves of budding technocrats leaving to study in the West, modern science came more and more into view as the key to strength for the nation-state. Oka's *shinkaron* not only offered access to this power in one of the established scientific disciplines most relevant to human affairs—evolutionary biology—but it amounted to a form of realpolitik in its own right. In fact, it can best be termed a form of evolutionary realpolitik that adapts organic state theory to evolutionary morphology and aspires for the national body to achieve a state of racial autarky.

Oka's realpolitik relies on the biopolitical premises of Haeckelian monism and initially attempts to offer its organicism as a template for scientistic reform. However, Oka's contribution should be thought of not so much as a direct derivation of Haeckel's scientistic paradigm as an innovative extrapolation on its basic organicist vision. Indeed, what makes Oka's evolutionism so intriguing is that it anticipates ideas that better-known European thinkers, who began from these same premises, would only develop to a similar extent in the aftermath of the First World War. In particular, the geopolitical thought of Ratzel and the Leipzig school, which culminated in the notion of living space, as well as the ideas of total war furthered by Ernst Jünger will come to seem far less original in light of Oka's earlier strategic ruminations based on Haeckel's organicist paradigm. In other words, the Russo-Japanese War provided Oka with a jumpstart in developing a biopolitical vision that would become, in different form, widespread in what Niall Ferguson calls the fifty-year "war of the world." The vision of total mobilization, *Lebensraum* and civilizational decline that appeared in Europe after the First World War, had their debut—though certainly not their origins— in Japan in the aftermath of World War Zero.

Oka enunciated his evolutionary realpolitik in two wartime essays, "War and Peace" and "Mankind's Struggle for Existence." While the former article was more polemical and the latter more systematic, they both focus on the same themes and share an attitude characteristic of reformist scientism: a sense of enlightening the readers to the underlying reality offered by evolutionary science in order to disabuse them of potentially self-defeating delusions. Together these articles set out to metapolitically ground the geopolitics of the nation-state in the ecology of superorganisms. In what follows, we will carefully delineate Oka's wartime political biopolitical vision, drawing on these two articles as if they constituted a single systematic description. However, it will first be necessary to briefly say something about each article separately in order to specify its audience and clarify its intent.

Published during the second month of the war in the youth magazine *Seinenkai* (Youth world), "War and Peace" was meant to counter, as we have already intimated, Tolstoy's humanitarian pacifism. Espousing a corporatist ethnic nationalism which was to be advanced by an unambiguous embrace of technological civilization, "War and Peace" warns its student readers that the peace and happiness promised by an international order founded on humanitarian morality (*jindō*) represents a dangerous illusion. Instead of being misled by chimerical pacifism or distracted by materialism, individualism, or literature, the Japanese must accept that human life is a perpetual struggle for autarky between inherently expansionist collectivist racial entities. Because modern technology is essential to this struggle, Japan must commit to the development of science to outcompete other ethnic nations (*minzoku*).

Appearing at the conclusion of the war, and, in fact, just after the Treaty of Portsmouth, "Mankind's Struggle for Existence" brought a more succinct, systematic, and pointed version of the same reasoning to a much larger audience. *Chūō Kōron*, the venue in which this bold statement of evolutionary realpolitik was featured, testifies to Oka's rising stature: it was the premiere intellectual journal of the day and the article is an indication that Oka was quickly becoming the public spokesman for modern biology and evolutionary science in Japan. "Mankind's Struggle for Existence" was, as it turned out, the first of ten articles carried by the publication between 1905 and 1912[68] and, along with the anthologies and collections of his writings these *Chūō Kōron* articles stand as one of the primary reasons Oka's influence was so manifold in the early twentieth century.

What this inaugural article espoused was not only electrifying but tone-setting for Oka's latter contributions: Japan, Oka enjoined his readers to grasp, must gird itself for the future inevitability of race war. While he admitted that the struggle for existence is pervasive throughout human existence, he argues that the primary and therefore proper echelon at which this struggle occurs is between race nations. Though the internal concord that prevails within these collective entities may seem to suggest that civilization has enabled humans to transcend the struggle for existence and separate themselves from other animals, Oka warns that each nation functions like a lone predator and therefore the competition for humans is actually more intense than it is elsewhere in living nature. As he did in "War and Peace," Oka worries that alliance between nations might confuse his compatriots into sacrificing national self-interest for the sake of ephemeral justice, sympathy, and internationalism. Not only, did he warn, were alliances merely temporary expedients and world government an impossibility, but

---

68   Migita, *Tennosei to Shinkaron*, 35.

nation-states of mixed ethnicities were impermanent and doomed to fail. Only nations comprised of a single race would endure mankind's struggle for existence.

As our brief overview of these two wartime articles—we will deal with a third in the next chapter—suggests, Oka's metapolitical identification of the nation-state with superorganisms became especially prominent in the "Mankind's Struggle for Existence." Though the earlier "War and Peace" did express fears that individuals might "give free rein to their selfishness alone" and disregard "the interests of the entire society"[69] which he depicted as a racial collective, it was the later article that explicitly portrayed the ethnic nation as a higher individuality. The wartime slogan *Kyokoku itchi* (National unity) could be understood, Oka explained, as a subordination of the "countless levels" of evolutionary struggle within human society to "the highest ranking level at present"[70] which he identified (at least initially) as the nation. Such "internal concord"[71] served to "limit the competition within the nation between individuals or between small groups to the degree that we have no worries about our nation being put in jeopardy by enemy nations."[72] At their supreme state of integration and self-organization, such nations would approach "ideal groups, in which there is not the least bit of external strife" in order that they "can direct all their power against their enemies."[73] In Oka's view, nation-states constitute solitary individuals in a hostile nature: they should be thought of as predators, like lurking tigers or lone wolves, self-interested living beings whose bodily functions coordinate together to ensure the survival of the organism as a whole.

It is with the model of such organic individuality in mind that Oka amends himself toward the end of his essay, explaining that "there remains a level above that of the nation where the struggle for existence occurs. This is race [*jinshu*]."[74] For Oka, true nations, nations with long-term prospects for survival, are *minzoku* (ethnic nations), a term which he construes on a racial basis. Because "whatever the race, the natural inclination to exclude other

---

69 Oka, "Sensō to Heiwa" [War and peace], 95.

70 Asajirō Oka, "Jinrui no Seizon Kyōsō" [Mankind's struggle for existence], in *Shinka to Jinsei* [Evolution and human life], (Tokyo: Yūseidō Shuppan, 1968), 78.

71 Ibid., 79.

72 Ibid., 78.

73 Ibid., 79.

74 Ibid., 82.

races is something basically bred from birth and it cannot be possibly wiped away by means of reason,"[75] mixed-race nations are not viable and only exist on a temporary basis to meet external, mutual threats. Ultimately, the natural aversion which causes races to treat one another like foreign bodies and "get to the point of driving one another away"[76]—an aversion, he points out, is on display in the discrimination toward blacks in North America and Chinese in South Africa—will "naturally" result in such multiracial nations breaking up into "many nations,"[77] each of a racially homogeneous constitution. In short, "the foundation of mankind's struggle for existence is the competition between races."[78] Construed as racial superorganisms, predatory nation-states, such as Japan, should, as Oka says in "War and Peace," "prepare for war without end rather than for coexistence with others."[79]

LIVING SPACE

The various features of Oka's evolutionary realpolitik follow from this conjoining of organic individuality and race nationalism. The first such feature is the drive for racial autarky that characterizes the geopolitical stance of nation-state organisms. Oka's conception of the national body here has much in common with that of the contemporary school of geopolitics that conceived of nations as space-organisms. Significantly this school not only formed in the 1890s at the very same Leipzig University,[80] where Oka was a graduate research student in Rudolf Leuckart's laboratory, but its founder and early spokesman, Friedrich Ratzel began his academic career as a zoologist, developed a close relationship with Ernst Haeckel, and even published a popular account of Darwinism in 1869, *Being and Becoming in the Organic World*,[81] based largely on Haeckel's *General Morphology*. In keeping with this background, the field of "biogeography," which Ratzel developed in his *Political Geography* and other influential works, began with a vision of the nation-state as "an earth-bound living organism."[82] Such organisms would, as a natural

75   Ibid., 83.
76   Ibid.
77   Ibid.
78   Ibid.
79   Oka, "Sensō to Heiwa" [War and peace], 87.
80   Herman, *The Idea of Decline in Western History*, 197.
81   Weikart, *From Darwin to Hitler*, 112.
82   Dorpalen, *The World of General Haushofer*, 50.

feature of their process of growth, augment in size and, as their more and more numerous individual persons spilled into surrounding territory, start to clash with nations in a "struggle for space" or *Kampf um Raum*.[83] Guided by an "expansion drive, colonizing talent [and] gift to rule" that Ratzel called "space sense,"[84] the stronger and healthier of these growing, earth-bound superorganisms came to require living space, or *Lebensraum*, a term that became synonymous in the coming decades with the attainment of economic and political self-sufficiency by aspirant modern empires.

Working from similar Haeckelian premises, Oka's evolutionism devised its own account of such an inherent expansionist drive for superorganic autarky. "Each human race," Oka explained, "as long as it does not incur extreme pressure, possesses a nature that should always be expanding and projecting itself forth in the direction of least resistance. Because this audacity is never checked, it is certain that circumstances will arise one after another in which a particular race's individual existence are threatened due to the expansion of another race."[85] In Oka's version of biogeography, not just the natural process of growth but conditions of Malthusian scarcity contribute to expansionist tendencies. Overpopulation, Oka believes, is endemic to the human condition and leads inevitably, as it does with other animals, to survival struggles: "As a rule, living things, whether they are plants or animals, give birth to several tens, hundreds or tens of thousands of times the number of offspring that should be in reality able to survive. On top of this, due to the geometrical increase with each additional generation, although the fewest kinds of offspring are born, if every offspring survives and breeds, it means that numbers will at once become excessive, and the struggle to survive cannot possibly be avoided. Though compared to other animals the number of offspring which humans give birth to is very small, it is computed that each woman gives birth to four and a half children. For this reason, the unavoidability of the struggle for existence is absolutely the same as for other flora and fauna."[86] Such unsustainable increases in population growth put a strain on resources—and it is this which causes the rivalry between nations to exacerbate:

---

83 Weikart, *From Darwin to Hitler*, 193.
84 Dorpalen, *The World of General Haushofer*, 58.
85 Oka, "Sensō to Heiwa" [War and peace], 88.
86 Oka, "Jinrui no Seizon Kyōsō [Mankind's struggle for existence], 76–77.

The intensity of the struggle for existence must in general be proportional to the level of imbalance between supply and demand. If you give two dogs two pieces of meat to divide between them, no conflict will ensue. However, if you produce a single piece of meat, a fight will begin right away. If there are twenty applicants when just ten new students will be allowed, then competition cannot possibly be avoided. Yet if the applicants number fifty, the competition must be even more intense. The competition between one human nation and another is the same.[87]

On this basis Oka concludes that "the competition between the largest units, nations, in the human struggle for existence is very difficult to avoid and it is appropriate to regard it as something which will become more and more violent in the future with the rise in population and the development of land."[88] To underscore the truth of his evolutionary realpolitik Oka points to the contemporary geopolitical situation under the New Imperialism. In the open, underpopulated areas of the world map, "the vast territories still to be seized in Africa and Asia" there is no necessity yet for "intense competition."[89] However, as attempts are made "in every corner" by imperialist nations "to divide it up and manage this land," a "still more intense competition from here on in perhaps cannot be avoided no matter how things turn out."[90] In Oka's estimation, "the increasing world population"[91] will inevitably pit individual against individual, group against group, and nation against nation across the globe. A universal intensification of the struggle for existence is inescapable.

Given the humanitarianism espoused during the war not only by antiwar activists but, in a different fashion, by the government itself, Oka was eager for his readers to understand the dangerous folly involved in attempting to temper international struggle with principles of universal morality. He expressed a special wariness for "nations who proclaim a peace policy wherein they will never attack another nation."[92] Alluding most likely to the United States and Great Britain, Oka argued that "such countries, due certainly to their large land areas and small populations, merely have inherited na-

---

87 Ibid., 80.
88 Ibid., 80–81.
89 Ibid., 80
90 Ibid.
91 Ibid.
92 Ibid.

tional circumstances which do not require the seizing of other countries."[93] In the future such self-satisfied moralists were destined to learn a hard lesson: "When their populations become dense, and their circumstances alter, they will, before they know it, inevitably come to forget this peace policy and go on the attack against other nations."[94] In short, while Oka acknowledges that "nations that advocate a peace policy should be praised" he believes "it is an enormous mistake to think that this peace can continue on forever. Such nations must adequately ready themselves for the coming day when another nation qualifies as an enemy."[95] In other words, nation-states must never forget that "contrary to relations between individuals, where legal and moral sanctions hold sway, between nations there are no such things at all."[96] The harsh reality is that "weak nations merely fall into adversity and are destroyed by others."[97] Though some of the weaker nations may "retain their independence"[98] for a time while the strong nations focus on battling one another, the fate of the weak is either to be annexed or eliminated.

Oka's geopolitical vision, most of which is articulated in "Mankind's Struggle for Existence," not only became a central feature of his evolutionism but underwent refinement in later years, particularly in his "Ideal Group Life," which we discussed in the introduction. As will be recalled, Oka, in this essay from 1907, mused that gazing down into a pond where moss animals reside "gives one the same feeling as when one looks at a geopolitical map."[99] Representing the ideal superorganism because of their "true national unity,"[100] these moss animal colonies exhibit the innate expansionist impulses that Oka identifies at every level of organic individuality: "Since there is only peace within the nation and its power is exerted in an outward direction, if a case arises where there is something which disturbs the forward progress of the particular nation, the nation musters up all its strength, and fights violently to try to conquer whomever or whatever is in its way. When we see many moss animal nations arrayed sided by side in a narrow space, each country fiercely pushes up against the others along their mu-

93 Ibid.
94 Ibid.
95 Ibid.
96 Ibid.
97 Ibid.
98 Ibid.
99 Oka, "Risōteki Dantai Seikatsu" [Ideal group life], 73.
100 Ibid.

tual borders."[101] While a case can certainly be made that Oka's presence at Leipzig University in the 1890s exposed him to this mode of analysis, a more fertile explanation for the similarities between Oka's vision of racial autarky and Ratzel's biogeography is that both took Haeckel hierarchy of organic individuality as axiomatic and derived their biopolitics on its basis. The quest for autarkic living space (*Lebensraum*) by healthy nations that possess a strong "space sense" follows directly from the conceptualization of such nations as superorganisms, the highest echelon of this hierarchy.

The possible connection with Leipzig biogeography is especially intriguing because Ratzel's most influential disciple, Karl Haushofer, held up Japan as a "model geopolitician"[102] whom Germans should study for the "almost unrivalled degree" of their "space sense."[103] Haushofer's enthusiasm for the "deep-rooted geopolitical instinct of the Japanese people" was sparked during a visit to Japan in 1909 as an army attaché. Sent to inspect the Japanese army and teach artillery techniques, Haushofer was not only introduced to prominent military and political figures—which included an audience with the emperor—but toured the Japanese empire in Manchuria and Korea. In a series of book-length studies on the Japanese and their geopolitical situation which appeared just before and after the First World War, Haushofer developed his own school of geopolitics to focus on the notion of *Lebensraum* that would become, according to Niall Ferguson, the virtual ethos of the empire-states of the Second World War. By the term *empire-state* Ferguson refers to the "new empires of the twentieth century" that "inherited from the nineteenth-century nation-builders an insatiable appetite for uniformity."[104] Rejecting the ungainly pluralism and "haphazard administrative arrangements" of their imperial predecessors, empire-states such as Italy, Japan, Germany, and the USSR sought to overcome economic volatility and ethnic discord by filling the space vacated by the old, declining empires with homogeneous populations under the command of a streamlined political and economic authority. In their quest for *Lebensraum* and its concomitant uniformity, these empire-states "made a virtue of ruthlessness" and proved "willing to make war on whole categories of people, at home and abroad."[105]

---

101 Ibid.
102 Dorpalen, *The World of General Haushofer*, 29.
103 Ibid., 30.
104 Ferguson, *The War of the World*, lxvi.
105 Ibid., lxvi.

While Oka's evolutionary realpolitik never endorsed the kind of revolutionary program Ferguson ascribes to these empire-states—he retained a reformist stance even as he advanced generative ideas—his vision of racial autarchy based on the superorganismic expansion of the nation anticipates the conjunction of ethnic violence and imperial conquest that would become the signature of *Lebensraum* thought after the First World War. That Oka arrived at his own brand of empire-state logic as early as the Russo-Japanese War suggests evolutionary biology—especially its construal of organicism—may have more complex and pervasive links to twentieth-century politics than previously thought.

Total Mobilization

Ruthlessness and antihumanitarianism attain an even greater prominence in the second feature of Oka's evolutionary realpolitik, one that also anticipates strategic principles that would become broadly popular across the world only after WWI. This was his vision of total war. Of course, the provenance of total war doctrine in the aftermath of the Great War was extremely varied and, unlike the *Lebensraum* concept, it cannot be traced definitively back to evolutionary biology. Nevertheless, perhaps the most prominent theorist of this doctrine, Ernst Jünger, studied zoology at the University of Leipzig in the aftermath of the First World War and became a renowned entomologist as well as a famous writer and philosopher. Jünger's grim celebrations of the "front experience" written in the 1920s not infrequently invoke superorganisms to depict the collective struggle across no man's land.[106] It is in an essay from 1930, "Total Mobilization," that Jünger, according to Richard Wolin, "argues forcefully" that "in an age of total warfare, the difference between 'war' and 'peace' is effaced, and no sector of society can remain 'unintegrated' when the summons to 'mobilization' is announced."[107] In a follow-up book, *The Worker,* Jünger underscored that the permanently

---

106 Jünger's adherence to corporatist evolutionism is explicit in his 1922 "chronicle from the trench warfare of 1918" entitled *Copse 125*: "Wars are bound to occur from time to time. In them is manifested that determination of nature to intervene directly in the evolution of the greatest organisms of the earth." In the same volume he also wrote of the "higher social responsibility that lays less emphasis on the passing individual and his small concerns than on the race in whose history the individual is no more than an organic link binding the future with the past." See Jünger, *Copse 125*, 66, 182.

107 Jünger, "Total Mobilization," 121.

mobilized modern community he imagined would achieve its reintegration through an embrace of technology that transcended atomizing bourgeois individualism. Though it was certainly not the case that Jünger unwittingly rediscovered Oka, these three main features of his total war doctrine—complete integration, permanent war, and technological prowess—were already present in Oka's writings from the Russo-Japanese War. What Oka would come to call the "war in peace" prefigured European notions of total mobilization by as many as two decades.

One reason Oka readily appropriated the slogan *Kyokoku itchi* (National unity) and identified it with superorganismic life was the efficacious nature of mobilization during the war with Russia. In Oka's view, wartime measures had appropriately called on individuals to set aside their self-interest and coordinate their activities with the needs of the nation. In "War and Peace," for example, he approvingly cited the "wartime rules that a certain village is enacting" as recounted in the press. The rules included "not riding rickshaws except for sickness or urgent business, avoiding showy articles as best one can, and not spending money on unnecessary ceremonies."[108] He also mentioned "extreme measures such as having young women donate the cost of war out of their wages and getting elementary school students to ask their parents to contribute to the soldiers' relief fund."[109] As we saw in the introduction, Oka would ultimately imagine, in "Ideal Group Life," a state of such complete organic integration that parents on the home front would willing pack their flesh into cans for the sake of frontline fighters.

For Oka this complete subordination to the collective life was a precondition for success in the autarkic struggles between ethnic nations. In "Mankind's Struggle for Existence" he explains that "the competition a group exerts outward and the competition between each of internal parts stand in fixed relation to one another such that when one side increases the other decreases, forever waxing and waning in mutual opposition."[110] Thus, "in cases where one confronts the enemy as a group, internal concord is necessary above all else" and it is for this reason that competition between "ideal groups" is so "extremely violent"[111]: the individuals within the nation func-

---

108 Oka, "Sensō to Heiwa" [War and peace], 91.
109 Ibid.
110 Oka, "Jinrui no Seizon Kyōsō" [Mankind's struggle for existence], 79.
111 Ibid.

tion like the cells and internal organs of a predator, subordinating themselves utterly to the well-being of the organism.

The problem Oka had with wartime mobilization was that it was misunderstood as a merely temporary measure. "With the onset of war [mobilization] regulations are quickly established, and when the end of the war is upon us, they are once again discarded."[112] The "unity of the nation" that he thought he saw in the self-coordinating activities of the population—and perhaps also in the lantern parades and other manifestations of wartime chauvinism that Shimazu cites—were treated simply as wartime expediency. However, for Oka, the comprehensive social cohesion that is instituted during war should never be abandoned because in all circumstances "ordinary life must always be understood to resemble war conditions."[113] No "special preparations different from those of everyday life are required in time of war"—and, even when the struggle abates, "one must not lose wartime resoluteness."[114]

What Oka is really saying is that war never goes away: "With so many different races squaring off against one another, war does not really cease."[115] War is the permanent predicament of human beings and superindividual national unity is an evolutionary mobilization measure needed to survive it. Peace, in contrast, is an illusion. In apparent response to Tolstoy and the Japanese peace movement, a great deal of his essay "War and Peace" is devoted to making this simple point. Peace represents one of those phenomena "in this world" that "merely have a high reputation but lack reality."[116] He likens peace to the alleged existence of ghosts: whichever nation one visits, there is not a place where ghosts are not popular, but, in actuality, not even once have we heard of such a thing being caught. So-called peace is, in truth, such a thing."[117] Oka is especially cynical about how this phantasm is conjured up in order to mask the ruthless pursuit of self-interest, especially in the racial conflicts which comprise the main part of mankind's struggle for existence:

---

112 Oka, "Sensō to Heiwa" [War and peace], 91.
113 Ibid.
114 Ibid.
115 Ibid.
116 Ibid., 86.
117 Ibid.

While such a thing is in reality null and void, it is quite common to hear its name mentioned. In nearly all cases where something is perpetrated between different races, there is an instant where the act is dubbed to be "for the sake of peace." Wars are started "for the sake of peace." Adversaries are defeated and annexed "for the sake of peace." Forcing the abandonment of another country's spoils is done "for the sake of peace." Suddenly taking up what you were preparing to abandon is done "for the sake of peace." In short, in the present situation all and sundry is deemed to be "for the sake of peace"—and then one does just exactly what one pleases.[118]

Those who are duped by this rhetoric of peace, Oka warns, will become akin to "the merchant traveling on the Arabian Desert who spies a mirage thickly grown over with palm trees and eagerly rushes off thinking there will be refreshing shade and cool waters waiting for him once he arrives there. The closer he approaches the more the mirage recedes. However far he continues on, he cannot reach it."[119]

Oka's primary metaphor for the futility and danger brought on by the aspiration for an illusory state of peace comes from the theater. "So-called peace is like the intermission at a stage play: it is merely a word to express the period of preparation for the next war."[120] He elaborates: "War and peace are not originally two fundamentally contradictory conditions, but signify two different mutually alternating periods from within a single continuous life process. That is to say, when the curtain opens, there is war, when the curtain closes, there is peace. From the audience's vantage point, the leisure of intermission feels dull, but those behind the curtain will not be ready for the next act if they do not work diligently at this time."[121] In Oka's view, "though there is no doubt that from the beginning of history there have been some periods of peace wedged in between one war and the next, these times of peace are merely an interval in which one can prepare until the next war commences. For all that, whenever there is peace, it is limited only to the outward appearances: never is there peace behind the curtain."[122]

In order to draw a stark contrast between his total war doctrine and contemporary pacifism and humanitarianism, Oka invokes a proverb: "We

---

118 Ibid., 92.
119 Ibid., 87.
120 Ibid., 86.
121 Ibid.
122 Ibid., 90.

must not forget the war in peace."[123] It is indicative of Oka's metapolitical technique and his outlook of reformist scientism that he deems this "ancient admonition" to be "among the first rank" from "the standpoint of racial survival."[124] Like Haeckel's enlistment of Christian altruism for his monist philosophy which was discussed in the previous chapter, Oka's approach is to reform the culture that has been handed down by affirming aspects of it that reflect the underlying reality of human life described by evolutionary science. In this case, "the war in peace" of "ancient" provenance spoken of in the proverb corresponds with the "single continuous life process"[125] of evolutionary struggle that constitutes the ontological bedrock of human existence. For him, "war in peace" refers not only to the continual war which occurs at "countless levels" within societies, but, more crucially, to the never-ending "all-out ruthless battle"[126] that recurs between race-based nation-states. It is, in Oka's estimation, with this ontological ground of martial struggle between superindividual nations in constant view that "we must prepare as best we can for the fact that, in a general sense, human wars in this world cannot possibly come to an end. Due to this an attitude that never forgets war in peace is always the most appropriate."[127]

The reality of perpetual war points to a final aspect of Oka's total war doctrine: the need for a scientifically astute nation. In the next chapter we will see that Oka will begin to imagine using evolutionary science to reconstitute humanity both biologically and nomically—devising a "human-way" that will instinctively unite the nation for evolutionary struggle. However, the two wartime essays we are considering here focus on the imperative to develop a technological civilization for the same end. The need for such technological prowess is obvious to Oka: during the "peaceful" intermissions in the continuing theater of war "forts are surely constructed, ships built, and, as much as possible, military forces readied."[128] In light of the "extremely high price" of such preparations Oka envisions an "arms race"[129] that might, in fact, constrain the outbreak of actual war. With an individ-

---

123 Ibid., 91.
124 Ibid.
125 Ibid., 86.
126 Ibid., 87.
127 Ibid., 93.
128 Ibid., 86.
129 Ibid., 87–88.

ual warship "worth tens of millions of yen" and even the firing of a single shell costing "several thousand yen"[130] war might even seem "impossible" to wage. Yet "in situations where one's own race comes into danger"[131] there is no choice but to completely embrace the "material civilization" that ensures success in modern warfare. Oka could not be more blunt in his assessment of Japan's predicament: "Looking at the state of today's world, the [human] species with high civilization are expanding day by day, and those with low civilization are disposed toward decline due to the increasing pressure they are under."[132] In his estimation, "whether or not a species progresses toward civilization is a life-and-death issue."[133]

It is in this context that Oka denounces "Tolstoy and his kind" who "in triumphant tones call today's civilization the civilization of masters."[134] In contrast to such pacifists and humanitarians, Oka regards "intellectual power as the mightiest weapon in mankind's struggle for existence."[135] For Japan to become "a first-rank nation" and "plan the development of our race": "it should try to be properly informed of values of civilization in the struggle for existence, and to possess for our nation such things as the most sturdy battleships, the fastest locomotives, the best museums our country can put together, and the most complete experimental labs. If we do not show this degree of ambition, immediately the civilization divide with various other countries will increase. The less we pursue civilization the further behind we will find ourselves."[136]

In order to clarify what he has in mind, Oka distinguishes his notion of material civilization from the bourgeois civilization of "the so-called gentleman's luxurious life."[137] For him "civilization is never a luxury for the sake of increasing the happiness of all humankind, but rather a necessary condition which must be relied upon if the species is to be able to survive."[138] He openly admits that "human happiness does not increase at all"[139] with the

---

130 Ibid.
131 Ibid., 88.
132 Ibid., 93–94.
133 Ibid., 94.
134 Ibid.
135 Ibid.
136 Ibid.
137 Ibid., 93.
138 Ibid.
139 Ibid.

advance of civilization. Unmistakably referring to the hardships and dislocations attendant to industrialization, Oka asserts that "however much civilization has advanced, it is clear that the majority of people must, as is usually the case, endure lives of suffering."[140] In a similar vein, Oka concedes that, ethically speaking, less civilized people's may actually be equal or even superior to the contemporary Westerners who possess material civilization in such abundance: "Even among aborigines who live in the deep mountains of Africa or along the rocky coasts of the South Seas there are people who are not at all inferior to Europeans when it comes to displaying fearless courage before an enemy or a chivalric spirit of self-sacrifice for the sake of one's race."[141] For Oka, however, evincing such courage and chivalry has little benefit in circumstances such as those encountered in the Russo-Japanese War: "Yet when they are shot at with machine guns and attacked by torpedoes there is nothing they can do. No matter how certain the spiritual aspect alone is, if the material aspect is considerably inferior, races cannot possibly hope to win in today's struggle for existence. Civilization is a word which indicates intellectual power. Human beings defeating other animals and civilized men conquering savages are primarily examples of this intellectual power."[142]

In the coming chapters we will see that Oka not only modifies his assessment of this self-sacrificing "spiritual aspect" but comes to question, in his own way, the mode of modern life implicated in material civilization. However, his estimation of "intellectual power" as the mightiest of evolutionary weapons will remain a major aspect of his *shinkaron*. Throughout *Evolution and Human Life* and his later writings, Oka subscribes to the central scientistic belief that, as Todorov puts it, "the world is transparent" and "that it can be known entirely and without residue by the human mind."[143] Unraveling "all the secrets of nature" and identifying "the causes of all facts and beings," science can "modify processes involved and steer them in a more desirable direction."[144] Not only is Oka's "War and Peace" written to warn the up and coming generation that the nation "will fall into irreversibly dangerous circumstances" if, in the manner of Tolstoy, "we look down on science

---

140 Ibid.
141 Ibid., 94.
142 Ibid.
143 Todorov, *Hope and Memory*, 19–20.
144 Ibid., 20.

and civilization even just a little,"[145] but the major preoccupation of his literary output will become the creation of a scientifically astute population that simultaneously harnesses the processes of nature and conducts itself according to its inner workings. To express it in the language of organic individuality: Oka's metapolitics imagines that knowledge of nature will enable worker bees to maximize their efficiency while aligning their activities to the needs of the national hive.

The third section will explore how Oka's failure to make evolutionary science a fixture of the national school curriculum contributed to bringing out the generative potential in his scientistic organicism. Essays that reiterate the essential need for education in natural science, in fact, figure large in *Evolution and Human Life* as well as the anthologies that come after it. Oka returned again and again in the coming years to the point that "the aim of education," which "those working in education" should "never forget ... even for a moment," was "to cultivate upcoming generations of a nation's people who have the capacity to do just what it takes to stand up in the arena of competition among the nations of the world and thrive on its own."[146] "An ethnic nation (*minzoku*) that is indifferent toward ordinary scientific knowledge and does not adequately plan its development will be quickly bypassed and perhaps cannot escape defeat in the war of peace."[147] Oka's model for national development in science education was the nation that had taken the global lead in both commerce and technology: Wilhelmine Germany. In Oka's estimation the Germans had managed to strike an ideal balance between pure research, technological application, and public education. While "the newly established Kaiser Wilhelm Institute for the Encouragement of Science and other organizations like it, aim at advancing scientific research without any necessary connection to present-day applications,"[148] the education system ensures that "scientific knowledge spreads to workers and they actually understand the logic of [applications] and do not merely imitate the outward appearance."[149] The result is that "Germany is the best of the best at exten-

---

145 Oka, "Sensō to Heiwa" [War and peace], 97.
146 Asajirō Oka, "Kyōiku to Meishin" [Education and superstition], in *Shinka to Jinsei* [Evolution and human life] (Tokyo: Yūseidō Shuppan, 1968), 117.
147 Asajirō Oka, "Minzoku no Hatten to Rika" [Science and the development of the race-nation], in *Shinka to Jinsei* [Evolution and human life], (Tokyo: Yūseidō Shuppan, 1968), 115.
148 Oka, "Kyōiku to Meishin" [Education and superstition], 121.
149 Ibid., 119.

sively applying the knowledge of chemistry, achieving the ability to create as they will, in various areas, manufactured products by artificial means from only what were until now select natural resources."[150] Visiting the Ginza district of Tokyo, Oka marvels at the high quality of even German toys: "many German-made products are laid out and, moreover, these are intricately and solidly constructed yet inexpensive. Models of steam engines, electric generators, and electric lights are set up on a single stand and can be purchased for only about 10 yen."[151] The fact that "Germany is at present superior to England and succeeds in each area of world commerce"[152] Oka attributes to this combination of a research elite adept at unlocking the secrets of nature and a general population of workers scientifically educated to manipulate the world.

In the aftermath of the war with Russia Oka frequently blamed Japan's technological inferiority on the absence of such an educational system. In Oka's view victory had lulled his compatriots into a false sense of complacency that it was a "first-rank" nation when, in fact, it might be called "inferior to nations of even the third or fourth rank when looking at aspects other than war."[153] Japan's famous export products are "raw silk and tea" which remain "unaltered from their natural state."[154] Though foreigners condescendingly praise it as a "fine arts nation"[155] for its handicrafts, the few technological items Japan has to offer are mere imitations: "The inventions and machinery at our nation's exhibitions and fairs are so pitiful that one is almost brought to tears. The things thought to be a little better are Western-made items which have been slightly altered. Not a single one is seen that was invented from scratch in Japan."[156] The one example of original "machinery that is representative of civilization" and attracts the attention of people at international expositions is "a noodle machine" which, Oka believes, is "no better than a toy."[157] As a consequence Japan remains dependent on Western nations for technology and industrial products: "Machinery that is assembled through the use of human intellectual power is valuable—crushed

---

150 Oka, "Minzoku no Hatten to Rika" [Science and the development of the race-nation], 115.
151 Oka, "Kyōiku to Meishin" [Education and superstition], 119.
152 Ibid.
153 Oka, "Minzoku no Hatten to Rika" [Science and the development of the race-nation], 112.
154 Ibid., 109.
155 Ibid., 111.
156 Ibid., 110.
157 Oka, "Kyōiku to Meishin" [Education and superstition], 118.

into ground metal it is worthless. In other words, our nation sells natural resources according to their value as raw materials, and buys at a high price
from foreign nations items which have added intellectual power to natural
products."[158] To acquire this intellectual power, the "brainpower to invent
mechanical devices"[159] which Oka also calls "new civilized knowledge," and
become a "real first-rank nation" Japan must not only be "strong in war, but
in education and learning."[160] Like Germany, it must, in the spirit of scientistic reform, produce a nation of workers who can efficiently manipulate the
mechanisms of the natural world uncovered by the ongoing activity of scientific research.

AUTARKY WITHIN INTERNATIONAL ANARCHY

Oka's warnings about the inevitable costs of educational and technological
neglect are in themselves rather pedestrian—typical of the statements of late
developers. Yet considered together with what Oka says about the "war in
peace" they add up to an espousal of total war that is strikingly prescient. It
would take the cataclysm of world war for similar visions of a technologically
primed, permanently mobilized national body to achieve international currency. When combined with his portrayal of empire-state logic at play in the
innate drive of these bodies for racial autarky, Oka's evolutionary realpolitik
begins to look like something more than a rejection of the humanitarian nationalism that Shimazu describes. Anticipating—and perhaps shaping—an
outlook that would become national policy three decades hence, Oka repudi-
ates the notion of a liberal global order based on international governing bodies and the rule of law. Although his emphasis on autarky and total war are
contributing factors, it is primarily in his organicist conception of race that
the vision of international anarchy that he puts forth has its genesis.

The determinative importance of race in international relations becomes
evident in how Oka readily dismisses any sense of common cause between
nations and peoples. In "Mankind's Struggle for Existence," for instance, he
takes strong exception to "a particular magazine" that had attacked a style of
realpolitik much like his own. Oka quotes this unnamed magazine in a short

---

158 Oka, "Minzoku no Hatten to Rika" [Science and the development of the race-nation], 109–10.
159 Ibid., 111.
160 Ibid., 112.

passage: "There are those who say that because there is no law or morality between nations, let us strive for victory, by using whatever means are available to us without reserve. However, this outlook is gravely mistaken. In actuality, since present-day Japan is fighting for justice, and Russia is a country indifferent to truth or falsehood, doesn't everyone in the world express sympathy for Japan? Justice is in truth the strongest weapon of all."[161] Oka regards such reliance on abstractions like justice and sympathy as "extremely misguided." This "thing called" sympathy is "only a word" and it "does not at all have the effect of making weak nations victorious."[162] To drive home his point he reminds his readers of how little international sympathy really meant in the recent Boer War. In the case of the Japanese, for instance, "we, for a time, fancied praising Transvaal, yet it was never hoped for this reason that Transvaal would defeat England."[163] This is because "when the victory of a particular nation does not profit one's own, it is not expected that one should be pleased."[164] In the case of the Boer conflict, Japanese could not support Transvaal due to the alliance with England. In similar fashion he suggests that "though there were many nations who were happy that Russia lost"[165] in its conflict with Japan, this sympathy was motivated either by self-interest, as in the case of England, or meaningless emotional indulgence. "Perhaps Japan alone enjoyed the victory for its own sake, apart from financial gains and losses. While we must be tremendously grateful for the sympathy and kind intentions conveyed today to our nations from various nations abroad, what value this sympathy holds in truth will perhaps gradually become clear based on the behavior of various foreign nations toward us in the future."[166]

The most bewitching of the abstractions that occlude the strategic acumen of the nation is "humanity" (jindō)—a term which can also cover morality and, as we will see in the next chapter, "the way of humans." It is to a common humanity that Tolstoy and the peace movement appealed in their protests to the war. In Oka's view "for use between nations the meaning of

---

161 Oka, "Jinrui no Seizon Kyōsō" [Mankind's struggle for existence], 81–82.
162 Ibid., 82.
163 Ibid.
164 Ibid.
165 Ibid.
166 Ibid.

this term is very vague."[167] Indeed, because it is "so vague and noncommittal, it is supremely suitable when used as an excuse for something one needs to do,"[168] such as wage war. Thus, "the extent to which up until today barbarian peoples have been attacked and destroyed by civilized nations 'for the sake of humanity' is not known. Even among like-minded civilized nations, the phrase 'for the sake of humanity,' because it comes across as being used like an embellishing sign on occasions when one must plainly speak for the sake of our species, is indeed the same as 'for the sake of peace'—best regarded as a kind of prescribed formal phrase."[169]

Oka's concern was that these formalities, necessary as they were, might be taken to heart and end up encumbering the pursuit of national interest. Clearly aware of the great pains Japan was going to during the war to establish that it was a civilized nation in the humanitarian sense, Oka worried that his compatriots did not grasp the significance of being lectured by other nations "to treat enemies with kindness, either by loving peace, respecting humanity or advocating peace conference."[170] In his view, even those nations who spoke out for the sake of humanity and against the enemies of peace understood that these humanitarian expressions "do not reflect reality."[171] It was imperative that Japanese comprehend the self-aggrandizement that drives ethnic nations and grasp that "phrases such as 'enemy of peace' or 'enemy of humanity,' if we were to translate them plainly, are merely interlopers impeding the development and expansion of our race."[172]

Oka insisted that this vigilant awareness of racial advantage must be carried even into relations with purported friends. Despite his multilingual, multinational early education and the close bond he formed with his mentor, Rudolf Leuckart, at Leipzig University, Oka, perhaps alluding to his experience in Germany, asserted that "kind treatment toward a foreign traveler does not at the same time mean that the traveler's race is loved. Even though countries show kindness to a few travelers, the treatment is certainly the opposite toward many immigrants."[173] Oka was particularly adamant

167 Oka, "Sensō to Heiwa" [War and peace], 92.
168 Ibid.
169 Ibid.
170 Ibid., 93.
171 Ibid.
172 Ibid.
173 Oka, "Jinrui no Seizon Kyōsō" [Mankind's struggle for existence], 84.

that his fellow Japanese remain cognizant of the underlying racial self-interest at work in friendships with other nations. In both "War and Peace" and "Mankind's Struggle for Existence," Oka underscores what for him is a central truth of international relations: "Strife between nations is endemic and alliances are merely a temporary expedient"[174] to "protect against common enemies."[175] As he explains, "searching through the historical record, no matter which century, no matter which country, there are no examples of more than two different races joining into a union when there was no common enemy. The conditions under which more than two different races agree to form an alliance due to a common enemy resembles a wooden tub which is kept together by an encircling hoop. Accordingly, once the common enemy is gone, the union breaks apart—which is not at all different from when the hoop around the tub is cut."[176] Oka also likens alliances to a wolf pack that has come together on an ad hoc basis:

> Even wolves join forces at times in which it is not suitable to go it alone. For instance, in situations such as when a large bull is seized upon, only then will more than forty or fifty wolves band together. A united league between nation and nation is the same. Even though wolves will fight each other to the death to capture a lone rabbit that they have come across, many will prepare to cooperate in the face of a large bull. Not only at times when individuals attack, but also at times of defense the same thing occurs. In this way, even solitary animals form unions for a while when faced with a powerful foe—and human nations are not an exception to this rule.[177]

From the standpoint of Oka's biological corporatism, once the task is completed and the common foe vanquished, the superindividual nations revert to their usual natural state: "the different races all become enemies to one another with the result that new alliances can once again be forged. The sequence in which alliances are made and unmade is roughly like this: the alliances are never permanent."[178]

Oka seemed particularly wary of Japan's friendship with two of the champions of internationalist humanitarianism, England and the United States.

---

174 Ibid., 81.
175 Oka, "Sensō to Heiwa" [War and peace], 89.
176 Ibid.
177 Oka, "Jinrui no Seizon Kyōsō" [Mankind's struggle for existence], 81.
178 Oka, "Sensō to Heiwa" [War and peace], 89.

Japan had entered into an alliance with England in 1902 and both countries had provided Japan financial and moral support during the war with Russia. It was with England in mind that he warned: "that certain alliances seem to be long standing is, after all, because we cannot see very far into the future due to our brief, individual lives. Various powers do form such alliances despite the fact that there is no common foe. Nevertheless, it must be stated that from the standpoint of human nature such alliances can never continue on permanently."[179] Oka's primary apprehension, however, was not just with the compromises that would ensue by treating the alliance like the one with England as permanent but with the liberal international order that these advocates of humanitarian civilization hoped to construct out of the system of alliances. According to Oka, "there are those who argue that each one of the presently independent nations will form a union, all the countries of the world will combine into a single, unified state, and that war between nations will come to an end."[180] Only the "insufficient development"[181] of society and the imperfection of nations prevents the formation of such a global superstate. In Oka's estimation, acceptance of this viewpoint could have disastrous consequences: "if a large number of people honestly came to believe such theories, it might have a terrible influence on the nation in its usual preparedness."[182]

The precedent for such an "international union" is "the increase, one after another, of united international enterprises such as an international post, an international exchange, and international health and fishery conferences."[183] Yet the transition to an actual global government would come with the organization of "a single high court for trials or mediation" designed to "judge disputes among the nations of the world before all countries."[184] In order to expose not only the impossibility of such an arrangement but the self-serving hypocrisy of those proposing it, Oka asks his readers to consider the results if such a court had attempted to adjudicate the conflict between the British Empire and the Boers. "Supposing on the occasion of the dispute in South Africa a few years back a high court of all the world's nations united to-

---

179 Ibid.
180 Oka, "Jinrui no Seizon Kyōsō" [Mankind's struggle for existence], 76.
181 Oka, "Sensō to Heiwa" [War and peace], 90.
182 Oka, "Jinrui no Seizon Kyōsō" [Mankind's struggle for existence], 76.
183 Oka, "Sensō to Heiwa" [War and peace], 90.
184 Ibid., 89.

gether had justly decreed that the Transvaal belonged to England—would the Boers have respectfully approved of it? Despite a small population, insufficient funding, and a clear knowledge that they would lose, it is certain that the dispute would never have been allowed to end without war."[185] Though such a court might work just fine when it comes to mediating "insignificant incidents"[186] between nations, "in important affairs, concerning the life and death or the rise and fall of one's own race, no one in the end can consent to accepting a disadvantageous outcome."[187] The implication is clear: like the Boers, the Japanese should never subordinate their vital interests to courts set up by "humanitarian" powers, such as Great Britain and the United States, who are already in possession of autarkic empires. "If we think about who the advocates of international peace conferences are, it is clear that such organizations cannot possibly be of service to one's true character."[188]

In the end, Oka's evolutionary realpolitik rejects a liberal global order founded on humanitarian values because he does not believe in a common humanity. Just as nations that are comprised of more than one race are destined to fall asunder, an international order can never remain intact due to innate interracial aversion. For Oka, "the white race which occupies Australia and proclaims such things as 'blood is thicker than water'" in order to "block the immigration of colored races"[189] is only giving voice to an ineluctable "natural inclination" that must be accepted as indicative of all human races. As a consequence, Oka believes "we must always think only in terms of our own power, and strive to the fullest measure to make the nation strong."[190] Human life is a perpetual winner-take-all struggle between expansionist nations for racial autarky. Those nations that achieve conditions of permanent mobilization, racial homogeneity, and technological proficiency will prevail in this ceaseless war. Not "eternal peace" but the international anarchy that has always characterized mankind's struggle for existence lies in store for the races that constitute "humanity." Accepting and preparing for the future reality of an intensifying global race war is Oka's ultimate message of evolutionary realpolitik.

---

185 Ibid., 90.
186 Ibid., 89.
187 Ibid., 90.
188 Ibid.
189 Oka, "Jinrui no Seizon Kyōsō" [Mankind's struggle for existence], 83.
190 Ibid., 84.

INCOMMENSURABLE SPECIES OF MAN

Oka's admonitions concerning the incompatibility of races received swift confirmation in the aftermath of the war. In "Mankind's Struggle for Existence" he suggested that "should a nation of the yellow races come to gain some measure of power, the white nations would naturally become increasingly wary toward this nation, and countries which had been antagonistic toward one another over other issues would come together over this one."[191] Something like this had in fact occurred in 1895 with the Triple Intervention by Russia, Germany, and France that had deprived Japan of its territorial gains in Manchuria, transferring them to the Tsar "for the sake of peace" in East Asia. Now, once again, in the wake of the Portsmouth Treaty, Japan became the target of a fresh wave of yellow peril hysteria, this time emanating from the most vociferous proponent of liberal humanitarianism and a nation that had recently established an autarkic empire in North America—the United States.

The most severe outbreak of racial animus occurred in San Francisco just a year after the victory over Russia. Although the Japanese Red Cross, in yet another gesture of humanitarian goodwill, had just donated a quarter of a million dollars in relief funds to aid victims of the recent earthquake, the San Francisco Board of Education used the devastation within the city as a pretext to segregate all Chinese, Korean, and Japanese students in special "Oriental Public Schools."[192] The reasoning of the board was that "Our children should not be placed in any position where their youthful impressions may be affected by association with pupils of the Mongolian race."[193] Backing the Board, the San Francisco Chronicle left no doubt that the primary target of this racism were Japanese children, whom the paper referred to as a "moral poison"[194] in the classrooms. Such statements were nothing new in the San Francisco press, which had responded to the influx of Japanese immigrants after 1900 with headlines such as "The Yellow Peril—How Japanese Crowd Out the White Race" and "Japanese a Menace to American Women."[195] In total the Japanese population in the United States rose from

---

191 Ibid.
192 LaFeber, *The Clash*, 89.
193 Boyle, *Modern Japan*, 147.
194 Ibid.
195 Ibid.

24,000 to 72,000 in the first decade of the twentieth century, and the actions of the school board were in many ways the culmination of rising calls from organized labor, nativist groups, and farmers to curtail immigration and protect the white identity of northern California.

The Japanese press responded to what was happening in San Francisco with outrage. A leading Tokyo paper even called for a military response: "Stand up, Japanese nation! Our countrymen have been HUMILIATED.... Why do we not insist on sending [war]ships?"[196] President Roosevelt, who had negotiated the Portsmouth Treaty the year before, also responded in disgust, publically calling the school board "fools" and their actions a "wicked absurdity."[197] After summoning members of the board to Washington, he worked out a deal designed to satisfy both sides: the school board was made to rescind its segregation order and in return the Japanese government promised that it would no longer give passports to peasant farmers and other laborers bound for the United States. This so-called, "Gentleman's Agreement of 1907" was not a treaty but, as the name indicates, an informal arrangement. The message it conveyed about the unequal status of Japanese as a race was writ large for people back in the home country.

This message was reinforced by bellicose overtures from the American government during these same years. Roosevelt had moved so quickly and publically to thwart the school board because of a new wariness toward Japanese power after the war with Russia. He complained that "those infernal fools in California insult the Japanese recklessly ... and in the event of war, it will be the nation as a whole that will have to pay the consequences."[198] "During 1905 to 1908," according to Walter LaFeber, "the possibility of war between Americans and Japanese was much in the air."[199] Although he had personal ties with Japanese, famously celebrated the samurai spirit by handing out copies of Nitobe's *Bushidō*, and enthusiastically cabled Tokyo after the Battle of Tsushima that "neither Trafalgar nor the defeat of the Spanish Armada was as overwhelming,"[200] Roosevelt privately worried that with a Japanese victory "there will result a real shifting of the center of equilib-

196 LaFeber, *The Clash*, 89.
197 Boyle, *Modern Japan*, 147.
198 Ibid.
199 LaFeber, *The Clash*, 89.
200 Boyle, *Modern Japan*, 147.

rium as far as the white races are concerned"[201] and in a meeting with his Harvard acquaintance, Baron Kaneko, expressed his fear that Japan "might get the 'big head' and enter into a career of insolence and aggression."[202] The decisiveness of Japanese land and sea victories caused Americans to undergo a reevaluation of their nation's strategic position and by 1906 Roosevelt and his military had drawn up War Plan ORANGE, which revealed the vulnerability of its Pacific holdings and, as a result, initiated preparations for a future conflict with Japan. As Japan began to consolidate its position in Manchuria during 1907 in defiance of the Open Door Policy, Roosevelt, sensing that American interests in Asia were becoming dependent on Japan, decided to send the US fleet on a cruise that would circumnavigate the world and thereby demonstrate America's unilateral power. This "Great White Fleet" arrived in Tokyo with sixteen first-class cruisers in October of 1908. Although it was welcomed by large crowds that not only waved the Stars and Stripes but sang the American national anthem in English,[203] the sixteen first-class cruisers that comprised the fleet communicated a message not dissimilar to that of the school board back in San Francisco.

American discrimination, yellow peril racism, and gunboat diplomacy certainly had everything to do with the success of *jinshuron* after the Russo-Japanese War. Though "domestic public opinion" during the conflict "had assumed the Yellow Peril was the dominant Western perspective on the Japanese struggle against Russia,"[204] there was a hope that the nation would "integrate fully with the West, simply by accepting the code of 'civilized' international conduct, regardless of racial, cultural and religious difference."[205] However, with the lifting of wartime censorship and the realization "that the West was not willing to accept the Japanese as racial equals,"[206] *jinshuron* racial arguments began to gain ground and a hardening of attitudes toward the West took hold. As we have discussed earlier the special issue of *Taiyō* published in 1908 was entitled "The Clash of the Yellow and White Race" and helped establish "'race' as one of the principal determinants of Ja-

201 LaFeber, *The Clash*, 80.
202 Ibid.
203 Ibid., 90.
204 Shimazu, *Japanese Society at War*, 160.
205 Ibid., 164.
206 Ibid.

pan's self-identity in the international arena."[207] Perhaps echoing Oka's wartime writings, the contributors emphasized that the rivalry between "racial stocks" was not only inevitable but intensifying.

Oka's own evolutionary realpolitik, however, should not be understood as a reactive stance. Instead, as the final paragraph of "War and Peace," written just two months into the war with Russia, testifies, Oka considered the situation for the Japanese race to be fluid and full of possibility. "Standing in the arena of existential struggle," the Japanese, Oka believed, "must do whatever is required to overtake other races."[208] This advancement can be achieved by "striving" and not neglecting "for a single day" the "development of science and the progress of material civilization."[209] Technological prowess and the martial benefits that follow from it are not the exclusive possession of the now dominant West. It is something that the Japanese can and must strive to acquire. This insight from the Russo-Japanese war experience, which Niall Ferguson identifies with a profound shift in global affairs resulting in nothing less than the rise of the East and the relative decline of the West in later decades of the twentieth century, leads Oka to offer the following musings at the close of the conflict: "Up to now the powerful nations of the world have been created by the white races despite the quarrels among them. If in the future a powerful nation were to emerge from the yellow races, and reach a point where it occupied an equal position with the nations of the white races, wouldn't it bring about a new variation in the state of international competition?"[210]

As the next chapter will explore, part of Oka's confidence in racial advancement derives from his Lamarckian faith that the appropriate habits could engender new traits and with them new capacities. However, at an even more basic level, Oka's ambition for Japan rests on his vision of an order of "international competition," one articulated by an elaborate ranking of races. As he describes it in "Mankind's Struggle for Existence," "among the classifications called races, there are various levels. If there are the classifications of the German race, the Latin race and the Slavic race, there are also, among others the classifications of the Japanese and Chinese races. Just as the former are

---

207 Ibid., 166.
208 Oka, "Sensō to Heiwa" [War and peace], 97.
209 Ibid.
210 Oka, "Jinrui no Seizon Kyōsō" [Mankind's struggle for existence], 83.

all included as part of the white race, and the latter are somehow included in the yellow race, there are great distinctions and small ones."[211] Though Oka is vague about how particular ethnic peoples relate to one another within larger categories, it should be obvious based on what we have said up until now that Oka subscribes to a belief in a basic incommensurability between races due to their innate aversion to one another. In fact, not only are the distinctions between the terms nation (*kuni*) and ethnic nation (*minzoku*) blurred together with that of race (*minshu*) but at times all three terms are treated as the equivalent of "species"(*shuzoku*). His evolutionary realpolitik, in other words, paints a picture of a global contest for autarky between human species—species-specific nations expanding into empire-states.

While similar ideas were in wide circulation in the early 1900s, the most probable source of Oka's biopolitical vision with its emphasis on human speciation was the one Haeckel provided in his *History of Creation*. Not only was the hierarchy of human species that Haeckel described at the end of this book included in the numerous reprintings of this text well into the twentieth century but it also inspired other visions of racial hierarchy including that of Chamberlain in 1899. Haeckel's hierarchy would have been especially intriguing to Oka for a simple reason beyond the fact that it appeared in one of the founding texts of evolutionary morphology: it accorded the "Mongol species," of which the Japanese were thought to be a subspecies ("race"), a special place of precedence in the global evolutionary struggle. Japanese were not evolutionary also-rans, according to Haeckel, but the leaders of the "second dominant variety of man."

Haeckel's account of human speciation was entitled "Hypothetical Sketch of the Monophyletic Origin and of the Extension of the Twelve Races of Man from Lemuria over the Earth." Lemuria was a mythical "lost" island that Haeckel conjectured must have existed in the Indian Ocean. On this island resided a hypothetical creature that Haeckel dubbed "*Pithecanthropus alanus*, the speechless ape-man."[212] The *History of Creation* provided, among other things, a reconstruction of the pedigree of contemporary humans beginning from the first ancestor, "single cell without a nucleus,"[213] that Haeckel called the monera, and ultimately included a total of twenty-

211 Ibid.
212 Gould, *Ontogeny and Phylogeny*, 173.
213 Ibid., 483.

two stages. *Pithecanthropus alanus* represented the penultimate, twenty-first stage and, according to Haeckel, "very probably existed toward the end of the Tertiary period."[214]

These "apelike men" were significant for human evolution because the twelve primary human races that Haeckel identified had their origins in twelve separate migrations from Lemuria. In other words, race predates the appearance of human beings and each race evolved to the human stage of evolution, the twenty-second stage in Haeckel's grand phylogeny, along a distinct path—and, most importantly, with distinct, unequal results. Such unequal results were most apparent with regard to the trait that defined man: the "higher differentiation"[215] of the brain as he referred to it in his follow-up to *The History of Creation*, *The Evolution of Man*. While *Pithecanthropi alanus* had distinguished themselves from their immediate ancestors, "the Man-like Apes, or *Anthropoides*, by becoming completely habituated to an upright walk" still "did not possess the real and chief characteristic of man, namely, the articulate human language of words development of a higher consciousness, and the formation of ideas."[216]

Language, in fact, plays the preeminent role in Haeckel's explanation of human speciation. Influenced by the Hegelian philologist, August Schleicher,[217] Haeckel presented language as integral to the evolution of the brain: "[T]he origin of human language must, more than anything else, have had an ennobling and transforming influence on the mental life of Man, and consequently upon his brain. The higher differentiation and perfecting of the brain and the mental life as its highest function developed in direct correlation with his expression of means of speech. Hence, the highest authorities in comparative philology justly see in the development of human speech the most important process which distinguishes Man from his animal ancestors."[218] Given this inseparability of linguistic development and human evolution, the "multiple, or polyphyletic origin"[219] of human language meant that "human speech, as such did not develop probably until the genus of Speechless or Primeval Man, or Ape Man, had separated into

---

214 Haeckel, *The History of Creation*, vol. 2, 293.
215 Haeckel, *The Evolution of Man*, 181.
216 Haeckel, *The History of Creation*, vol. 2, 293.
217 Di Gregori, *From Here to Eternity*, 98–106.
218 Haeckel, *The History of Creation*, vol. 2, 301.
219 Ibid., 302.

several kinds or species."[220] Though the convention is to regard these species as all human, they, in fact, evolved on parallel paths at uneven rates. Some, in other words, developed more sophisticated languages and complex brains to go with them, while others were not so different from their ape-man ancestors. It is in light of this alleged differentiation of men into distinct species of unequal value that Haeckel makes his frequent assertion that "the gulf between [the] thoughtful mind of civilized man and the thoughtless animal soul of the savage is enormous—greater than the gulf that separates the latter from the soul of the dog."[221]

This speciation of mankind based on philological accounts of the linguistic past finds vivid illustration in *The History of Creation*. A plate featuring a map of the world depicts the historical migration of the races on to the continents as twelve fernlike branches, extending from their primeval root in hypothetical undersea Lemuria. Using hair texture because, according to Haeckel it was, like language, a more reliable measure of heredity, Haeckel initially divided these twelve species into two groups: the woolly haired "Ultrichi" and the straight-haired "Lissotrichi." After quickly writing off the Ultrichi—which included Papuans, Hottentots, Kaffres and Negros—as destined for extinction or subjugation because of their supposed simian nature which rendered them incapable of "true inner culture" or "higher mental development,"[222] he concentrates on using a combination of linguistic and follicle analysis to show how it is from among the remaining human species categorized as Lissotrichi—which include Australians, Malays, Mongols, Arctic men, Americans, Dravidians, Nubians and Mediterranese—that a single subspecies of man, the "Indo-Germanic," has emerged as the crown of creation.

The racialist reasoning that elevated Caucasians above all other human varieties is spelled out in a chilling passage from *The History of Creation*:

[T]he Mediterranean species, and within it the Indo-Germanic, have by means of the higher development of their brain surpassed all the other races and species in the struggle for life, and have already spread the net of their dominion over the whole globe. It is only the Mongolian species which can

---

220 Ibid.
221 Haeckel, *The Wonders of Life*, 407.
222 Haeckel, *The History of Creation*, vol. 2, 309–10.

at all successfully, at least in certain respects, compete with the Mediterranean. Within the tropical regions, Negroes, Kaffres, and Nubians, as also the Malays and Dravidas, are in some measure protected against the encroachments of the Indo-Germanic tribes by their being better adapted for a hot climate; the case of the arctic tribes of the polar regions is similar. But the other races, which as it is are very much diminished in number, will sooner or later completely succumb in the struggle for existence to the superiority of the Mediterranean races. The American and Australian tribes are even now fast approaching their complete extinction, and the same may be said of the Papuans and Hottentots.[223]

In predictable fashion Haeckel goes on to explain why the specifically Germanic peoples should be deemed superior even among the "Indo-Germans":

The various branches of the Indo-Germanic race have deviated furthest from the common primary form of ape-like men. During classic antiquity and the Middle Ages, the Romanic branch (Greco-Italo-Keltic group), one of the two main branches of the Indo-Germanic species, outstripped all other branches in the career of civilization, but at present the same position is occupied by the Germanic. Its chief representatives are the English and Germans, who are in the present age laying the foundation for a new period of higher mental development, in the recognition and completion of the theory of descent. The recognition of the theory of development and the monistic philosophy based upon it, forms the best criterion for the degree of man's mental development.[224]

Perhaps no intellectual has ever paid himself such an extravagant compliment: Haeckel himself by dint of his monistic philosophizing claims to have so elevated the German branch of Indo-Germanic race that it now stands at the very pinnacle of all organic life. *The History of Creation* concludes with the suggestion that its own author represents the most perfect creature that has ever graced planet Earth with its presence.

Haeckel's vainglory and white supremacism should not, however, cause us to overlook the fact that his account is, in a backhanded manner, encouraging if not flattering to East Asians, and Japanese in particular. Though the "Mediterranese" species is awarded pride of place as the first dominant va-

---

223 Ibid., 324–25.
224 Ibid., 332.

riety of man, Mongols are not far behind: they are "the second dominant variety." As we have just seen they alone are capable of competing with the Mediterranean. Aside from whites, Mongols alone have had an "actual history"[225]—that is, they have contributed to the overall epigenetic development of mankind as a whole. In the last chapter we saw what this relatively elevated status meant in Haeckel's later extrapolation of this hierarchy into an account of the value of life: Japanese came to constitute one of the "higher civilized races," a species of man on a par, in Haeckel's historicist schema, with the Romans of the classical period world and Western Europeans of the early Renaissance. While not yet possessing the prowess and "value" of the "cultivated races" that fostered modern scientific civilization, Japanese, nevertheless, were not that far off the pace. The fact that they possessed an "actual history" meant they might one day become the front-running "cultivated race" in the world-historical unfolding of human species into higher echelons of health, power, and integration.

Oka's frequent insistence that Japan must aspire to "become a nation superior to all others"[226] follows in part from the fluidity of the racial rankings offered by evolutionary morphologists. Separate and unequal could be taken as a strength, especially if your race was a conferred "second dominant" status and accorded living space that encompassed the entire eastern half of the Eurasian landmass. However, along with this separateness came a sense of incommensurability between races. The most sinister and destructive element of the "war of the world" that Ferguson describes is the treatment of other humans as aliens—as separate species. Imperial Japan would play an unfortunate role in the violence implicated in this speciation of humankind: a little more than a quarter century after Russian prisoners were greeted as honored guests at Matsuyama and other prisoner of war camps by a government eager to establish its humanitarianism before the world, Japan began to conduct biological experiments on local populations in Manchuria. Over the next fifteen years large-scale atrocities were carried out across China and Southeast Asia. By the end of the Second World War live vivisections were being conducted on allied military personnel by Japanese medical teams.[227] The process by which Japan went from offering a

---

225 Ibid., 231.
226 Oka, "Minzoku no Hatten to Rika" [Science and the development of the race-nation], 112.
227 Ienaga, *The Pacific War*, 189.

model for humanitarian treatment of prisoners at the Hague Conference of 1907 to exhibiting a genocidal disregard for human life only exceeded by Hitler's Germany and Stalin's USSR remains in many ways a mystery. As we will suggest in the conclusion, Oka's regenerative vision of national destiny may have helped provoke the radicalization of emperor-centered ultranationalism along organicist lines. The extent to which the evolutionary realpolitik that this vision contained played a similar role in the transmogrification from humanitarianism to race war is a question for future scholarship.

In the next chapter we will see that his rejection of humanitarianism not only extended beyond geopolitics and into relations within the ethnic nation-state, but became a pretext for completely reengineering humanity itself. It is this reengineering that will prove integral to the transformation of Oka's scientism from a reformist stance to a generative one that seeks to regenerate the national body within a cosmic scheme.

CHAPTER 5

THE HUMAN-WAY:
NOMIC INSTINCTS AND
THE TRANSFORMATION OF HUMANITY

Our previous chapter explained how Oka's evolutionary realpolitik was premised on his identification of wartime "unity of the nation" with the collective life of superorganisms. In Oka's view, the condition of superindividuality ensured social harmony and cohesion because "for animals," such as humans, "which lead a group existence, the struggle for existence occurs mainly between groups and the struggle between individuals is just one small part of the whole. The struggle for existence between groups makes for the most complete group—that is to say, the struggle for existence between groups is everything for that animal, and there is no strife at all between individuals that belong to the same group."[1]

The benefit of this strife-free internal cohesion was, as we saw, the capacity it provided the homogeneous ethnic nation-state to project maximum power in the expansionist pursuit of racial autarky. Nonetheless, even as Oka sang the praises of a racialist "unity of the nation" he admitted that such nations were also in jeopardy of succumbing to internal strife which would prove geopolitically paralyzing. As he explained:

[H]umankind's struggle for existence, whomever it occurs between, has countless levels, whether it is between individuals or groups, the largest and the smallest parts within the group, or between groups of various levels. There is competition between candidates who want to become members

---

1   Oka, "Jinrui no Seizon Kyōsō" [Mankind's struggle for existence], 77.

of the city or prefectural assemblies. There is competition between one store and another doing the same business within the same city. There is competition between the established enterprise which has held a monopoly over a certain business for a long time, and the newcomer who has established the same kind of enterprise. And there is competition between political parties trying to take over as much as they can and quickly extend their power. All of these forms of competition can usually be seen right before one's eyes, and because they show up even on the pages of the daily newspaper, it is not necessary to provide particular examples.[2]

What limited "the competition within the nation between individuals or between small groups to the degree that we have no worries about our nation being put in jeopardy by enemy nations"[3] were laws and morality. According to Oka, "if the people within a nation disregarded all the laws and morals and fought one another with utter abandon, that country would be taken advantage of by enemies and in no time would cease to exist."[4] In this manner Oka placed a tremendous burden on the normative disposition of the people. "War and Peace," for instance, included frequent references to national morale: "limitless forbearance," "durability of spirit," "wartime resoluteness," "self-sacrifice," "resolve"[5] will all be required for the ethnic nation-state to remain unified, mobilized, and primed for autarkic struggle. A lack of such preparedness or any manifestation of internal discord during the "war of peace" could conceivably be attributed to a failure not just of collective willpower but of the underlying system of norms, conventions, and laws that maintained the "unity of the nation"—that is, as a breakdown of nomos.

Such a breakdown seemed to occur in early September 1905 with the announcement of the terms of the Treaty of Portsmouth. Though, as James McClain argues, victory over Russia "represented the consummation of the Meiji Dream, a grand achievement that simultaneously confirmed the success of Japan's modernization efforts, certified the nation's release from semicolonial status, marked acceptance into the comity of great powers, and offered the prospect of a more secure future,"[6] the lack of an indemnity

---

2 Ibid., 78.
3 Ibid.
4 Ibid.
5 Oka, "Sensō to Heiwa" [War and peace], 88, 91, 94, 96.
6 McClain, Japan, 283.

in the Portsmouth settlement incited violent protest against the government in the very same public space—a newly opened park situated adjacent both to the Imperial Palace and Tokyo's government district—where privately sponsored rallies had been held to revel in Japanese military success:

> Surprisingly, the thirty thousand or so craftsmen, shop clerks, and factory work-ers who came to Hibiya Park on 5 September intended not to praise the treaty but to protest it. To their way of thinking, the government had not extracted nearly enough concessions from Russia; rather, "clumsy" and "weak-willed" negotiators had settled for a "shameful" peace. As firecrackers exploded, bal-loons floated into the air, and brass bands banged out patriotic songs, speaker after speaker urged the cabinet and the emperor to "reject the humiliating treaty" and order the army to resume "the brave fight to crush the enemy." As the rally drew to a close, some flag-waving participants began marching toward the Imperial Palace. When the police attempted to block their way, tensions mounted, tempers flared, and fights broke out. The people had only clubs and stones to use against police swords, but they enjoyed an advantage of numbers, and soon they ran wild, sacking police stations and setting fire to government buildings. The authorities declared martial law the following day, and by the time a heavy rain extinguished the violence on 7 September, some 350 build-ings had been destroyed, five hundred police and at least an equal number of protesters had suffered wounds, and seventeen demonstrators lay dead.[7]

McClain regards this violence as an affirmation by the rioters of their status as *kokumin*, citizens of the nation, who had earned the right to be heard due to the hard work and personal sacrifices which were integral to the "nation's collective achievements since the restoration."[8] Despite the fact that the crowd set fire to the home minister's residence, which was lo-cated across the street from Hibiya Park, McClain finds a "commonality of interests"[9] uniting the protestors and the government, an honorific nation-alism that not only bound the people to the state but envisioned a future of imperial expansionism. However, for some scholars, Hibiya did not indi-cate the unity of the nation but its opposite. In fact, in her recent *Japanese Society at War*, Shimazu Naoko portrays this unity as largely fictional even

---

7   Ibid., 284.
8   Ibid.
9   Ibid.

during the war itself. Instead of a monolithic state orchestrating solidarity Shimazu sees a society characterized by "diverse constituents" that evinced "multifarious manifestations" of nationalism—and more often than not did so on their own initiative. In Shimazu's view the precedent for the Hibiya mayhem were the "raucous, boisterous and demonstrative" wartime lantern parades which contained "seeds of political and social instability" because of their "potential for radicalization."[10] Ostensibly celebrations of victories in the war with Russia, these "outbursts of popular energy" became occasions for the masses to vent their pent-up frustrations. Unable to control the crowds, the Home Ministry placed a police ban on lantern parades during the early months of the war, from "late February to May 1904."[11] When the parades resumed in early May, the result was violence: a parade on 8 May claimed twenty lives—including some children—and caused the police to set strict rules for future gatherings. Along with the antiwar movement and the general sense of war-weariness, these volatile expressions of popular patriotism revealed the ambivalent "cacophony of voices" that comprised Japanese society. Indeed, in Shimazu's estimation, far from exhibiting an idealized unity, wartime Japanese society was "a society in conflict with itself as much as it was in conflict with others."[12]

Thus, the radicalization of latent dissent not only at Hibiya but at a similar riot the following year, 1906, "overturned the semblance of social order that the state had desperately tried to maintain during the war"[13] and "underlined the vulnerability of a political system that rested on a narrow balance of power between powerful political elites, excluding not only dissenters, whether socialists or chauvinistic nationalists, but also the majority of kokumin from the political process."[14] Shimazu's views contribute to the consensus among scholars that September 1905, "the first time that the crowd acted as a political force," represents a "turning point,"[15] an inauguration of "heightened political consciousness," which "presaged the emergence of a new political community."[16] In his *Labor and Imperial Democracy*,

---

10 Shimazu, *Japanese Society at War*, 8, 15, 43.
11 Ibid., 44.
12 Ibid., 19, 21.
13 Ibid., 50–51.
14 Skya, *Japan's Holy War*, 190
15 Ibid.
16 Pyle, "The Technology of Japanese Nationalism," 56.

Andrew Gordon constructs a periodization of modern Japanese history around this watershed moment: depicting it as the beginning of a movement by the excluded *kokumin* to challenge the Meiji system of imperial bureaucracy through which "civilian bureaucrats and the military ruled the nation on behalf of the sovereign emperor"[17] without accountability to the people. In Gordon's account the popular protests, labor activism, and factional politics of compromise that typified the period after the Russo-Japanese War culminated, by 1918, in imperial democracy, a new structure of rule through which bourgeois democratic parties wielded state power under the aegis of a sovereign emperor and his imperial order.

Walter Skya depicts this "politicization of the masses" after the conflict with Russia as a result of an awakening to their "subjective freedom," that is, to the sense that "the individual, reflecting on his own consciousness" could serve as "a law unto himself"[18] apart from the group, nation, or state. Though Skya focuses on how this new self-awareness enabled individuals to "have their own knowledge of the emperor's 'true desires'"[19] and thereby defy the ministers of state who claimed to act in his name, it was perhaps in the area of customary "socio-moral bonds"[20] that this potentially destabilizing new freedom from authority was most powerfully felt. For instance, Kakehi Katsuhiko, the Todai professor and radical Shinto ultranationalist ideologue whom we will discuss in the epilogue, experienced this postwar period as a time when "the spiritual foundations underpinning the Japanese nation began to crumble."[21] In Carol Gluck's view, "the vanguard of intelligent civil concern"[22] shared this perception and regarded it as confirmation that "the social results of Japan's plunging rush toward modernity"[23] had finally caught up with the nation. As we will describe in detail in the next chapter, these social moralists described a contagion of "social fevers" sweeping the nation, which, justified by ideologies alternative to that of the state, were eroding the traditional customs and mores that had held society together. What these so-called fevers really indicated was that the individ-

---

17 Gordon, *Labor and Imperial Democracy in Prewar Japan*, 13.
18 Skya, *Japan's Holy War*, 156–57.
19 Ibid., 156.
20 Gluck, *Japan's Modern Myths*, 110.
21 Skya, *Japan's Holy War*, 190.
22 Gluck, *Japan's Modern Myths*, 28.
23 Ibid., 27.

uals who could question political authority were also now able to contemplate a new spirit of experimentation and inventiveness toward social roles, values, and conventions. There was, in other words, a growing realization that not only political arrangements but the nomic foundations of society were constructed—that they were malleable and, therefore, could be contested and, indeed, even rejected altogether. In short, the awakening of subjective freedom brought with it a new unsettling prospect: that of anomy, the possibility that norms and conventions might break down completely and all social cohesion be utterly lost.

Karl Popper in his *Open Society and Its Enemies* warns of the tendency for such fears to accompany the awakening of subjective freedom or what he calls critical dualism—the rejection of the monistic identity of nature and convention. For Popper, the insight that norms are made by human beings served to liberate individuals, enabling them to forge their own lifestyles, and rendered ethical decisions autonomous from the inexorable forces of nature. For many, however, this autonomy of the individual and his ethical disposition promised only a "loss of organic character"[24] in interpersonal relations and the emergence of a merely abstract society that tended toward internal anarchy. Instead of being internally regulated by something like a customary "ethical life" that fostered cohesion by preserving the concreteness of human community, the individuals of this new open society employed their own faculties of critically informed self-interest to select the social relations into which they wanted to enter. Such an "abstract" mode of existence was, as Popper emphasized, not only difficult to adjust to because of the strain of uncertainty and instability it brought, but it threatened—at least in the imagination of those who longed for the assurances of a closed society—to produce a completely atomized and anomic way of life, one in which people have "no, or extremely few, intimate personal contacts" and suffer "anonymity and isolation."[25] Separated off from their fellows, members of the nation relate to one another through competition and conflict, leaving society fragmented and weak.

As we discussed earlier in this study, the realpolitik-minded founders of the new Meiji state had been alerted to the prospect of such an untoward

---

24 Popper, *The Open Society and Its Enemies*, Volume 1, 174.
25 Ibid., 174–75.

eventuality as early as the 1880s, and the organicist state science they had appropriated from Germany was intended to preempt the unraveling of national cohesion by aligning the binding ethical life of the nation with inexorable ontological forces. For both those of a reformist bent, who regarded these forces as developmental, and those of a reactionary outlook, who identified them with an unchanging sacred reality, the internally conflicted society that made its appearance at Hibiya Park not only gave the lie to the vaunted "wartime consensus of the 'unity of the nation,'"[26] but seemed, in the coming years, like the advent of anomy. Chapter 6 will explain how the sense that the "social foundations"[27] of the nation were under fundamental threat in the final years of the Meiji era led to a plethora of ideological schemes to shore them up—conflicting efforts which only increased the perception that a geopolitically disastrous loss of all sociomoral bonds was in the offing. It was against the background of this "nomic crisis" that the reactionary statism, articulated by Hozumi, would embark on a program of administrative and spiritual activism in the name of the family-state.

Oka's reformist response to the perceived advent of anomy would be remarkable: he would reconceive nomos as instinct and, in doing so, redefine humanity itself. Whereas the two wartime essays that we have discussed thus far had focused on the outward manifestation of the organic nation-state, its holism, his groundbreaking postwar essay, "The True Character of Humanity: The Human-Way," filled out his metapolitical vision by turning to the inner workings of this organicism and, in particular, to the interdependent nature of its spontaneously participating components. Rejecting laissez-faire social Darwinism and its disembedding individualism, Oka ascribed this "soft organicism" to what he called *jindō*—a term that can be translated as humanity, morality, or, literally, as the way of humanity or human-way. Oka identified this normative term for being human with altruism and, more specifically, with altruism toward other members of one's ethnic nation. In place of the humanitarian fraternity of mankind of Tolstoy and the antiwar movement, Oka endorsed engendering the true human-way through the Lamarckian mechanism of use-inheritance. Practicing a strategic, race-specific altruism would, in other words, ingrain instincts that

---

26　Shimazu, *Japanese Society at War*, 51.
27　Gluck, *Japan's Modern Myths*, 157.

would reintegrate the differentiated persons of the human collective into the kind of interdependent organic whole that was an evolutionary precondition for survival. While such altruistic instincts are usually called social instincts, here they will be referred to as nomic instincts to underscore Oka's preoccupation with the basis of the "unity of the nation." Oka's human-way, which, we will see, seamlessly connects to his evolutionary realpolitik, daringly and originally proposed binding the national superorganism through the biological and nomic reconstitution of *jindō*—humanity itself.

Before tackling "The True Character of Humanity: The Human-Way," this chapter will explore how Oka's wartime speech "Evolutionary Theory and Hygiene" set a precedent for his eugenic approach to his organicist metapolitics. Although not published until 1906, in the first edition of the *Evolution and Human Life* anthology, this address to the National Conference of the Medical Sciences in June 1905 not only illustrates Oka's antihumanitarianism, hostility to individualism, and the impetus of his Lamarckism. It also provides a first taste of what will become the most radical aspect of his evolutionism in later years: the positing of future growth as the measure of ultimate value. As we will see in the final part, "Regeneration," it is this futural orientation that will define his generative scientism and facilitate its subtle interplay with the emerging orthodoxy.

COLLECTIVE HYGIENE

Oka's attack on humanitarianism and the universalist notions of human nature that underwrote it represents a subtle, if not devious, piece of argumentation. Standing up before the National Conference of the Medical Sciences shortly after the Battle of Tsushima and at time when, though peace talks had begun, Matsuyama and twenty-seven other POW camps were still in operation, Oka faced an audience that was at the forefront of implementing the civilized "humanitarian nationalism"[28] that Naoko Shimazu says characterized the "moral diplomacy of the Japanese government."[29] At the start of the conflict the government, through the Japanese Red Cross, had tasked the medical community to "demonstrate to the world our hu-

---

28 Shimazu, *Japanese Society at War*, 195.

29 Ibid., 15.

manitarian mission" through the expression of "sympathy to our side as well as the enemy."[30] As Shimazu explains, the Red Cross had managed to grow exponentially from its founding in 1887 to include 900,000 members at the war's inception by presenting humanitarianism "as one aspect of nationalism": "one could only be a good humanitarian if one were a good patriot because love for one's country was fundamental to all proper conduct, including love for others."[31] Oka's stratagem in his speech was to pry nationalism free of humanitarianism by using evolutionary theory to illustrate the inadequacy of received notions of hygiene and health. Even though the medical community, confused by "empty theories such as respecting human rights,"[32] thought it should be applied to individuals, "artificial aid"[33] was in fact, something best suited for groups. The health of the ultimate human groups, races, and nations were not only supremely paramount but they could be improved by the techniques that evolutionary science, especially in the new fields of race and social hygiene studies, made available.

The technological potential of evolutionary theory was a main facet of Oka's message. In his view, "the late nineteenth century was the period in which the theory of evolution of living things, or theory of natural selection, was researched and the coming of the twentieth century perhaps should be regarded as the arrival of an era when we should devise an application of this theory."[34] In this new era "the prosperity of the nation and the happiness of the people" would be gauged by "enacting applied schemes with the theory of evolution as a basis."[35] Though it was understandable that "there was not a direct connection at all between the theory of evolution and the study of hygiene"[36] while the former was still being researched, Oka believed the time had come when evolution had been established and must be fully accepted. Nevertheless, some scholars of a traditional bent "passionately take a stand against the theory of natural selection."[37] Believing these medical

---

30 Ibid., 173.
31 Ibid., 176.
32 Asajirō Oka, "Shinkaron to Eisei" [Evolutionary theory and hygiene], in *Shinka to Jinsei* [Evolution and human life] (Tokyo: Yūseidō Shuppan, 1968), 192.
33 Ibid., 188.
34 Ibid., 187.
35 Ibid.
36 Ibid.
37 Ibid.

professionals have not only misunderstood evolution but "the reasoning behind applying natural selection to humans,"[38] Oka focused his argument on illustrating that the mechanism of evolutionary descent did not bring about the moral outcomes they imagined.

Oka's subtlety and cleverness come through in how he sided with these humanitarian critics on the question of social Darwinism—that is, the laissez-faire survival of the fittest within society. It is this classic social Darwinism that "specialists of the traditional study of hygiene"[39] have in mind with their "vigorous" opposition to the theory of natural selection. "To them the advocates of natural selection are saying that the survival of the superior and downfall of the inferior is the cause of the evolution for each species of living organism. Thus, if we wish for racial improvement even in human society it is good that inferior beings are in this way allowed to be naturally disposed of and destroyed. If such a thing is done, over generations only the superior will survive and, as a consequence, it is certain that the physical constitution of the organism also improves."[40] From the standpoint of traditional "scholars of hygiene,"[41] advocates of natural selection are calling the very practice of medicine into doubt by suggesting that humanitarian hygiene obstructs both the evolutionary mechanism and the progress it makes possible: "Due to medical science and hygiene, a point has been reached where the workings of natural selection are denied so that succor is provided even to the inferior to let them survive and leave behind offspring on equal terms with those who are superior. Therefore, medical science and hygiene are not only actually useless but harmful things."[42]

In short, because the one sees the "downfall of the unfit" as "the one overriding cause of the progress of all things" and the other believes "artificial aid" should be administered to the "weak and inferior," allowing them to "live and breed," the conclusion drawn by these humanitarian opponents of evolutionism is categorical: "[T]he theory of natural selection and [the practice of] hygiene do not seem at all compatible."[43]

---

38 Ibid. 188–89.
39 Ibid., 188.
40 Ibid.
41 Ibid.
42 Ibid.
43 Ibid.

In Oka's estimation, these medical practitioners "are fighting an imaginary enemy."[44] "It cannot simply be argued," Oka insists, that protecting the weak stymies progress and humans, therefore, "should immediately leave everything to natural selection" so "the weak should all be allowed to die off."[45] What humanitarian nationalists have failed to grasp is that "the unit of competition" in the struggle for existence is "not at all the same" for "different kinds of flora and fauna."[46] Among animals in which "each carries on with an independent life" it is indeed the case that something like social Darwinism holds: "[T]he superior individuals survive and the inferior individuals perish" because "each individual comprises one unit in the struggle for existence."[47] Yet for gregarious creatures that lead a collective life "the unit in the struggle for existence is the group."[48] This means that "groups that are fit for existence triumph and survive while those that are unfit for existence lose out and perish."[49]

By once again invoking Haeckel's hierarchy of organic individuality Oka is able to redefine evolutionary fitness in a manner contrary to social Darwinism. In particular, if the survival of the fittest and other such things comes to be carried out with regard to groups"[50] the evolutionary worth of individual persons is evaluated much differently: "[E]ven those groups which are stronger than their enemies when analyzed individual by individual will certainly die out if they are weak as a group, while even groups that are extremely weak when analyzed individual by individual will certainly triumph if they are stronger than their enemies as a group."[51] Not only are weak persons countenanced if they happen to strengthen the higher individuality of the group, but they can possess "characteristics or structures which are disadvantageous to its own self and of benefit to the group as a whole."[52] To drive home this critical point Oka cites the example of the ultimate soldier-worker in the consummate group or superorganism:

---

44 Ibid., 189.
45 Ibid.
46 Ibid.
47 Ibid.
48 Ibid., 190.
49 Ibid.
50 Ibid.
51 Ibid.
52 Ibid.

Insects, such as bees, live in groups they have formed and their unit in the struggle for existence is the group. Yet when we try to take each individual, bees have stingers which are disadvantageous to themselves as individuals yet which are useful to the group. Since for bees these stingers were originally employed for both offensive and defensive purposes, groups of bees must have prospered by triumphing over many enemies. Yet looked at in another way this stinger is a hook. Once it pricks a human or some other creature the stinger remains there and cannot be drawn out. If the bee tries to extract it by force, the stinger breaks off at the base, entrails gush forth from the wound and the bee expires. Because animals that live group lives in such conditions and animals that lead individual lives are greatly different on various points, even when we come to discuss natural selection, we must always take care to not to forget that groups are the unit at which the struggle for existence occurs where animals which lead group lives are concerned.[53]

As we have seen many times already and will see many times again, Oka invokes the equivalent of the hive and the expendable worker bees that comprise it to intimate the metapolitical ground upon which viable human communities actually function. Though it may have astonished his audience of medical practitioners, it will not surprise us to hear Oka announce that "in mankind's struggle for existence the unit of competition consists of groups such as races and nations."[54] To illustrate the collective nature of human struggle and the "unreasonableness" of the theory that humans should merely be "left to the mercy of natural selection and the weak allowed to die without a care,"[55] Oka asked his wartime audience to imagine "cases of military conflict"[56] and, in particular, the kind of beach landing that often occurred in the battle with Russia: "Figuratively speaking this irrational argument is no different from the case where a military force lands at a certain place and allows the soldiers to drink as they please without examining whether the water of that place is good or bad; the weak, who seem to have imbibed bad water and died, are allowed to perish without a care; only those soldiers remain who have not died even though they drank water; the result is that the entire army gradually becomes robust. Yet even if only robust in-

53 Ibid.
54 Ibid., 194.
55 Ibid., 190–91.
56 Ibid., 191.

dividuals remain the extreme decrease in numbers of people will result in them not being able to pull through in battle."[57]

For Oka the disadvantages that would ensue from randomly allowing those with weak constitutions to be selected out far outweigh the benefits of a more fit and "robust" fighting force: not countenancing the weak in these circumstances will result in "decreasing the group's battle strength" and "often it will, in the end, come about that the group must perish."[58]

Merging in this manner beehive collectivism with his musings on total mobilization for racial autarky, Oka redefined "hygiene from the point of view of the theory of natural selection" as a necessity for "the self-defense of one's own group."[59] Viewed properly, "those who research hygiene pay attention to the health of individuals but they are mindful for the sake of the entire group to which they themselves belong."[60] The "health and prosperity" of their own group, in fact, takes complete priority, becoming the overriding "goal."[61] Yet, Oka insinuates, this approach is not that different from the pre-evolutionary practice of hygiene: it still "consists in maintaining the health of individuals and strengthening the body"—it is thus "needless to say that individual hygiene is a necessary thing."[62] The "importance of facilities, such as the water supply or sewage" concerned with "infectious diseases"[63] do not need to be rethought. Most importantly, a population of healthy individuals is essential to national prosperity. "Groups such as nations and races" which consist of "natural gatherings of individuals each of whom is robust" can have "many hopes" that the group as a whole will "triumph in the struggle for existence."[64] Self-defense of one's group—in this case the ethnic nation—and individual hygiene are seemingly one and the same project.

While this emphasis on group health is not inconsistent with a concern for individual well-being, Oka's regards the correct practice of hygiene as endorsing neither humanitarianism nor individualism. This is evident from how he summarizes the goal of hygiene toward the end of his speech: To "do research on the means and methods by which to achieve the present

---

57 Ibid.
58 Ibid., 190.
59 Ibid., 191.
60 Ibid., 192.
61 Ibid.
62 Ibid.
63 Ibid.
64 Ibid.

and future health and prosperity of the group to which we ourselves belong, and to promote as hard as we can the life and health of each individual in so far as doing so does not collide with group interests."[65] Later in this chapter we will see that Oka eventually comes to regard individualism itself, in the form of egoism, as on a collision course with the group. However, in this speech Oka's stress is on those individuals whose "life and health" are apparently beyond repair. Despite what he says toward the beginning of his remarks about proposals to eliminate the weak being a misrepresentation of evolutionary progress, Oka now, toward the conclusion of his talk, suggests that even at the collective level the workings of natural selection do not, in general, allow the weak to survive. One reason for this is that "in present-day society, there is no room to live but for more than a part of those who are born."[66] With each generation "from the many children who are born only a small number are able to survive."[67] Defying nature and "trying whatever artificial means one can" in order to "keep alive, one way or another, humans that are weak in body, feeble in mind, and only a burden to the group" is, according to Oka, "very disadvantageous to the group."[68] Such misguided "artificial assistance" amounts to "taking up the existential space of others who would be able to work well for the group."[69] In short, efforts to "keep everyone alive" do not just help the weak but take space and resources from the strong. In this way humanitarian medical hygiene diminishes the overall power of the nation-state.

Even more hostile to humanitarianism than this application of living-space logic—which we introduced in the last chapter—to the life of the nation is a eugenic argument out of which Oka's generative scientism will eventually emerge. Though "keeping alive by compulsion humans who will leave inferior offspring" may be a "great job" which is "suited to a philanthropic spirit," doing so "will trouble our comrades in the future with their weak constitutions."[70] In his view, "the improvement of the race cannot at all be wished for when artificially protecting inferior and harmful hu-

---

65 Ibid., 194.
66 Ibid., 193.
67 Ibid.
68 Ibid.
69 Ibid.
70 Ibid., 191.

mans and then allowing them to live and breed."[71] The "weak people, who can be kept alive only by artificial treatment" will "leave behind children" and "they too, like their parents will not be healthy at all."[72] Thus, acting on the basis of "empty theories such as respecting human rights"[73] really "means placing an extra burden on people living in the future" and represents "a case of offering to sacrifice the future for the sake of the present."[74] In short, "disregarding future matters by considering only what is before one's eyes and ignoring the benefits to tens of millions of other people by thinking only about oneself are in fact like an inversion of things light and heavy, big and small."[75]

It is in the midst of this argument that the specter of degeneration makes its first appearance in Oka's writings. Degeneration is the ultimate "inversion" because it thwarts "natural selection," which represents not only "the great cause of evolution for living things"[76] but a "principal" within which "all of human society is also clearly contained."[77] By Oka's reasoning, causing natural selection to "cease" and allowing the "superior and inferior" to "survive and breed" in equal numbers would bring about "the opposite of progress—degeneration."[78] After describing how the vision of "fish that live all year round inside dark caves"[79] degenerates to the point of blindness, Oka explains how a similar process can take hold among humans: "Humans too by this same logic, if they protect through artificial means even those with weak bodies who cannot endure the struggle for existence, or those who do society harm by harboring a terrible illness to live and breed and then allow these to live and breed the same as individuals with sound, healthy bodies, the result will no doubt be the degeneration of the entire human race."[80] The very low point of such degeneration would, according to Oka, be a situation in which "the entire group might not be able to survive if it does not have artificial protection."[81]

---

71 Ibid.
72 Ibid., 193.
73 Ibid., 192.
74 Ibid., 191.
75 Ibid., 192.
76 Ibid., 191.
77 Ibid., 189.
78 Ibid.
79 Ibid.
80 Ibid.
81 Ibid., 193.

For the positive application of "artificial aid" Oka looks to two new disciplines discussed in Chapter 3: racial hygiene and social hygiene. Again, Oka views his contemporary early twentieth century as a "stage where, from here on, we try to apply what was previously researched as mere theory and thereby promote the improvement of human society."[82] The task taken up by racial and social hygiene is to "research the hygiene of the group based on the principle of natural selection."[83] Concentrating on "promoting the health of the group" above all else, these fields preoccupy themselves with "the question concerning which method must be adopted to prevent"[84] degeneration taking hold. It is from "among people who do research in these studies"[85] that we get the theory which has so upset humanitarian medical practitioners, turning them against natural selection itself. This "so-called racial degeneration theory" allegedly argues simply that "artificially assisting inferior humans by means of medical hygiene will bring about the degeneration of the race because it interferes with natural selection."[86] Oka, of course, largely agrees with this position and, as we saw earlier, has already craftily sidestepped humanitarian objections by allowing that in some cases the "weak" can actually contribute to group cohesion and strength in a manner that a homogeneous nation of the "robust" might not. Though Oka admits that "extreme views" may at times emerge from these fields, such anomalies do not undermine his conclusion that "hygiene and the theory of natural selection are not at all antagonistic."[87] The fields of racial and social hygiene studies, as they conduct more research and theoretically settle on a method of application, should accordingly serve as future guides for the correct application of "artificial assistance."

Oka's own degeneration theory, which we will discuss at length in Chapter 7, borrows from race and social hygiene its moral orientation toward future generations. In Oka's version the healthy development of the ethnic nationalist superorganism through the stages of the growth cycle will become the measure of ultimate value—and degeneracy evinced by anomic disintegration indicative of senescence and eventual extinction. Though Oka

---

82   Ibid., 193–94.
83   Ibid., 194.
84   Ibid., 193.
85   Ibid., 194.
86   Ibid.
87   Ibid.

makes frequent overtures to "future generations," such historicism—which we will associate with generative scientism—is otherwise absent from "Evolutionary Theory and Hygiene." Instead his focus is on reinforcing the message of his other wartime essays about holistic organicism by arguing that collective health is of supreme importance to the ethnic nation. He is especially eager to decouple nationalism from humanitarianism with the reasoning that, because the "unit of competition" among humans is the group, all individuals—including, on occasions, healthy ones—are expendable. Like worker bees whose entrails gush out once they have planted their stingers in enemies of the hive, the members of the nation-state do not exist for their own health or their own self-interest but for the prosperity and "self-defense" of the group.

Before turning to consider the most complete statement of Oka's organicist metapolitics, "The True Character of Humanity: The Human-Way," we should clarify that the artificial alterations and hygienic methods Oka has in mind to "promote group health" do not rely on selectionism as we presently understand it. As P. J. Bowler has argued, the decades around the fin-de-siècle were characterized by an "eclipse of Darwinism" during which non-Darwinian mechanism of evolutionary descent either rejected natural selection or combined with it. The triumph of selectionism did not take hold in scientific circles until the 1920s[88] with the result that seminal figures in the promotion of evolutionary theory, including not only Haeckel but Darwin himself, allowed for nonselectionist mechanism such as Lamarckism. Oka, in fact, like Haeckel and Darwin, mixed Lamarckism and selectionism together, often referring to both under the blanket term "natural selection" in his sociopolitical writings. In "Evolutionary Theory and Hygiene" this combined approach is reflected in "the three characteristics" he attributes to natural selection in the opening sections of the essay. While two of these, heredity and the tendency for unlimited breeding, do reflect a strict selectionism, a third characteristic, "change"—the fact that there are "difference and alterations even between children born from identical parents"[89]—allows for both natural selection and Lamarckism. Despite his championing of natural selection, Oka includes vague statements in the essay that seem

---

88 Bowler, *The Non-Darwinian Revolution*, 125–30.
89 Oka, "Shinkaron to Eisei" [Evolutionary theory and hygiene], 185.

to indicate that the individuals' own actions contribute to produce the traits they need for survival: "individuals who have best developed characteristics fit for existence come to command victory, at all costs, when competing. At times in which they exist and breed, such creatures come to pass along to their offspring, also through heredity, characteristics which have been proven superior in competition."[90]

This ambiguity is reinforced by Oka's admission toward the end of the essay that "the range of ways which we promote the present health of the group is becoming extremely wide."[91] Not only strictly biological disciplines but sociopolitical institutions are involved in ensuring national health: "[I]n addition to fields of study such as hygiene studies, pathology, physiology, and biology," Oka believes "the health of the group is connected to law, police work, education, and other various spheres of life."[92] It is precisely this interface between sociopolitical action and inheritable biological traits that will open an avenue for Oka to propose a transformation of humanity. Collective health will be ensured not just by recasting human biology but engineering the instincts that facilitate sociopolitical cohesion. The centerpiece of Oka's reformist scientism, the "human-way," will fit nomos to nature by ingraining social instincts into humans.

INTERNALIZING THE WAY

"The True Character of Humanity: The Human-Way," the essay where Oka enunciates the human-way, stands out among Oka's sociopolitical writings on several fronts. It is with this contribution that Oka seems to first hit his stride as an essayist: his argument is tight, the rhetoric sharp, and the phrasings memorable. The essay is also distinguished for being perhaps the most unabashedly Haeckelian of his literary efforts. Toward the close of the piece Oka, in fact, quotes Haeckel's statement of ethical naturalism from *The History of Creation* that, we will see, justifies the application of violence by the biologically superior. Just as significantly, Oka frames his essay as a discussion of the "riddle" of humanity: because "human undertakings are full of contradictions" human beings "appear to be a riddle within

---

90 Ibid., 186.
91 Ibid., 194.
92 Ibid.

a riddle."[93] Without question Oka has in mind here Haeckel's global best seller *The Riddle of the Universe* and its equally popular follow-up piece, *The Wonders of Life*, which we touched on in Chapter 3. That Oka's riddles play off those posed by Haeckel can be seen not only in Oka's focus on "riddles concerning behavior,"[94] but the manner in which he relies on evolution to solve riddles: "[A]fter the grand principle of the evolution of living things was discovered and we tried to think about the human body in terms of this principle, we came to understand some of the impenetrable riddles of the past, we gradually solved freshly emerging problems, and, still more, we have now reached a stage where we are working to try to solve the next riddle one step up ahead of us."[95] One of the two examples of such a solved riddle that Oka cites are the fishlike gill slits that "during the period of growth within the womb" appear "on the sides of the neck" only to later "completely close up and disappear."[96] Of course, it was the "grand principle" of biogenetic law—"ontogeny recapitulates phylogeny"—that Haeckel devised in his *General Morphology* (1866) that was famously used to pictorially solve the gill slit conundrum in his *History of Creation* and subsequent writings. Not only, as we have seen, was recapitulationism the guiding insight of the discipline in which Oka was trained—evolutionary morphology—but Haeckel's chart illustrating the comparative embryology of vertebrates was actually featured prominently in *Lectures on Evolutionary Theory*.

The example of Haeckel's system and its biopolitical applications may be why this essay also stands out as a statement of Oka's metapolitics. The reformist organicism of his wartime writings is synthesized with new clarity into a vision that explains how racial autarky and total mobilization are brought to bear on morality and interpersonal relations internal to the ethnic nation. As we will see, Oka's astonishing statements that "war and the human-way seem to be identical, front and back" and that "wars are made possible by the human-way alone"[97] could serve as mottos for the biopolitical conception pervading all the essays in *Evolution and Human Life*—that of the nation-state as a permanently embattled superorganism. The closing section of this chapter will explore the extent to which this identification of

---

93   Oka, "Jindō no Shōtai" [The true character of humanity: the human-way], 57.
94   Ibid.
95   Ibid.
96   Ibid.
97   Ibid., 63.

war and the human-way—all in the name of the most seemingly humanitarian of all principles, altruism—represents the introduction of totalitarian thinking to the Japanese reading public.

The impact of Oka's essay on this public cannot be doubted. "The True Character of Humanity: The Human-Way" was the lead essay in the New Year's issue of Japan's premiere intellectual journal, *Chūō Kōron* (The central review).[98] In the course of his literary career, Oka, according to Migita, published a total of ten articles in this journal, six of which were granted the prestige of opening the issue. Writing the lead essay for the New Year's issue was an especially high honor which reflected the great popularity which *Lectures on Evolutionary Theory* had achieved since it was published at the start of the war. By January 1906 Oka was the public authority on evolutionary theory in Japan and the "Darwin boom" which would ensue in the following years would be largely due to the popularity of his writings. "The True Character of Humanity: The Human-Way" represents Oka's first wide-reaching pronouncement on the application of evolutionism to human affairs. It is the culmination of the first edition of *Evolution and Human Life* which later that year first anthologized Oka's speeches, articles, and essays through 1906.

The January publication was also significant because it was the first essay written in response to the immediate aftermath of the war. While "Mankind's Struggle for Existence" appeared just after the Hibiya disturbances, it was clearly composed during the final months of the war. Only in "The True Character of Humanity: The Human-Way" do we see Oka grappling with the "disunity of the nation," which wartime mobilization and its attendant hysteria had concealed. The "ideal society united in patriotic sacrifice"[99] which the slogan *Kyokoku itchi* was meant to encapsulate was exposed as a myth. The wartime lantern parades had morphed first into a patriotic anti-government demonstration and then into complete mayhem that revealed the tensions and disillusionment that had long been rankling beneath the surface of society.

In "The True Character of Humanity: The Human-Way" Oka depicts this postwar milieu as an anomic dystopia. Scanning the human scene of

---

98   See the introduction for a discussion of Chūō Kōron.
99   Shimazu, *Japanese Society at War*, 40.

postwar Japan, he sees a society suddenly torn to pieces by rampant egoism, one in which "people operate on the principle that it is all right if another person gets into some type of trouble just as long as we ourselves are fine."[100] Scoffing at humanitarians who longingly anticipate a "strife-free, peaceful golden age of paradise on earth," Oka has concluded that "the imperative for humans is to advance forward and attain their goals even if doing so means other people are pushed aside and trampled down."[101] It is a world that "teems everywhere with people who cannot shy away from beating another person to death in order to lay hands on the polish they put on their shoes."[102] Harkening back to his wartime evolutionary realpolitik, Oka laments that "if each individual within the group vigorously pursues his own selfish impulses, there will be no survival for the group."[103]

As we will see in the next chapter, Oka's voice was but one of a chorus of pundits who attributed the coming anomy of the postwar era to an enflamed individualism. With the apparent victory over Russia, Japan had attained the goals of national independence and great power status which had justified all of the sacrifices the population had been called on to endure since the early Meiji era. The consensus in support of these goals came to an end and a new consensus, directed toward imperial expansion, had not yet come together. In the interim individualism began to assert itself for, according to the scholar Oka Yoshitake, "the sense of crisis that had subjugated the national spirit ever since the late Tokugawa period faded, and the release of tension provided the individual with an opportunity to liberate himself from the state."[104] The most visible indicator of this unterhered individualism and the most significant threat to evolutionarily requisite "national unity," was the new vogue for success (*seikō*) after the war. Although *risshin shusse* (getting ahead in the world) had been a rallying cry since the Meiji Restoration, success during those years had adhered to conventional paths: it was associated with attaining a government post and it had been pursued to increase the honor of one's family or village. Now getting ahead came simply to mean getting rich: not only did acquiring material wealth become the final measure of success but the ambitious strivers

---

100 Oka, "Jindō no Shōtai" [The true character of humanity: the human-way], 55.
101 Ibid.
102 Ibid.
103 Ibid., 59.
104 Oka, "Generational Conflict after the Russo-Japanese War," 201–2.

who had left small towns for the modern metropolis seemed to pursue this wealth for themselves alone. As Tokutomi Sohō complained in 1906, the customary ethos of *kanson minpi* (respect the officials, despise the people) had been supplanted by the vulgar notion of *kinson kanpi* (respect money, despise the officials).[105]

Where such egoism seemed to pose the most vital threat, however, was not to the authority of the state and its officials but, as we saw in the opening of this chapter, to that of traditional morality—to the customary nexus of norms and conventions that enabled the nation to cohere. Oka, however, was not at liberty to simply dismiss egoism for its alleged immorality. Celebrations of *risshin shusse*, after all, were often presented after the war as a manifestation of the Darwinian struggle for existence, the survival of the fittest at work in human society. The problem for Oka was that he agreed with this social Darwinism—or at least with its fundamental insight that life forms instinctively strove for self-preservation by "actualizing selfishness"[106] which he calls "paramount characteristic of life."[107] In Oka's estimation selfishness or egoism is "the common property of all animals"[108] and, according to evolutionary morphology, it was akin to the vital force that drove organicism through epigenetic stages of growth toward an integrated unity-in-difference. As a consequence, "existence without selfishness is like wind that does not blow, or fire that does not burn: it seems we cannot conceive of it at all."[109]

To illustrate this endemic egoism he cites the example of doves "which the public usually regards as symbols of peace."[110] Instead, they "turn out to be competitive through and through if one examines the circumstances of their lives. Every day they eat, one by one, a countless number of seeds, each of which should become a single, complete plant. It is only by robbing these seeds of their plant lives that doves preserve their own lives. Moreover, because when an individual dove eats seeds, it is deducting just that amount of feed from both other doves and other seed-eating animals, it naturally brings it about that some individuals somewhere are most likely starving to

---

105 Ibid., 198–99.
106 Oka, "Seibutsukai ni okeru Zen to Aku" [Good and evil in the animal world], 49.
107 Oka, "Jindō no Shōtai" [The true character of humanity: the human-way], 59.
108 Ibid., 58.
109 Ibid.
110 Ibid.

death. Because doves lack claws and tusks and do not shed blood, people, looking only at the surface, have the feeling that the lives of doves are extremely peaceful. However, viewed from the totality of nature, this selfishness on the part of doves is of an intensity not at all inferior to that of other animals."[111]

Thus, unlike other contemporary moralists, Oka had to reconcile his disdain for a contemporary society based on the individualistic pursuit of wealth with a discipline, evolutionary science, which affirmed egoism and competition even in the most seemingly pacifistic quarters of the natural world. His morality, in other words, had to follow through with the Haeckelian project of seeking "the foundations of ethics in ecology" by finding a means to redirect the impulse to actualize selfishness toward the building up of instincts necessary for a permanently mobilized nation-state. Social Darwinism as a justification for egoism had to be exposed a basic distortion of evolutionism.

Oka's response to the problem was extraordinary: he reconceptualized the traditional device for aligning normative imperatives with ontological forces, the "way," as an instinct which he then identified with humanity itself. Just as Shinto, Taoism, and Bushidō constituted the "ways"—*michi* or *dō*—or nomoi of Shintoists, Taoists and samurai respectively, *jindō*, the "human-way," stood for the nomos of *Homo sapiens*, the human normative response to the ontology of organic evolution. Although Oka still regarded "actualizing egoism" to be indicative of this ontology, the proper "way" for humans involved transcending the individualist egoism of laissez-faire social Darwinism and embracing the higher individuality of the group. We have already encountered this move many times in this study—most recently in the first subsection of this chapter—yet what made Oka's use of the "way" so exceptional in this context is how he took the extra step of imagining norms, conventions, and laws becoming literally embodied as biologized social instincts. These nomic instincts, as we will call them, would define humanity and do so in a manner that performed the triple task of dispelling the false *jindō* of the humanitarians, matching the conservative pundits who wanted to restore "civic morality"[112] and, once again, vigorously

---

111 Ibid., 58–59.
112 Gluck, *Japan's Modern Myths*, 102.

counteracting the social Darwinist individualism that was threatening to tear the nation asunder. Unlike the universalist "humanity" of Tolstoy and the peace movement, and in stark contrast to the success-obsession of post-war egoists, the human-way envisioned by Oka implanted the integrative, corporatist virtues—the very ones that fearful conservatives had begun to champion—directly into human biology. National cohesion would be preserved not just by fitting human conventions to nature but by eradicating any separation between the two. In Oka's reformist scientism, *Sittlichkeit* would become flesh.

In Chapter 3 we saw that Oka developed the notion of an "ape-way" in order to intimate what an evolutionarily based ethics for human beings might entail. Employing Haeckel's hierarchy of organic individuality, Oka's "Good and Evil in the Animal World" situated primates between "solitary egoists"—persons in Haeckel's schema—and "consummate groups"—corms or superorganisms. Where conduct at either of these echelons of individuality can be said to be amoral—the actions of lone wolves and worker bees both being matters of self-maintenance, the equivalent of eating boiled rice—primates are burdened with moral responsibilities because they are forced to choose between these two, self-interest and commitment to the group. Following Darwin, Huxley, and, most especially, Haeckel, Oka identifies these two choices with "egoism" and "altruism": the former acts for the "individual self alone"[113] while the latter serves the "collective will [*Volitio cormi*]."[114]

In "The True Character of Humanity," Oka returns to this mode of analysis but radically transforms it through the addition of two elements. Firstly, he boldly elaborates on the "ways" of social animals by conceiving the way as a "method for actualizing selfishness."[115] Each type of "group-oriented animal"[116] has "endowed" its members "with some spirit of altruism and compassion"[117] and practices "some altruistic, sympathetic deeds."[118] According to Oka, "it is due to the conduct of this 'way' that groups can cohere, and display their egoism as a group to the world."[119] In other words, "the al-

113 Oka, "Seibutsukai ni okeru Zen to Aku" [Good and evil in the animal world], 46.
114 Ibid., 51. Latin used in the original text.
115 Oka, "Jindō no Shōtai" [The true character of humanity: the human-way], 59.
116 Ibid.
117 Ibid., 60.
118 Ibid., 59.
119 Ibid.

truism between individuals inside a group can be regarded as a form of ex-
pressing the heart of collective self-interest."[120]

In order to demonstrate the functioning of altruistic instincts not only
does Oka return, as we will see in a moment, to the ape and the "ape-way"
but he explores a variety of other social animals and their respective "ways."
For instance, Oka cites the example of elephants: "[W]hen a herd of elephants moves forward, the robust elephant males form a perimeter, making
the females and children stand inside it. They thereby manage to help the
weak and guide the infants as the herd advances. This is what we might call
the "elephant-way."[121] An analogous case is that of black-tailed seagulls. Oka
describes how "if an enemy draws near when a flock of black-tailed seagulls
is on the beach, the first gull to discover this beats the water with its tail. The
other members of the flock who hear this sound dive into the water to save
their lives." This behavior would be an example of the "black-tailed seagull-
way."[122] The most perfectly integrated example of altruistic coordination
among social animals is exhibited among insects such as ants or bees whose
nests and hives approximate the "consummate group life":

> Looking at the behavior of so-called social insects such as ants, we should be
> surprised to a degree by the advancement of an "ant-way" or a "bee-way." Not
> in their capacity as individuals is it necessary that worker ants and bees labor
> all day long without rest, breaking their bones for the benefit of others. Since
> just a bit of food is sufficient for the individual self, one would expect that
> they should not have to work so vigorously every day from dawn until dusk.
> However, it is for the sake of supporting infants and their fellow workers that
> they go out every morning to search around all day for food and carry it back
> with all their might to the nest. The dutiful manner in which attendants at
> an orphanage care for their wards can only compare unfavorably to the zeal
> with which these worker insects retrieve food to their hives.[123]

Because Oka believes "the 'human-way' is merely one way among others,"[124]
he proposes to solve the "riddle of humanity" by explaining how the normative disposition of humans had its origins in the altruistic instincts common

---

120 Ibid., 61.
121 Ibid., 60–61.
122 Ibid., 60.
123 Ibid.
124 Ibid.

to all social animals. Metapolitically grounding "ethics in ecology," however, will not be easy because humans have evolved into "contradictory creatures" who "simultaneously possess both selfishness, which only thinks about the self, and altruism, which takes other people into consideration."[125] For Oka the war provided especially vivid examples of this contradictory quality of humans, waxing and waning between egoism and altruism:

> Though we vigorously manufacture torpedoes on a daily basis in order to sink instantly a large warship with a single shot and simultaneously kill one hundred officers and men, we also make plans to nurse, as a courtesy, even the wounded soldiers of our enemies. While tormenting other people in business competition to the point where they are psychologically affected, we provide public funds to build hospitals for the sake of housing mental patients. If, on the one hand, we consider whether there are scholars who argue that the enemy must be attacked and destroyed wherever he is to be found and who complain that is a disgrace that lectures are being given on peace in a time of war, there are, on the other hand, also teachers who teach that we and our enemies are both human, and we should love one another on this basis. To the extent that these alternatives are not limited to the examples we have given, human undertakings are full of contradictions.[126]

At the strictly individual level what concerns Oka is that little of the original binding altruism that made community possible seems to remain: "[H]umans seem to have so crystallized into selfish entities that it feels as if one must doubt whether this human-way exists anywhere at all."[127] However, "taking a broad view of human action and examining our own minds," he believes that we can see that there "also exists an altruistic spirit in humans."[128] This spirit makes itself evident in many areas of human life: "[W]hen we hear of another's sorrow we are sorrowful with them, and when we see another in pain we feel we want to help them. If we listen to stories of unhappy people in miserable circumstances, tears naturally fall, and a spirit that yearns to somehow save them from their plight takes hold. Seeing a painful sight, such as a horse hauling a heavy pack up a slope, heartfelt pity arises in us,

---

125 Ibid., 56.
126 Ibid., 56–57.
127 Ibid., 55–56.
128 Ibid., 56.

and we feel inclined to want to lend it assistance."[129] According to Oka these reactions are not mere cultural or social epiphenomena but point to something more basic and permanent in the human constitution. They are emanations of instinct: "[T]he spirit of sympathy is neither a false show for outward adornment, nor the result of being taught and trained, but, in truth, it is an instinct we have possessed from birth. Though individuals never possess this instinct to the same degree, it must never in any case be doubted that everyone has been left with some measure of it in their hearts. This is, in other words, the source of this thing called humanity, or the human-way."[130]

It is with regard to this remaining "measure" of altruistic instinct in the human heart that we come to the second area where Oka goes beyond his earlier account of the way. In "The True Character of Humanity" Oka's ultimate emphasis is on scientistic activism: "[T]o make the effort to assist artificially in the germination of a faint human-way, which we have possessed from birth, in order to solidify artificially the unity of our group, and to develop our group's might in the face of rivals."[131] Intrinsic to the large-brained "contradictory creatures"—suspended between echelons of organic individuality and therefore forced to choose between egoism and altruism—that humans have become, this capacity for artificial assistance is also integral to the human-way: "The essence of man consists in artificially enhancing whatever is deficient in nature, creating through his own wisdom things which are better than those obtained as a result of the natural selection other animals undergo, and overcoming rivals."[132] Such improvements on nature can be seen everywhere in how humans apply their scientific knowledge to technological innovations: "Though they also lack tusks or claws, humans can make torpedoes and heavy cannons, and then they can kill several hundred men in an instant. Though they lack legs which are adequate for sprinting, humans can lay down railroad track and run several hundred *ri* in one day."[133] As we saw in Chapter 3, Todorov described scientism as an outlook according to which science unravels "the secrets of nature," identifies "the causes of all facts and all beings," and then modifies "the processes involved … to steer them in a more desirable direction." In

129 Ibid.
130 Ibid., 56.
131 Ibid., 62.
132 Ibid., 60.
133 Ibid. A single *ri* was measured in the Meiji era as approximately 2.4 miles or around 3.9 kilometers.

this manner, science comes to underwrite "techne, a tool for changing the world."[134] It is in this sense that Oka's metapolitics amounts to a technology of the normative disposition, one through which he hopes to engineer a new humanity (human-way) by fashioning the instincts.

What makes Todorov's description of scientism particularly relevant is Oka's propensity to turn the freedom to artificially enhance into a facet of necessity. As Todorov says: "The world is entirely homogeneous, entirely determined, entirely knowable, on the one hand; but on the other, man is an infinitely malleable material, whose observable characteristics are not serious obstacles to the chosen project. Everything is *given* and at the same time everything can be chosen: the paradoxical union of these two assertions comes by way of a third, according to which everything is knowable." Wedding in this manner "a systematic determinism and a boundless voluntarism," scientism imagines a perfectly transparent reality in which "everything is necessary, of course, but one has the freedom to accelerate necessity in order to follow the direction of history or the direction of life."[135] In Oka's case necessity was defined by mankind's collective existence and the ability to "accelerate" it facilitated by Lamarckism, the evolutionary mechanism which translated acts of will into inherited traits. Though humanity was malleable, survival demands placed constraints on the possible: "human beings" are "fated to engage in group competition" and for humans to live as humanitarian individualists is like a crab trying to "walk upright" instead of "crawling horizontally."[136] Oka's task was thus to accelerate the necessity of group life by employing the voluntarism of Lamarckian use-inheritance. The altruistic instincts required for collective cohesion would be artificially enhanced through habitual acts of will.

Employing Lamarckism use-inheritance in place of natural selection was necessary due the size of human groups and the long duration of human life. Oka clarified that "altruism is not something that existed from the beginning" but was "a secondary characteristic that gradually evolved from selfishness with the advance of group existence."[137] For most creatures this evolution occurred on the basis of "natural selection between groups."[138] Oka

---

134 Todorov, *Hope and Memory*, 20.
135 Todorov, *Imperfect Garden*, 23–24.
136 Oka, "Jindō no Shōtai [The true character of humanity: the human-way]," 65.
137 Ibid., 61.
138 Ibid.

cites the example of the ants and bees, consummate groups in which altruism is "ideally practiced"[139]:

> [S]ince for insect species such as ants and bees the vicissitudes of life and death come rapidly on, the workings of natural selection are sufficient for the duration of their existence. Groups that are fit for survival triumph and prosper, while those who are unfit are defeated and die out. Before one knows it, generations of groups pile up and the results of natural selection are revealed. Characteristics suited for group life gradually develop and spread to descendants as instincts. Finally, the level they are at today, where they are able to carry on an ideal group life, is reached.[140]

For most creatures this cross-generational evolution of altruistic instincts had occurred in small group units. To underscore this point Oka cites the examples of apes and the ape-way. In Chapter 3 we saw that in 1902 Oka had used the "ape-way" as a means to offer suggestions about the nature of human morality. In "The True Character of Humanity" the ape-way reappears, but this time it is brought in to contrast the altruism of primates to the egoism of men. Oka describes the altruistic propensities of primates in glowing terms:

> Among monkeys, when a member of the group is injured, fellow monkeys gather together and tenderly nurse the injured party. Even in cases where that monkey dies, it happens that, after great numbers have gathered around and wept, the corpse is carried off and secreted away to a place unknown to the others. In the diaries of those who have hunted in the African interior, it is often mentioned that slain monkeys could not in the end be taken because, although they had been shot, their companions had come and carried their corpses off. Moreover, if infant monkeys remain after the mother has passed away, another female monkey will immediately take the child on and raise it just as if the child were its own. Because this is "the way" by which groups of monkeys conduct themselves, it should be dubbed the "monkey-way."[141]

According to Oka these instincts evolved due to the small size of ape groups: "[T]hey gather together in small numbers to form groups; when

---

139 Ibid.
140 Ibid.
141 Ibid., 59.

there is an intense struggle for existence between the groups only those groups fit for existence survive; those groups which are unfit die out and vanish; natural selection starts to operate with the group, perhaps with the result that one arrives at the stage where there is the instinct necessary for collective life—that is, altruism."[142]

For humans the evolutionary pressures on small groups with short life spans have been lifted. Thus, in contrast to other social animals, "with human beings, because the number of individuals within the particular group is large and because their lives are comparatively long, the vicissitudes of life and death come on quite slowly and there is very little room for natural selection to operate during their lives. Especially in accordance with the advance of civilization and the opening up of the remaining communications and transportation, the ability of a number of individuals to combine together as a group is gradually increasing. Because groups are gradually getting larger as compared to the age of savagery, the workings of natural selection are becoming less and less."[143] The result of this lack of natural selection is that "once these primates become human, it seems that progress nearly comes to a halt."[144] In other words, the "instinctive altruism, which was once acquired during the monkeylike era, is handed down nearly unchanged until today."[145] This lack of development amounts to a "piecemeal degeneration in this process."[146] In contrast to our primate ancestors, Oka believed that the contemporary "human spirit possesses ninety-nine parts selfishness to one part altruism."[147] Humankind had degenerated to the point where "scanning present-day circumstances" the instinct for "altruistic sympathy, when compared to selfishness, is little known among humans."[148]

It is to reverse this degeneration that Oka turns to Lamarckian voluntarism: "[M]an must assist in the burgeoning of the naturally weak human-way by practicing it."[149] In his view humans have little choice in the matter: even though "the altruism which humans have possessed from birth" is "a

---

142 Ibid., 61–62.
143 Ibid., 61.
144 Ibid., 62.
145 Ibid.
146 Ibid.
147 Ibid., 56.
148 Ibid.
149 Ibid., 62.

paltry thing" it is "a necessity in the existence of group-oriented animals."[150] Because humans cannot wait for a natural "increase in altruism among individuals" as it occurs in "the workings of natural selection over a long period of time" for other species such as ants and bees, "we must find another method that is able to obtain the same results."[151] It is in this context that Oka speaks of the "effort to assist artificially in the germination of a faint human-way."[152] Though the "kind of social cohesion" contemporary humans want will not be obtained "in a single leap,"[153] his metapolitics imagines an order in which the practice of altruistic habits engender the instincts of the human-way and thereby reverse the degeneration of the human superorganism.

In our last chapter we will see that Oka eventually devises a theory of degeneration that places the development of the nation-state in a cosmic framework and seeks its regeneration by a palingenetic return to an earlier condition of healthy cohesion. Such generative scientism, which we will argue is a form of programmatic modernism, yields its first glimmerings in this call to reverse the degeneration of the human-way. However, the main thrust of Oka's scientism in 1906 is still reformist, as can be seen in how he merges the instinct-engendering practice of altruism with the exercise of state legal authority. For him it is a vital "necessity that the human-way be adopted by means of laws, morality and coercion."[154] Augmenting altruistic instincts through habitual practices should be adopted "either through the special establishment of an artificial system for enforcing sanctions, or through the use of bonuses and flattery."[155] Though in this essay Oka does not elaborate beyond these vague suggestions, his main point is clear: "[L]aws and morality are needed in the life of the group"[156] and the state should reform itself so that system of norms, conventions, and laws are embodied in the instincts of the ethnic nation. For the human-way to revive nomos must become an inheritable trait—it must be permanently internalized. Nomic instincts are the precondition for national cohesion. The organic interdependence of Oka's metapolitics emanates from this instinctual substrate.

---

150 Ibid.
151 Ibid.
152 Ibid.
153 Ibid.
154 Ibid., 63.
155 Ibid., 62.
156 Ibid., 63.

Sanuki Masakazu, focusing on Oka's essays from the 1920s, has construed Oka as subscribing to a form of "republicanism" based on "spontaneous democracy." Though Sanuki is correct that Oka envisioned the full participation of the people in national projects and imagined this occurring in an unreflexive, almost automatic fashion, the suggestion that Oka specifically endorsed democracy and all that implied is misguided.[157] In fact, Oka's politics seem to lean heavily toward the organic statism described in Chapter 1, an outlook which found tremendous encouragement during his student years in Germany where an "organicist consensus"[158] had come to inform sociopolitical questions. However, the very fact that scholars are forced to speculate on Oka's politics is the best indication that it was not in the specific form of politics but in the preconditions for an evolutionary viable political order that Oka was invested. The political order under the Meiji Constitution was not even seventeen years old when Oka wrote about the "human-way" and given the unstable and volatile nature of Meiji politics and the dangers involved in questioning orthodoxy it should not be surprising that Oka emphasized reforming the metapolitical substrate that he believed made possible the organic cohesion of a "spontaneously" participatory, homogneous population. This was, in a sense, a version of the "technocratic anti-politics"[159] that his contemporaries in Europe endorsed, though in Oka's case the spread of correct ideas about evolution through society via education and the press became the critical factor in implanting the collectivist instincts of the human-way. As we will see in the next chapter, the distortion of evolutionism by disparate ideologies and its implicit denial by an emerging religious orthodoxy will be what inspires him to stress the

---

157 Sanuki, "Kindai nihon ni okeru kyowashugi." Oka's understanding of the national superorganism as a kind of republic or democracy is strikingly close to that of his contemporary evolutionist, Ishikawa Chiyomatsu (1861–1935). Ishikawa not only studied under August Weismann in Freiburg a few years before Oka, writing a series of influential textbooks upon his return, but performed research on invertebrate superorganisms in their natural habitat. An article of his from 1923 entitled "The Human Body and Democracy" argues that the manner in which "the body's cells achieve a diverse division of labor and take on specialized functions" represents the "true democratic spirit." Eschewing the extremes of communism and capitalism yet countenancing differences in station within society, the organicist "cellular organization" of livings beings literally embodies "the way the nation-state should be." According to Hayashi Makoto this appropriation of cell theory by both Oka and Ishikawa connects them with "totalitarian social theory." I will address the relationship between Oka, Ishikawa, and several other members of their generation in an upcoming project. See Hayashi, "Cell Theory in its Development and Inheritance in Meiji Japan"; Ishikawa, "Jintai to demokurashii," 178–80.

158 Weindling, *Health, Race and German Politics*, 27.

159 Ibid., 20.

historical dimension of his organicism and thereby bring out the generative aspect of his scientism.

Education would figure especially large in Oka's reckonings not just because it was his chosen profession but because he had begun to suspect that self-interested individualism was the source of anomy. Oka's writings on education often reiterate the need for pure science, free enquiry, and science education. Yet, Oka's intent was not to liberate individuals' will but to inform them of evolutionary necessity. Once members of the ethnic nation understood that a substrate of nomic instincts was vital to its collective survival they would subordinate their individual egos to the needs of the nation-state through instinct-engendering altruism. The anomic potential of awakened subjectivity would be averted by enlightening the population to the organicism of interdependence. The diverse, differentiated body of the ethnic nation would reintegrate when its members turned their newfound freedom not to self-interested ends but collective ones. Natural selection and, most especially, Lamarckism provided a technique by which the nation could literally transform its normative disposition into a feature of the natural ontology. The chaos evinced at Hibiya could be overcome via the self-coordinating technology of the human-way.

MONIST TOTALISM

Implicit in this subtle self-abnegation of individual persons and, indeed, in Oka's program to preempt anomy through the promotion of an instinctual nation-state there can be found a rebranding of humanity itself, one that picks up where the wartime essays left off. At the very beginning of "The True Character of Humanity: The Human-Way," Oka explains that "when commonly used between individuals, the word 'humanity' comes across as meaning 'expending some effort or money in order to decrease the suffering of another human or a creature dear to humans'—that is to say, it refers to acts performed out of altruism and sympathy."[160] As the essay draws to a close and Oka has finished explaining how this human-way needs to be revived through "artificial assistance" he places a qualifier on this altruism and sympathy: "According to what has been said above, it should be ex-

---

160 Oka, "Jindō no Shōtai" [The true character of humanity: the human-way], 55.

pected that there is no human-way, in the true sense of the word, to be found in the struggle for existence between one ethnic nation and another."[161] In fact, because the ethnic nation is "the primary unit in competition"[162] for humans, the human-way "is never practiced at this level either."[163] While "individual altruism" may "perform altruistic acts for members of another group at times," doing so is analogous to "the tongue, which evolved in order to sense the sweetness of nourishing sugar, experiencing nutritionally lacking saccharine as sweet."[164] "Showing humanity [the human-way] toward another race-nation to get a feeling of satisfaction" in this manner "is not at all a bad thing."[165] However, in the end, Oka insists that "a notion of humanity [the human-way] which affords advantages to another ethnic nation, while damaging one's own, is greatly misguided. This is never the true human-way. Through thick and thin the true human-way should place paramount emphasis on one's own race."[166]

Oka's race-specific rendering of the human-way not only reminds us of the notions of human speciation which evolutionary morphologists developed—notions which rejected the humanitarian tradition of a fraternity of man in toto—but indicates a common confusion concerning the opposition of individualism and collectivism. In his *The Open Society and Its Enemies*, Karl Popper describes how for many thinkers—going at least as far back as the pre-Socratics—individualism has been equated with egoism and collectivism with altruism. This has resulted in a skewed view of moral questions, one in which individualism is always opposed to altruism and collectivism opposed to egoism. Oka can be understood as engaging in this misguided analysis with his dismissal of humanitarianism: as we have just seen, altruism toward other individuals who do not belong to one's group is seen as either an empty indulgence or, more likely, a perversion. It is not the "true human-way" because there is no humanity that is common to all ethnicities. There is only the ethnic nation—and allegiance is owed to this "species of the nation" alone.

Interestingly, Oka's entire metapolitics rests on a possibility that Popper says is, like altruistic individualism, usually denied by moral philosophers:

---

161 Ibid., 63.
162 Ibid.
163 Ibid., 63–64.
164 Ibid., 64.
165 Ibid.
166 Ibid.

egoistic collectivism. As Popper points out, "collective or group egoism, for instance class egoism, is a common thing."[167] In *Evolution and Human Life* the egoism of the ethnic nation is not an analogy but something quite literal: the nation-state is a consummate group or superorganism, a "higher self" as he calls it in his early "Good and Evil in the Animal World."[168] The altruism of the members of this ethnic nation—that is, their subordination to collectivist needs through the human-way—is what makes this national egoism possible. As he explains: "altruism between individual members of a particular race-nation is something which is needed by that race-nation to actualize racial self-interest in an outward direction. These two things can be regarded as two faces of the same coin."[169] It is based on this insight that Oka is able, at the end of his essay, to turn humanitarianism on its head and equate the human-way, morality, and humanity itself with war-making: "Waging war requires national unity and because national unity is first made by way of individual altruism, war and the human-way have an extremely intimate relationship. That is to say, racial self-interest, which appears on the outside as war, is on the inside a quest between individuals for the human-way."[170] It is just this ruthless group egoism, the outward expression of the human-way, that Oka observes in the evolutionary realpolitik of world affairs:

Opening a map of the world, one sees that to the furthest reaches of America, Africa, and Australia all has been divided up and conquered by a few powerful nations. Yet if we try to compare the people indigenous to these territories with the conquering Europeans, right and wrong are indistinguishable. All this means is that, like a wolf devouring a sheep or a fox killing a hen, one side is strong and the other is weak. Haeckel also recognized this phenomenon, declaring in one of his books that, "As a rule, for organic life the utmost violence justly triumphs." In our country the proverb "Winners become authorities, losers outlaws" [Losers are never in the right] even more succinctly expresses the same idea. Thus, each ethnic nation should rely only on its own power in mankind's struggle for existence.[171]

---

167 Popper, *The Open Society and Its Enemies*, Volume 1, 100.
168 Oka, "Seibutsukai ni okeru Zen to Aku" [Good and evil in the animal world], 47.
169 Oka, "Jindō no Shōtai [The true character of cumanity: the cuman-way]," 63.
170 Ibid.
171 Ibid., 64.

The quotation in this passage from Haeckel's *History of Creation*, with its stress on the strong justly triumphing over the weak, brings us back to the statements with which we began our discussion of "The True Character of Humanity: The Human-Way": "[W]ars are made possible by the human-way alone" and "war and the human-way seem to be identical, front and back." The notion of justice being espoused in this identification of successful warmaking and the normative disposition of humans—the human-way—was portrayed by Karl Popper in another section of *The Open Society* as exemplary of a "biological form of ethical naturalism."[172] Along with the closely associated position of ethical positivism, this ethical naturalism displays a "tendency toward monism, that is to say, toward the reduction of norms to facts"[173]—or, as we have referred to these relations, of nomoi to nature. For evolutionists like Haeckel and Oka this monism of norms and natural processes elevated successful outcomes to a moral ideal and validates the kind of "might makes right" doctrine espoused in the above quoted passage. Just as individual egoists, such as wolves and foxes, justly triumph over their prey due to superior strength, so do collective egoists, such as "powerful nations," become the instinctive authors of a naturalistic ethos used to justifiably subjugate "indigenous peoples." The so-called human-way serves this "just" end.

It is, however, in how this monism of "nature and convention" translates into the internal workings of powerful nations that the human-way betrays its totalitarian hostility to both humanitarianism and individual persons. As we have argued, Oka's reformist scientism aimed to refashion the existing societal nomos to fit the organic independence found in successful social creatures. Such instinctual altruism was necessary not for the welfare of individuals or the good of humanity but as a coordinating device to fortify the higher self of the superorganism. In other words, the health and fighting capacity of the group completely overrides the value and usefulness of individual persons to the extent that these persons are thought to be almost entirely insufficient apart from collective life. Popper calls this collective egoism an example of "political hygiene" and identifies it with the "totalitarian theory of morality."[174]

The potential for totalitarian ethics is intrinsic to proposals to reform the nation-state along the lines of a superorganism. Conceiving the nation as a

---

172 Popper, *The Open Society and Its Enemies*, Volume 1, 68.
173 Ibid., 73.
174 Ibid., 107.

literal collective body could always lead to reducing its respective parts to a perfectly subordinate status. The hygiene of such a body was to be maintained by treating any parts that did not support the health, harmony, and goals of the overindividuality of the nation as diseased and potentially excisable. What especially distinguishes Oka's human-way is that this hygienic condition of healthy unity is to be achieved by the activities of the parts or cells themselves. Through education of the race-specific ethos of the human-way, the parts would coordinate themselves into the larger organism—each, it is implied, taking its proper place in the division of labor to bolster the national body. The national entity would only be able to function in a healthy and effective manner in its inevitable struggle with other ethnic nations when individuals are made to willingly render themselves utterly transparent to the needs of the collective.

It is in what would happen if this self-coordination did not occur that we can begin to get a sense of how fears of nomic breakdown nudge Oka's organicism toward totalitarianism. A nation in which everyone pursued their own self-interest or their own separate version of the good would not build up the necessary instincts for healthy cohesion. Without any built-in self-regulation there would be no unifying normative disposition, no nomos. Anomy would reign. Oka's response to anomy is to draw on the normative exemplars and transformative techniques rendered transparent by evolutionary science and employ these to internalize an instinctual nomos within the physical constitution of individual persons. Enlightened to the truths of evolutionary science, they would adopt altruistic habits toward their compatriots and these habits, through the Lamarckian mechanism of use-inheritance, would implant normative responses into their instinctive makeup. The health requirements and survival imperatives of the totality would become part of the involuntary response mechanism of its constituent parts—and this would be achieved by a voluntary submission of individuality to collective life. Wayward subjectivity would be tamed—perhaps permanently—by the internalization of the human-way—the literal creation of a new *jindō* or humanity.

In her *Origins of Totalitarianism*, Hannah Arendt famously asserted that "totalitarianism is never content to rule through external means."[175] She

---

175 Arendt, *The Origins of Totalitarianism*, 431.

goes on to explain how a totalitarian order does not necessarily seek control through the exercise of power but by means of a symbiosis through which the rulers and subjects are so profoundly identified with one another that they act as one. In Chapter 3 we saw this same apolitical ideal at play in the soft organicism of reformist scientism. Though these technocrats ostensibly only set out to reform the existing order, their "corporatist biology"[176] began to envision "the potential for creating a society corresponding to a total institution."[177] Along with circumventing messy party politics and internal factionalization, the totalistic concept of the social organism lent transcendental technocrats unlimited access to the lives of the differentiated persons who comprised the national body. The cells of the superorganism could be administered to and made to healthily reintegrate into the collective. For Oka this technocratic utopia is embodied in the human-way, a new mode of humanity that instinctively achieves organic unity with the totality of the nation. In addition to the perceived pressures of imperial encirclement, what distinguishes Oka from his contemporaries abroad was that the techne used to achieve this internalization relied on the active consent of the very same anomic society he was trying to reform. Despite what we have said about Oka's espousal of eugenics and racial hygiene, his program at the beginning of 1906 in "The True Character of Humanity: The Human-Way" primarily entailed enlightening the populace. His totalitarian aspirations— if that is what they can be called—were, somewhat paradoxically, still part of an educational effort and thus remained dependent on the egos or lower selves that he hoped to sublimate into the higher self of the national body.

As the next chapter will reveal, Oka's frustrations in realizing such a scientistic "total institution" through the dissemination of the normative truths of evolutionary biology would tease out the generative potential of this organicist scientism. Offering evolutionism as a metapolitics—ontological preconditions to which existing political orders should be reconciled—and relying on education and, to a lesser extent, the press as the means by which to implement this technocratic reform were always going to be problematic. However, the primary obstacle would turn out to be individuals themselves. It was their new assertiveness during and after the war

---

176 Weindling, *Health, Race and German Politics*, 45.
177 Ibid., 19.

that led to both the perception of anomy and the totalitarian measures to reverse the degenerate condition it seemed to express. In a sense, what Oka and others who worried about the dire consequence that would befall the nation if it sacrificed its nomic cohesion to competing individuals and internal factions were confronting is the emergence of the open society. As Popper describes it, an open society is one which has begun to experience the "loss of its organic character" and become an "abstract society"[178] typified by depersonalized relations of rational exchange and self-interested cooperation. Though Popper admits that the loss of concrete connections can isolate and atomize individuals, he portrays the coming of the open society as a moment of human liberation from the oppressive monism of "facts and decisions."[179] Freed from the taboos of the tribal past through which nomoi became sacralized manifestations of a sacred ultimate reality, a "critical dualism" develops by which human beings come to understand that ontologies are contested and that norms, conventions, and laws are humanly constructed. For Popper, modern life was typified by the open society and its critical dualism. Totalitarianism, in contrast, was an attempt to return to the closed society by reestablishing the monism of facts and decisions, nature and nomos.

One way to interpret Oka's totalitarian metapolitics is as an ill-fated rationalist reversion to this monism of nomos and nature. Differentiated persons would be educated in evolutionary biology and adopt altruistic behaviors that would reintegrate them into the concrete relations of the tribe (ethnic nation) via Lamarckism. The engendering of nomic instincts would reestablish the monism of the closed society. Individuals would confine their freedom to unreflexively "accelerating necessity."[180] The problem with this reformist approach, however, was that it ultimately depended on getting individuals to willingly submit their newly awakened critical powers to the requirements of the whole. As Oka and the ideologues of state Shinto would soon discover, something more than abstract arguments (moralism) would be needed to win over the egoists of this alluring abstract society. For both Oka and the state Shintoists there was an understanding that a future-oriented cosmological element would need to be introduced in order to more

---

178 Popper, *The Open Society and Its Enemies*, Volume 1, 174.
179 Ibid., 62.
180 Todorov, *Imperfect Garden*, 24.

convincingly get individuals to identify with their respective monist visions. In Oka's case this would mean turning his organicism into a process of cosmic development that generated ultimate values: health would be measured not just by interdependence but the realization of future growth. It is through this generative scientism that, we will see, Oka converts his evolutionism into a form of programmatic modernism, one that seeks to regenerate the nation and vouchsafe its future epigenetic reintegration through a return to an earlier, healthier, and more propitious stage in the life cycle of national development.

PART III

Regeneration

Degeneration, when it reared its head in "Evolutionary Theory and Hygiene" and "The True Character of Humanity: The Human-Way," referred to a self-interested individualism that defies the organicist priority of wholes before component parts. While Oka echoed contemporary race hygienists and eugenicists in bemoaning the lack of national fitness due to the absence of natural selection, the unique feature of his reformist scientism was its emphasis on national cohesion as a product of what we have called nomic instincts. For Oka such instincts were formed through a Lamarckian process, one which demanded that members of the ethnic nation practice altruistic habits via the mechanism of use-inheritance. This altruism would engender a human-way—a normative disposition that would instinctively cause the nation-state to fulfill its collectivist nature and function internally as a single individual biologically primed for evolutionary struggle. Such antidegenerate organic cohesion was portrayed as the precondition for national survival.

Implicit in Oka's reformist, metapolitical program was the imperative that members of the ethnic nation embrace their proper place in the division of labor through an understanding of evolutionism. Oka's commitment to education and the popular dissemination of evolutionary biology stemmed from this imperative. However, it is precisely here that inflated individualism intervened to impede Oka's reformist scientism. As we have indicated, from at least the Hibiya Riot onward, subjectivity had been fully awakened and Japan had become what Gluck calls a complicated society. This advent of anomy—the possibility of nonconcrete, unregulated interpersonal relations accompanied by a critical grasp of the dualism of nature and nomos—

ushered in an era where the monism of norms and biological facts was not and perhaps could not be accepted in the way Oka wanted it to be. Despite a "Darwin boom" initiated by his writings, this awakened subjectivity interpreted evolutionism in a plurality of ways anathema to Oka's scientism. And more ominously factions within the state began to rethink and redouble their own administrative and ideological efforts to combat anomy. All of these factors forced Oka to reconsider whether the reformist and largely educational stance of his scientism had sufficient purchase on a national society that industrialism, urbanization, mass media, and the dissemination of radical ideologies seemed to be degenerating into anomic fragments.

Oka's answer to both anomy and the state ideological measures that attempted to combat it was a generative scientism that emphasized the temporal dimension of organicism. The impulse behind this hard organicism was continuous with that of his earlier metapolitics: to delineate the evolutionary preconditions of national survival and thereby initiate a reform of the existing nomos to fit the requirements of the natural ontology. The reformist scientism that Oka articulated during the war and its immediate aftermath imagined this organicism in atemporal terms as one of interdependence between parts. Members of the national community were to understand that they were not independent entities but interfused with the life of the nation-state and should therefore subordinate themselves to the needs of the national body. This was what he meant by *jindō*: humanity, morality, and the correct normative disposition—the human-way.

What Oka came to understand by the middle of 1907 was that, in the new postwar climate, rational appeals for adherence to such a "human-way" could easily fall on deaf ears even as so-called Darwinism grew in influence and popularity. Even if the public accepted the ontological truths laid down by evolutionary theory in Oka's books, it did not seem at all inclined to follow his lead in using this knowledge to construct a naturalistic nomos that would monistically close the gap between biological facts and human conventions. If anything, the spread of evolutionism exacerbated anomy by seeming to lend credence not only to individualism but to ideologies such as socialism, communism, and anarchism that were unabashedly subversive to the state. Faced with a free-for-all of responses Oka was at pains to establish the solemn necessity of his organicist metapolitics in a manner that distinguished it from other visions.

This task became especially urgent as the state's efforts to repair the frayed unity of the nation with state Shintoist indoctrination intensified. It is important to understand that these efforts shared a basic orientation with Oka's *shinkaron* (evolutionism), one that would become the terms of a tacit rapprochement between the *tennosei* (emperor system) and *shinkaron* decades later: they sought to counter the anomy of postwar individualistic society by cementing collectivistic norms, conventions, and laws to an ontological substrate that would render them beyond dispute. Though, like Oka, the promoters of orthodoxy attempted to shore up a real, concrete community on a consanguineous basis, the organic ethnic nation they described had its origins not in evolutionary development but in the imperial stem line that went back to the mythical founder of the universe, Amaterasu Ōmikami (the Sun Goddess). After the war with Russia the state aggressively augmented and intensified its program to instill this family-state ideology among the people. It was when these indoctrination measures began to encroach directly on education that the latent generative features of Oka's organicism emerged. To beat the orthodoxy at its own cosmicizing game Oka placed the life of the organic nation-state in a cosmic framework, stressing the temporal development of the national body through stages of growth, senescence, and extinction. This grand narrative of evolutionary growth invested the organicism of the ethnic nation with ultimate value in a manner that analysis of its internal interdependence alone did not. Regenerating the nation became not just a matter of political hygiene but of national destiny.

This historicist imperative to regenerate the *minzoku* (ethnic nation) was inseparable from Oka's belief that the human-way had degenerated and needed to be restored. However, under the influence of the theory of orthogenesis, a non-Darwinian offshoot of biogenetic law, we will see that Oka's generative scientism broadened into a critique not just of the absence of nomic instincts but of the modern mode of existence that was taking shape in the last years of the Meiji period. In the theory of degeneration which he articulates in 1910, the historicist schema of national development through cycles of life allows Oka to envision a palingenetic return to an earlier stage of health, one in which the overdeveloped "brains and hands" of the present would altruistically serve the superorganism and not individual egos. Coupling this pessimistic-sounding theory of degeneration with a reassertion of eugenic and racial hygiene, Oka's generative scientism amounts to a form of programmatic modernism. The alternate modern lifestyle that it seems to offer will hygienically reembed persons into the superorganism and through this rejuvenation promise to secure the future health, prosperity, and strength of the ethnic nation in a modern manner more convincing than the reactionary Shintoist orthodoxy.

The first chapter in this section, "Nomic Crisis," will describe the triangular relationship between postwar anomy, the fundamentalist response to it, and Oka's dismay at both these developments, especially the exclusion of evolutionary science from the increasingly Shinto-oriented school curriculum. Chapter 7, "Decadence and Destiny," explores how Oka's depiction of this late Meiji nomic dissolution as a degenerate phase of development facilitated his generative scientist program for national renewal. The epilogue, "Evolution and the National Body: An Unfinished Synthesis," suggests that Shintoist attempts to appropriate aspects of Oka's scientism and corporatist evolutionism indicates a partially completed accommodation between orthodoxy and evolutionary science in imperial Japan.

CHAPTER 6

NOMIC CRISIS

Religion and morality together try to prevent wrongdoing before it occurs. When this ideal is attained there will be a world without sin or crime. Moss animals, in other words, already inhabit such a world. The society of this species of moss animals have realized the ideal of religion and morality. As a consequence, this society is, when considered from this viewpoint, something extremely precious: it is valuable enough to be made the aim of our human advancement. Instead of listening to old-fashioned lectures on ethics and morals for one or two hours each week, it seems that it would be far more useful to show the students moss animal colonies under a microscope and have them hear detailed explanations on the circumstances of their group life. Furthermore, because humans, with their habit of saying "out of sight, out of mind," are apt to easily forget if they do not see something right before their eyes, Buddhism erects various images of the Buddha, arranging things so that the people will not be allowed to forget the Buddha night and day. At least this is what sect founders hold as an ideal. Because these sects cannot in the end attain the state which moss animal species actually exhibit, it would be more reasonable to construct enormous images of moss animals than to build statues of sect founders and the Buddha. Especially compared to the worthless bronze statues of humans which have been erected here and there as of late, I do not know how many times better it would be for the benefit of public morals to put up a bronze image of a moss animal and always have set forth before all eyes admonitions such as "Like this moss animal, do unto others as you would have others do unto you" and "Like this moss animal, escape the confines of the ego, proceed on to the level of the higher self."[1]

---

1   Oka, "Risōteki Dantai Seikatsu" [Ideal group life], 71–72.

As we described it in the introduction, this paragraph represents the culmination of Oka Asajirō's essay from July 1907, "Ideal Group Life." These moss animal superorganisms were thought to be "ideal" in the sense not only of consummate, organic integration but as objects of emulation: they are the proper "aim of human advancement." In the last section we argued that the outlook of reformist scientism that Oka shared with many other products of Todai regarded the superindividual life of the moss animal colony as a paragon after which human conduct should be modeled—a race-specific yet altruistic normative disposition, the human-way, which could be engendered through what we have called nomic instincts. For Oka the organicism of interdependence displayed by such superorganisms defined metapolitical preconditions for national survival. Adjusting the received laws, norms, and conventions of the nation so that they corresponded with and, ultimately, came to embody the human-way by which these preconditions would be met was the project of his reformist scientism.

By mid-1907, just over a year after Oka had articulated his human-way, this reformist project seemed to be failing. The conditions under which "wrongdoing" is prevented "before it occurs" seemed suddenly unattainable. This is yet another sense in which the group life of moss animals is "ideal": "everything that is labeled ideal must be, by definition, unrealizable in the immediate future" and "wherever one looks in today's world it is obvious that ideal things are nowhere to be found."[2] As a consequence, Oka despairs that "a perfect group life, such as we see in this species of moss animals, is not even a remote possibility for human beings."[3] While he ends by repeating the reformist conceit that "ideal things are needed as goals for advancement" that guide, "on a day-to-day basis, what direction progress should take," serving as a "reference point" for "cultivating ourselves or improving the social system,"[4] this essay marks a pivot away from this strictly reformist stance and the beginning of Oka's search for a scientism that will not just fit nomos to an ontological substrate but remake human beings to achieve a more perfect organic unity for the nation. The change in Oka's approach is evident in his suggestion that science education should supplant religion. Though half-mocking in tone, Oka's proposal that lectures on mi-

---

2   Ibid., 75.
3   Ibid.
4   Ibid.

croscopic observations should replace moral education and that bronze statues of moss animals should be erected where images of political and religious figures once stood testify that for him, like so many of his peers, the conditions of the postwar years constituted a nomic crisis, a period when the consummate cohesion of the ideal organic group seemed more and more remote. Measures more radical than mere scientistic reform would be required to reverse this apparent decadence and dissolution—ones that more forcefully connected the normative imperatives of evolutionism to cosmological processes in a manner not unlike religion.

In this chapter we will argue that this perception of nomic crisis in the period after the Russo-Japanese War was a shared response of the older generations of Meiji modernizers to the appearance of a less organic and more abstract social landscape. Unsettled by social change and the loss of national cohesion that manifested itself in the upsurge in urbanization, industrialization, and political and ideological pluralism, bureaucrats and other leaders of public opinion allowed the secular civic morality that they had devised to instill nationalism in the 1890s to become identified with the familiar communal mores and "beautiful customs" of the village and family. By 1907 this tribalist effort to retrieve the social foundations of the past in order to combat anomy had been taken over by a Shintoist-nativist narrative of *kokutairon*: an orthodoxy that conceptualized the Japanese national body (*kokutai*) as a family-state in which the emperor and imperial family were an unbroken stem-line that harkened back to the Sun Goddess and the *kokumin* (people) served as a dutiful and obedient extended branch family. Articulated by Hozumi Yatsuka as what Walter Skya has called "reactionary Shinto ultranationalism," this backward-looking, absolutist national ethos, which we first encountered in Chapter 1, came to be accompanied by an aggressive program of shrine consolidation and school indoctrination that together attempted to cosmicize the nomic bonds of the nation.

Oka would collide head on with these attempts to cosmicize "Japan's modern myths" as a member of the Ministry of Education textbook compilation committee. Assigned to the committee in 1904,[5] Oka found himself in a protracted struggle to have biology and evolution included in the cur-

---

5   Migita, *Tennosei to Shinkaron*, 106–7.

riculum for elementary schools during the very same postwar years that he presented the disappointed utopian vision of "Ideal Group Life." The failure of Oka's efforts on this committee—which culminated with the exclusion of evolution from the new textbook in 1911—was a primary impetus to his attempt to match the orthodoxy and more emphatically cosmicize the human-way. This would be achieved by invoking the historical process of organic development implicit in evolutionism. In order to counter Shintoist calls for restoration Oka would supply what we will see is not only a developmental but a palingenetic narrative of renewal. He too wanted the retrieve the solidarity of the past—yet in his case this did not involve arresting change but resituating the future of the *minzoku* within a restorative trajectory of healthy growth.

Oka's clash with advocates of orthodoxy should not cause us to overlook that both parties were reacting against the same anomic forces of social change and dissolution. For Oka, the decadent modern life of the postwar period was most apparent in the fickle individualism that followed its own whims in the pursuit of fads and fashions. Oka was especially distressed to see his successful efforts to disseminate evolutionary theory had resulted in a Darwin boom during which evolutionism was misappropriated for a variety of conflicting ends: for ambitious individuals, it became an ideology of success; for anarchists and socialists, a materialist justification for antigovernment activities; and for establishment-oriented bureaucrats and pundits who believed in the exoteric utility of the imperial myths, an esoteric doctrine, kept in parenthesis, away from the masses. Though Oka's response to this opening society was not to reverse change but to channel and control its wayward enthusiasms toward appropriate collective ends, his solution to its perceived degeneration, dissolution, and anomy involved, as it did with his Shintoist opponents, lending his normative prescriptions an ontological heft that would render them impervious to individual whim and ideological speculation. In other words, like the Shintoists—and religion in general—Oka aimed at a nomic restoration that prevented wrongdoing before it occurred. As we will begin to suggest at the close of the chapter, the expansion of his organicism into a value-generating, temporal vision of development would, even more successfully than Shintoism, serve, in the manner of religion, to cover up the constructed nature of the very norms, conventions, and laws he was involved in constructing.

ANOMY ASCENDANT

In her groundbreaking *Japan's Modern Myths*, Carol Gluck describes an attitudinal shift that occurred in the aftermath of the Russo-Japanese War among the generations who had promoted modernization during the Meiji period. Both an earlier generation, born in the 1830s and 1840s and which includes Yamagata Aritomo, Itō Hirobumi, and Katō Hiroyuki, and a later cohort, the "young men of Meiji," born in the 1860s and 1870s and which includes Oka Asajirō, grew alarmed that the modern order that had been created was enabling unintended "social change [that] might destroy the national gains Japan had achieved."[6] According to Gluck, these modernizers conceived of themselves as "reformers (*kaikakusha*)" and enacted their program of reform as "gradualists who preferred to pull the present out of the past without too radical a break." In keeping with what we have labeled, in Chapter 1, reformist statism, their earlier "aggressive pursuit of change" was meant to be "contained within the existing social system, which they assumed would be preserved."[7] One of their achievements had been to devise, in the years leading up to and following the initiation of the new constitutional order, a civil morality that deflected the urge to political participation into a new "nation-mindedness" or "sense of nation." To many, such as Oka Asajirō, the "unity of the nation" that had been mobilized during the war with Russia was this nation-mindedness made manifest. Yet now in the final years of the Meiji period the earlier "plunging rush into modernity"[8] seemed to be unleashing a contagion of social problems (*shakai mondai*) that undermined the tightly-knit organic polity that modernizers imagined they had constructed. "Confronted with a modernity that threatened to shake the social foundations of the nation, the ideologues turned to the verities of the past—the villages and the family, social harmony and communal custom—to cure civilization of its fevers so that society as they envisioned it might yet survive."[9]

This threat to the social foundations was not unanticipated. Not only, as we saw in Chapter 1, was the Meiji constitutional order erected in a statist manner intended to forestall dissent, but by the late 1890s modernist mis-

---

6   Gluck, *Japan's Modern Myths*, 274.
7   Ibid.
8   Ibid., 27.
9   Ibid., 178.

givings, which we touched on in Chapter 3, about the decadent and disembedding nature of material civilization began to reach Japan from Europe.
After the victory over China in 1895 Todai's Kanai Noburu and his disciples in the Shakai Seisaku Gakkai (Society for the Study of Social Policy)
began to fervently discuss the preventative actions that would be needed
in the areas of thought guidance and social policy to preempt the coming
social problems of the twentieth century[10] and soon there emerged, in the
early 1900s, among the "vanguard of civil concern," a stark "vocabulary of
social cataclysm":

> Society, they said, was in disarray, afflicted with ills, beset by economic diffi-
> culties, roiled by the struggle for survival, upset by labor problems, exposed
> to dangerous thought, threatened by socialist destruction, rent by gulfs
> between rich and poor, city and country, worker and capitalist. Localities,
> like youth, were delinquent; self-government lay in confusion. Cities were
> sinks of iniquity leading young people astray and fomenting social strife,
> even revolution. Customs were degenerating, morals in decline. And the
> middle classes, the "root and branch" from whom so much civic stability had
> been expected, had developed "social problems" of their own.[11]

According to Gluck "the ideological results of the social concerns that
began in the nineties assumed their full shape in the years following the
Russo-Japanese War."[12] By this time the creeping *shakai mondai* (social
problems) had come to be understood as part of a pandemic *bunmei byō*—a
civilization sickness brought about by the progress and development that
followed from the earlier reforms of *bunmei kaika* (civilization and enlightenment). This reversal in the status of material civilization—from a source
of enlightenment to a contagion—can be seen as an application of notions
of decadence—the "vocabulary of social cataclysm"—to the profound sense
of disorder that accompanied the rapid transformations within the political economy after the war. As we explored in Chapter 5, the Hibiya Riot
of 1905 marked the beginning not only of "mass participation in politics"[13]
connected with the coming of what Andrew Gordon calls "imperial democ-

---

10 Pyle, "Meiji Conservatism," 131ff.
11 Gluck, *Japan's Modern Myths*, 28.
12 Ibid., 41.
13 Skya, *Japan's Holy War*, 155.

racy," but of an "era of popular violence" that saw two additional Tokyo-wide riots in 1906 and another in 1908.[14] That the 1906 riots were aimed at hikes in streetcar fares and the 1908 uprising against tax increases indicates that the "politicization of the masses"[15] was resulting in, as Katsura feared in 1905, "mixing politics with social questions"[16] as industrialization intensified in the first decade of the twentieth century. Though the takeoff of industrial capitalism, which had begun after the war with China, had produced a great expansion of heavy industry and the world's most robust growth in percent of annual average GNP from 1870 to 1913,[17] Japan was also subject to cycles of economic volatility that contributed greatly to both this "awakening of the masses" and a perception of accelerating disintegration among those concerned with national cohesion. The year Oka published "Ideal Group Life," 1907, for instance, was particularly unsettling with a peak of industrial strikes across the nation taking place against the background of a deepening economic problems.[18] By 1908 a perception of social disarray had settled in: "[I]n the midst of the severe postwar depression, it appeared as if 'the pleasant dreams of victory' had faded in the face of increased tax burdens, economic hardship, fiscal incompetence at home, and 'anti-Japanese immigrant fever' abroad. The Russo-Japanese conflict, which had been a large and difficult foreign war, seemed to have bequeathed equally large and difficult problems in domestic postwar management [*sengo keiei*]."[19]

Most ominous of all was the picture that began to emerge as the precipitous changes in lifestyle and livelihood attendant to the transforming political economy began to be felt. Even though Japan remained a rural nation with a dual economy that was still primarily agricultural, steep growth in urbanization—the percentage living in cities with a population of over 50,000 doubling from 1888 and 1913—and the size of the industrial labor force—nearly a twenty-fold increase between 1888 and 1909[20]—contributed to a sense of the countryside being abandoned and the cities swelling with a deracinated proletariat. Rural youth, many of whom had taken ad-

---

14   Gordon, *Labor and Imperial Democracy in Prewar Japan*, 2, 28–29, 33.

15   Skya, *Japan's Holy War*, 154.

16   Gluck, *Japan's Modern Myths*, 175.

17   Ibid., 31.

18   Ibid., 31–32.

19   Ibid., 158.

20   Ibid., 32.

vantage of local investments in education, seemed especially susceptible to the lure of opportunity in the big city as tenancy in their villages increased to 45.5 percent in 1908 and large land holdings became more and more concentrated.[21] By "1911 only forty percent of Tokyo's inhabitants had been born there" and "Osaka doubled its 1897 population by 1916, reaching 1.5 million people."[22] Particularly problematic were the heterodox ideologies devised to entice this self-aware and individuated new urban workforce. On the one hand, a literature of success appeared that dispensed not only practical advice on how to increase one's job prospects in a difficult employment market, but a "social ideology of success" in the name of "rising in the world" (*risshin shusse*) that "enjoined not cooperative community spirit but personal striving."[23] On the other hand, the socialist and anarchist movements whose antiwar activities had, as we saw in Chapter 4, represented "social conscience in wartime society"[24] gained momentum in the rapidly industrializing, urbanizing conditions of the postwar period and began to shape the burgeoning labor movement.[25] In a word, the civilization that seemed to be materializing with these accelerating demographic transformations was not the organic polity that the Meiji modernizers had worked to construct. Instead, a potentially radicalized mass society had evolved, one in which the earlier achievements in nation-building appeared in jeopardy as individuals—in a sort of counterorganicism—placed their own interests above or on an equal par with that of the state.

The identification of this *bunmei-byō* (civilization sickness) with the centrifugal propensities of "subjectively free" individuals comes vividly across in the tendency among postwar commentators to portray Japan as a nation inflicted by an epidemic of social fevers.[26] For the inclination of postwar rural youth to leave their ancestral occupations for the jobs, education, and temptations available in Tokyo, Osaka and other urban centers, there was "city fever" (*tokainetsu*).[27] For the "numbers of nouveaux riches" successfully involved in speculation in the wake of the victory over Russia and who "pur-

---

21 Ibid., 33–34.
22 Ibid., 33.
23 Ibid., 206.
24 Shimazu, *Japanese Society at War*, 42.
25 Gordon, *Labor and Imperial Democracy in Prewar Japan*, 107.
26 Gluck, *Japan's Modern Myths*, 31.
27 Ibid., 159.

sued extravagance (*shashi*) and ostentation (*fuka*)" regardless of national well-being, there was not only "business fever" (*kigyōnetsu*) but the related "enterprise fever" (*jitsugyōnetsu*), "get-rich-quick market fever" (*ikkaku senkin no sōba netsu*) and even "go! go!-ism" (*yareyareshugi*).²⁸ And, finally, for the growing mania among large swaths of the population to transcend their station through the pursuit of higher education—a trend which was producing scores of educational idlers (*koutō yūmin*)—there was education fever. As Gluck concludes, these

> fevers represented a veritable catalogue of the attributes of a modernizing society. In the case of Japan they were but the economic, social, and technological results of the early Meiji reforms. It was as if the nation's eager pursuit of civilization had involved it in a process whose consequences lay far enough beyond the limit of contemporary vision that they now appeared to be a series of plagues unleashed upon Japan by some force that had not been reckoned with. Although the late Meiji ideologues did not regard cities, enterprise, education, and reading as social ills in themselves, they were nonetheless unprepared for the consequences of their diffusion, especially when these were associated with the breakdown of the agrarian order in the countryside and the emergence of new forms of social conflict in the cities and factories.²⁹

We might go further than this and argue that the attribute of modernization, the consequence of the pursuit of civilization that most unnerved the one-time reformers was the license that this opening and increasingly abstract society afforded individuals to evaluate the world around them after their own lights and self-consciously participate in forging the normative basis of their interpersonal existence. Whether joining industrial strikes, leaving their ancestral homes for urban opportunities, pursuing higher education, speculating on the market to get rich quick, reading newspapers and tantalizing naturalistic fiction, or entertaining radical political doctrines, members of the newly self-aware masses were beginning to decide on their own life courses with scant reference to the concrete relations of the traditional village or the needs of an expanding empire. As tentative as they may

---

28 Ibid., 159–60, 210.
29 Ibid., 177–78.

appear from the vantage point of more extensive transformations in later decades, for those who sought to maintain social cohesion in the aftermath of the Russo-Japanese War these first steps toward genuine individual autonomy looked like a disintegration into a chaos of unregulated designs and desires. The decadence of *bunmei-byō* was, in their estimation, a nomic crisis, an indicator that the integrating norms, conventions, laws, and customs that had always been taken for granted were now frayed and falling asunder.

Their correctives to the anomy ushered in by this perceived acceleration of socioeconomic change would determine the shape of orthodoxy for the next forty years. "For an industrializing economy they reinvigorated an agrarian myth, and in an urbanizing society they apotheosized the village. In the face of *Gesellschaft*, *Gemeinschaft* was invoked; confronted with increasing individuation and even anomie, ideologues enshrined the family."[30] What these pro-state ideologues sought to invoke, above all, were the concrete, organic values and relations of the communal past. The "socio-moral bonds"[31] of farms, villages, and patriarchal extended families would form the social foundations of the nation and "serve as bulwarks against the disintegration of society in the future" and "the negative social consequences of progress."[32] The final years of the Meiji period turned out to be a fertile time to establish these nomic foundations because of the "momentary congruence"[33] between these tribalist evocations and the rural upbringing of the majority of the *kokumin*. Postulating "the retrieval of a world that beckoned even as if it was disappearing,"[34] these familiar values would be "scrubbed and polished and enshrined" with more and more fervor during the coming decades even as continuing socioeconomic change rendered them less and less congruent with experience.

The origin of this orthodoxy, as we saw in Chapter 1, is the *Sittlichkeit* (ethical life) or civil morality devised to complement the new constitution that was being promulgated in 1889. A confluence of concerns both inside and outside the government about the politicization of the masses, the divisiveness of parliamentary partisanism, the lack of nation-mindedness, the insufficiency of moral education in the schools and, above all, the deteriora-

---

30 Ibid., 265.
31 Ibid., 110.
32 Ibid., 273.
33 Ibid., 267.
34 Ibid., 266.

tion of the integrating values and customs from the past resulted in the formulation of a civic ethos which was, like the constitution, handed down by
the emperor to people. As Gluck describes it the "Imperial Rescript on Education" was a "mixed and homogenized"[35] document that was readily accepted across the sociopolitical spectrum as a "national doctrine [kokkyō]"[36]
because it expressed what was already intuitively accepted as "familiar code
of customary social morality."[37] Presented as "the Way," this "civic creed"[38]
construed the continuity, unity, and obedience of the historical community
of Japanese subjects to be rooted in the virtuous spirit of loyalty and filial piety toward the imperial line and "Our Imperial Throne, coeval with heaven
and earth."[39]

The Rescript was "on education" not only because worries about moral
education had initiated the debate that led up to its codification but because Yamagata and others saw education, along with the military, as an especially effective "tutelary apparatus"[40] for turning national sentiments of
"unity and cooperation" into the "second nature"[41] of imperial subjects. Indeed, "the ideological message purveyed to elementary schoolchildren was
probably the most codified in content and single-minded in goal of any to
which late Meiji Japanese were exposed."[42] Despite the ideological unreli-
ability of many of its teachers and the interference of a stratified bureaucracy
not completely under its control, the Ministry of Education managed to establish the Rescript as the basis of moral education in 1891. Three compulsory hours per week were devoted to moral instruction (shūshin) with much
of the class time focused on manners and morals. Not only was the Rescript
memorized, recited and analyzed phrase by phrase in the classroom with
historical figures and folk legends invoked to illustrate its content, but it became the centerpiece of solemn school ceremonies which, with the help
of ministry directives that proscribed its ritual handling, conjured the authority of the imperial throne.[43] By 1903, when the government took over

---

35 Ibid., 121.
36 Ibid., 106–7.
37 Ibid., 127.
38 Ibid.
39 Ibid., 121.
40 Ibid., 147.
41 Ibid., 118.
42 Ibid., 147.
43 Gordon, *A Modern History of Japan*, 106–7.

the compilation of elementary school textbooks, the "Way" of the Rescript became the moral basis of "uniform and national texts"[44] that were not removed from the classroom until the end of the Second World War.

Although the Rescript was crafted as a secular document in order to satisfy the Western powers during the push for treaty revision that Japan had achieved a civilized separation of church and state, its language opened the door to the sanctification of this civic ethos of the "Way." In particular, the text included, along with gestures to Confucianism, the concept of *kokutai* (national body or essence) from Aizawa Seishisai's Mito writings and the nativist National Learning School.[45] In its opening sentence the Rescript had explicitly identified the "glory of the *kokutai*" with the historical continuity of "*waga kōso kōso*"—our imperial ancestors from Amaterasu and Jimmu through the unbroken line of historical emperors."[46] Satisfying the requirements to ground the nation in the imperial tradition and establish "national classics"[47] as an apolitical, nonreligious basis of education and government—requirements respectively stipulated by the two main compilers, Motoda Nagazane, a Confucianist,[48]and Inoue Kowashi, a student of Prussian organic theories of the state—this "emperor-centered historical view,"[49] as Migita calls it, provided the opening for Shinto to stage a comeback and begin to entwine itself into the civil morality. Though at the beginning of the Meiji period, as part of the effort to restore imperial power, a distinct Department of Shinto (*jingikan*) had been created, the secularizing policies of *bunmei kaika* in the 1870s and concerns with treaty revision during the subsequent decade resulted in the disestablishment of this department and a separation of rites and religion. Shinto was granted an ambiguous status as a nonreligion in charge of imperial rites which were deemed as a secular function of state. With the emphasis on what some in the press called "*kokutai-ism*"[50] in the Imperial Rescript on Education, Shinto gradually began to return to prominence, taking advantage of the role its ritual practices were accorded by Inoue Kowashi and others as "the foundation of the nation"

---

44 Gluck, *Japan's Modern Myths*, 147.
45 Ibid., 123. For Aizawa's writings, see Wakabayashi, *Anti-Foreignism and Western Learning in Early-Modern Japan*.
46 Ibid., 139.
47 Ibid., 123.
48 Ibid.
49 Migita, *Tennosei to Shinkaron*, 10–14.
50 Gluck, *Japan's Modern Myths*, 126.

and "the source of custom."[51] As the interpretation of the Rescript shifted from morality to loyalty and patriotism in the 1890s under the influence of the philosopher Inoue Tetsujirō—another enthusiast for German organic theory of the state and one of the reformist statits we discussed in Chapter 1—controversies concerning the political loyalty of Japanese Christians, fears of mixed residence, and, most of all, the Sino-Japanese War of 1894–95 raised the profile of shrines and Shinto theology as distinctively native and therefore intrinsic to authentic national sentiment. By 1900 a Shrine Bureau (*Jinjikyoku*) had been set up in the Home Ministry and while the priesthood still lacked full financial support, ideological preeminence and a ministry of its own, this position of administrative preference would supply the leverage needed to cosmicize the normative injunctions of the Rescript as a sanctified doctrine.

As we will see later in the chapter, this attempt at cosmicization intensified in the aftermath of the Russo-Japanese War. It was at this time that the idealization of the social past as represented by the concrete, communal relations of farm, village, and family began to combine with notions of the genealogically based *kokutai* and result in the conception of the nation as a *kazoku kokka* or family-state. Engaged in an "ideological offensive against social change"[52] after the war, Shinto, in effect, responded to the postwar anomy of *bunmei-byō* not just by extolling the organic mores and customs of rural life, but, by going further and identifying such norms and conventions with the cosmic narrative of the nation as a whole. The decadence that was evident in the break-up of villages, the rootlessness of city life, and the waning of patriarchal authority could be staved off by enshrining this nomos through the restorative function of imperial rites. Even if social fevers threatened to pull the national body apart, the sanctification of "socio-moral bonds" would conserve its primordial cohesion, returning it to a "former state of health."[53] The nation-state conceived as an extended family would resist the corrosiveness of modern "progress" by rendering its norms, conventions, and laws as changeless manifestations of a sacred ontology.

This tribalist vision can best be understood as a form of reactionary historicism. That is to say, it is a conception of history that regards change as

---

51 Ibid., 139.
52 Ibid., 186.
53 Ibid., 177.

decadent and the preservation of original conditions as a measure of timeless perfection and health. The primordial tribe of the family-state, identical
with the imperial ancestors and their extended family, the Yamato *minzoku*,
embodied communitarian virtues and any deviation from its ageless customs and conventions represented disintegration and decline. It was precisely in this reactionary manner that the term *kokutai* came to be regarded
in the aftermath of the Russo-Japanese War. Gluck explains how no less a
figure than Itō Hirobumi—perhaps the original reformist statist in Japan—
went from seeing the *kokutai* in 1884 as a "general name for the land, people,
language, clothing, shelter, and institutions of state, and as such it was only
natural that it change with the times"[54] to agreeing in 1908 with the emerging statist consensus that the *kokutai* is immutable, an unchanging essence
and, by extension, a verification of Japan's uniqueness. As we have seen, the
intervening years witnessed a growing sense of anomy, a perception that the
social foundations were decaying under the new modern constitutional order and needed to be solidified against corrosive change. The family-state
construal of the *kokutai* offered just the antidote to this "civilization sickness": "by generalizing the living emperor into a timeless series of emper-
ors-in-sequence, *kokutai* seemed to offer the abstract grandeur possessed by
such notions as *patrie* or *Vaterland* in the West. *Kokutai* provided a past that
was ageless, continuous, and secure in its ancestral tradition."[55] Immutable
and consecrated as coextensive with the national body, the nomos of Japan's
civic creed was immunized against the plague of modern decadence.

Anomic Evolutionism

As we will see at the conclusion of this chapter, the inadequacy of this reactionary statist response to change would soon become apparent even to
younger acolytes of the state Shinto movement who would began to transform its orthodoxy into a doctrine more amenable to the awakened masses
of early-twentieth-century Japan. Oka Asajirō, however, was not faced with
this problem. Though, as we saw in earlier chapters, he agreed that the nomic
basis of the sociopolitical order needed to be reengrained in the populace,

---

54 Ibid., 145.
55 Ibid., 145–46.

he was not hampered by a doctrine whose instinctive response to change was to try to arrest it. Instead, evolutionism conveyed a message of inevitable change and future development and thus was inherently more congruent with the fluid life experiences of the modern *kokumin*. Oka's primary challenge consisted in finding the means of controlling the change he saw around him by channeling it into the healthy, reintegrating process of future growth envisioned by evolutionary theory.

What Oka began to confront around 1907 was that gradual reform, or what we have called reformist scientism, was not up to this task. Itō Hirobumi may have reached a similar conclusion about the changing "national organization"—as he sometimes referred to the *kokutai*—and thus, as we have seen, opted to throw his hat in with the consensus that this "national polity" was immutable. For Oka the problem with reforming the nation to conform with the conditions set down by his metapolitics was that the "subjectively free" mass society had the option of either ignoring pronouncements on evolutionary necessity—such as the human-way—or, more often than not, misconstruing their purport. It was probably not until he was writing "Ideal Group Life" that Oka came to comprehend that his program to engender the human-way as instinct implied that humans would no longer possess the capacity to deviate from it—it would, like religion and morality, prevent wrongdoing before it occurs, preempting choice with a predisposition for moral conduct. His challenge then was the somewhat paradoxical one of presenting his necessary truths in a manner that ensured that they were necessarily accepted and internalized. In a sense, the *kokumin* were being asked to choose nomic instincts because they had, in actuality, no choice but to do so.

The obstacles to getting this subtle message across were, as Oka discovered in the complicated society of postwar Japan, daunting. As we pointed out at the beginning of this chapter, he had by 1907 come to despair that the superorganismic aim of human advancement was "hardly possible"[56] to attain in the present age. "Ideal Group Life," in fact, can be read as a catalogue of the metapolitical failures of his reformist scientism. Human beings have no choice but to "blush for shame" and experience "unbearable envy"[57]

---

56   Oka, "Risōteki Dantai Seikatsu" [Ideal group life], 74.
57   Ibid., 70, 74.

when they recognize that moss animal colonies do without the institutions that humans depend on to coerce and cajole individual persons into a virtuous collectivism. The very existence of things such as laws, religion, morality, government, lawyers, police departments, private property, and status distinctions speaks to the "extreme imperfection of human group life."[58] As we saw, in one of the more wry passages in this essay, Oka imagines passing the "loftily standing large and imposing judicial and legislative buildings in the capital"—which are surrounded by humans proudly "taking photographs of them and making picture postcards"—and whispering to himself that "to an insect's [moss animal *mushi* or zooid] way of thinking this is embarrassing."[59] Unlike moss animal nations where instinctual altruism predisposes individuals to automatically adhere to the Golden Rule with that result that "there is never any mutual strife,"[60] the human nation-state is characterized by "continual infighting day and night" because "humans are naturally self-interested, doing to others what they would not have done to themselves."[61] It is due to this innate egoism that "laws and police forces are necessary, and religion and morality cannot be abandoned."[62]

Although he concludes his essay by admitting that humans can never fully attain the perfection of moss animal nations, he continues to recommend the steps necessary for approximating the ideal life embodied in these paragons of nomic cohesion: "recasting human nature" and "eliminating selfishness."[63] A new humanity, one in which egoism has given way to an embrace of the higher self of the nation, remains the "aim of human advancement." However, what has become somewhat more pronounced by 1907 is how Oka holds individual egoism responsible, either directly or indirectly, for this anomy. It is the fading prospect that these self-interested and self-aware members of a contentious civil society would imbibe, appreciate, and internalize the necessities expressed by his metapolitics that goads Oka to contemplate more radical measures than mere reform.

At its most basic level Oka's disdain for modern individualism concerned the license to capriciousness and even frivolity that it afforded members of

---

58 Ibid., 72.
59 Ibid.
60 Ibid., 73.
61 Ibid., 74.
62 Ibid.
63 Ibid.

society. While his essays consistently championed the spirit of science and free enquiry, he did not do so, as some scholars have intimated,[64] to untether individuals and their personal preferences and desires from higher duties. Instead fee scientific enquiry and research were meant to expose the necessary conditions of group survival and lead to technological applications that would advance the prospects of the nation. In postwar Japan this "new civilized knowledge"[65] was, Oka believed, being neglected. According to him, Japan had become complacent[66] with its new status as a first-rank power after the victory over Russia. In reality, although Japan might be able to momentarily match the other powers in strictly military matters, "when looking at areas other than war, one regretfully wonders a great deal whether Japan is inferior to nations of even the third or fourth rank."[67] Japan was particularly far behind in the "war of peace,"[68] the technological and economic preparations that, as we saw in Chapter 4, occurred during the intervals between inevitable autarkic struggles. One only had to perform a cross-national comparison of the advertising sections of magazines and newspapers, which Oka regarded as "small mirrors reflecting the circumstances in a society,"[69] to grasp how backward Japan was. Whereas, "civilized knowledge is overflowing" in the advanced nations with a great deal of space "occupied by such things as automobiles, motorboats, gas-electric motor engines, jars of liquid oxygen and hydrogen, glassworks where quartz is melted, leasing radium, and many ticket offerings for flight examination places," Japanese advertisements focus on "patent medicines and cosmetics," and hardly include even "old-fashioned things like steam-engines."[70] Japan's facility with value-adding "new civilized knowledge" is so pitiful that its only original technological accomplishment is the "noodle machine"[71] mentioned in the last chapter—a device that is, in fact, inferior to the German toys on sale in the Ginza shopping district of Tokyo. Most of the domestic technology is either imported or, worse, poorly copied from the West, while Japan's exports consist in raw materials or handicrafts that, despite the condescending praise they receive from foreign-

---

64 Migita, *Tennosei to Shinkaron*, 42; Tsukuba, *Oka Asajirō Shū*, 437–47.
65 Oka, "Minzoku no Hatten to Rika" [Science and the development of the race-nation], 108.
66 Ibid., 114.
67 Ibid., 112.
68 Oka, "Sensō to Heiwa" [War and peace], 86.
69 Oka, "Minzoku no Hatten to Rika" [Science and the development of the race-nation], 109.
70 Ibid.
71 Oka, "Kyōiku to Meishin" [Education and superstition], 118.

ers who like to call Japan a "fine arts nation," are indistinguishable from the products of the most primitive nations or even "stone age men."[72]

Rather than concentrating on the essential task of absorbing the scientific knowledge needed for national cohesion and technological prowess, the individuals of the mass society allowed themselves to be enticed by alluring, yet intellectually questionable surrogates for science. Toward the end of this chapter we will see that the ultimate false surrogate proved to be the Shinto orthodoxy and its efforts at cosmicizing the "sociomoral" conventions of an idealized communal-familial past. Yet preliminary to susceptibility to such "superstitions," as Oka will allude to them, came, a fondness for fashionable ephemeralities among the individuated *kokumin*. Japanese society not only prefers cosmetics to the wonders of modern technology, but "advertisements for fortune-telling line the inside of trains and the pages of daily newspapers feature articles on astrology."[73] More crucially, when serious systems of thought appear, they are treated as mere fads.[74] As Oka explained in 1911, "just as a striped pattern which is the rage today in Tokyo will in a few months reach remote areas to become the rage there, it is certain, based on past examples, that theories which are being put forth in the West with great fanfare are in full flourish a few years later in Japan."[75] No matter its content there exists in Japan a "tendency to thoughtlessly prize and overestimate a theory while it is en vogue without plumbing its true value."[76] "Whatever the theory may be, while it is the rage in our country, everyone and his brother advocates it. Yet after a year or half a year it is as if there is a rule that the theory is forgotten and there is no memory of it."[77]

Darwin Boom

Although, as will be explored in the next chapter, Oka was anticipating in this passage the coming impact of the eugenics and racial hygiene movement in Japan, these generalizations about national fickleness really had to

---

72 Oka, "Minzoku no Hatten to Rika" [Science and the development of the race-nation], 111.
73 Oka, "Kyōiku to Meishin" [Education and superstition], 123.
74 Asajirō Oka, "Minshu Kaizengaku no Jissai Kachi" [The actual value of the study of racial improvement], in *Shinka to Jinsei* [Evolution and human life] (Tokyo: Yūseidō Shuppan, 1968), 197.
75 Ibid.
76 Ibid.
77 Ibid.

do with the theory of evolution. Oka believed this theory "should have a tremendous influence on the future of our ethnic nation [*minzoku*],"[78] and, in fact, it had also "taken the world by storm"[79] in the preceding years. In the aftermath of its war with Russia, Japan was, in fact, swept up in a "Darwin boom," a mania instigated, according to Migita, by the popularity of Oka's own writings. While disseminating evolutionism was the implicit goal of all Oka's endeavors, dismay at its fate in the marketplace of ideas coupled with fears over the prospect that evolution would be "in fashion temporarily and afterwards be forgotten all at once,"[80] motivated a fundamental transformation in how he attempted to actualize his metapolitics. Indeed, to a significant degree, Oka's sense of anomy can be attributed to the unwieldy ways that evolutionism was taken up and appropriated during this so-called Darwin boom. *Shinkaron* (evolutionary theory) came to mean many things to many people, and while, as I will argue, Oka's organicist scientism had a tremendous long-term impact in Japan, from 1907 onward it looked to him that a cacophony of interests was seizing upon his message and leaving the nation without the integrating metapolitical basis it needed to survive.

The mania for Darwin culminated in 1909, the centennial of his birth and the semicentennial of the *Origin of Species*. Arranged by organizations such as the Tokyo Academic Society for Animals and the Academic Association for Humanity, a cluster of celebratory events and exhibitions were held in that year across the country which included a "Conference to Commemorate Darwin" and a "Darwin Festival."[81] A controversial exhibit that was part of the Darwin Festival seems to have played an especially significant role in piquing interest in the English naturalist. From the early Meiji period rumors had circulated in Japan that the HMS *Beagle*, the British sloop-of-war Darwin had boarded on his voyage to South America and the Galápagos Islands, had been acquired by the Japanese navy and used as a practice ship. These rumors were confirmed by the journalist Shiga Shigetaka, editor of the magazine *Nihonjin*, who claimed that the ship had been dismantled and only its cabin remained intact. Darwin's cabin, accordingly, became the main exhibit at the Darwin Festival. In response to these sensational claims,

---

78 Ibid., 198.
79 Ibid., 197.
80 Ibid., 198.
81 Migita, *Tennosei to Shinkaron*, 29–30.

Watase Shousaburō, a professor of natural sciences at Todai who had started a Darwin Research Association in 1905, independently researched the matter and presented his findings at a Memorial Meeting for Darwin sponsored by the Tokyo Zoology Society on 24 November 1909 to mark the fiftieth anniversary of the *Origin of Species*. In Watase's view, the warship in question, the *Kenko*, whose cabin had been retrieved at Shinagawa wharf, may have once been an English ship called the *Beagle*. However, structural analysis of the Japanese ship revealed that it was not the boat on which the father of natural selection had sailed. It was, Watase concluded and newspapers across the country reported, a case of "same name, different vessel."[82]

Migita conveys the excited controversy that the Darwin Festival and its enigmatic sea cabin inspired by citing a passage from the diary of Takamura Mitsutarō, which recounts an episode that occurred the same day as Watase's lecture. Takamura describes attending the "Third Ministry of Education Exhibition" and, while standing before a statue representing "Primitive Man," suddenly finding himself surrounded by a gaggle of coeds who avidly launched into a discussion of Darwin's *Descent of Man*. Not only did these educated young women judge the statue according to the "philosophical" and "scientific" values delineated by Darwin, but they were familiar enough with translations of his writings that they were able to mimic his supposed manner of speaking.[83] In Migita's estimation, instances such as this one illustrate that "for late Meiji intellectuals" and would-be intellectuals "Darwin became an exceedingly bewitching intellectual symbol."[84] Though during the earlier phase of interest in evolution which occurred in the late 1870s and 1880s Herbert Spencer was the figure associated with evolutionary theory and the names of "outside specialists" such as Darwin were hardly known,[85] a survey of "318 intellectuals and members of the elite" conducted by *Jiji Shinpō* (News of current events) in 1909 make it clear that Darwin had, by this time, far eclipsed Spencer. Entitled "A Selection of 100 Foreign and Domestic," the survey ranked "The Social Philosophy of Spencer" eighty-third, but elevated the *Origin of Species* to the twenty-third position overall and fifth among foreign books. Migita cites this as evidence that

---

82 Ibid., 32.
83 Ibid., 58–59.
84 Ibid., 32.
85 Ibid., 28.

"intellectuals of the late Meiji worshiped and believed in Darwin and the writings on the evolution of living things."[86]

Yet Migita also admits that the "primary medium" for introducing "the shocking implications that the theory of organic evolution held" were "the successively published books and essays that Oka Asajirō produced from 1904 onwards."[87] In fact, another survey from 1909, this time published by *Taiyō* (The sun), a magazine for general readers, and focused on "up-and-coming" Japanese at the forefront of their respective fields, saw Oka garnering a large number of votes and being identified as a main authority in "the world of science."[88] Migita attributes Oka's prestige, which would only grow in the coming years and climax in his selection to the Imperial Academy in 1925, to *Lectures on Evolutionary Theory*, first published in 1904, and *Evolution and Human Life*, the 1906 anthology which is the main focus of our study. *Lectures on Evolutionary Theory* was, in particular, met with a "massive response"[89] upon its publication in January of 1904, selling out nearly 60,000 copies. Migita cites a passage from the diary of a female member of family of legal scholars who bought her copy at a well-known Tokyo bookstore on the last day of the year and subsequently spent the evening reading it aloud "with great rapidity to everyone present," covering "more than 100 pages" in a single breathless sitting.[90] The nineteen-year-old future anarchist Ōsugi Sakae, whom we will deal with later in this chapter, likewise obtained a copy as soon as he could and reported that it was "interesting beyond endurance. Each line was like an unknown, fantastically wondrous world that emerged before my eyes to the point that I was dizzy."[91]

The popularity of this general introduction to evolution and biology was perhaps most remarkable in how it was sustained over the decades: fourteen editions in all appeared between 1904 and 1940,[92] with expanded and revised eleventh and thirteenth editions being published in 1914 and 1925, respectively.[93] There are even reports that it was the one book that returnees from

---

86 Ibid., 29.
87 Ibid., 33.
88 Ibid., 35.
89 Ibid., 34.
90 Ibid.
91 Ibid., 36.
92 Matsunaga, "Evolutionism in Early Twentieth Century Japan," 221.
93 Migita, *Tennosei to Shinkaron*, 35.

Manchuria in 1945 regretted not being able to bring back with them.[94] Its sequel, *Evolution and Human Life*, was also a best seller which saw enlarged editions appearing as late as 1921. The essays from which this and later anthologies were comprised were, as we have previously stated, often featured in leading publications. In the late Meiji period alone "from his debut article in *Chūō Kōron* (The central review), "Mankind's Struggle for Existence," in October 1905 to the appearance of "Theories and Evidence for Heredity" in the May 1912 issue, he contributed a total of ten essays to the magazine. Among these were four that appeared in the opening pages and most are comprised of essays that deal with the theory of evolution."[95] One of his former students, Takakuwa Yoshi, related that Oka's publications in *Chūō Kōron* were met with great fanfare, "absorbing the attention"[96] of the readership.

The combined effect of the Darwin boom and his own engaging and accessible writings appeared to be just what Oka had hoped for: converting the younger, school-age generation to the evolutionary worldview. And, indeed, another survey carried out in 1909 seems to confirm his success in the meeting his objective: when 900 members of the younger generation, most of whom were in the twenty–to–twenty-one-year-old range, were asked "Is the theory of the evolution of living things true?" a full 70 percent answered in the affirmative with only 3 percent rejecting the theory outright.[97] However, as we have seen, what concerned Oka was that this popularity was fleeting, yet another passing fad, and that the intrinsic value of evolutionary theory was not being appreciated or absorbed. In particular, the social and political conclusions drawn from the theory not only stood in stark variance with his interpretation of its significance for humankind but actively subverted what he was trying to achieve as a scientist, educator, and author. For Oka the message that evolutionary necessity conveyed was that individuals must subordinate themselves to the concrete whole of the ethnic nation by practicing a race-specific, altruistic "way." Inculcated in the population through education, this organicist "way" would engender a normative disposition through what we have called nomic instincts and thereby turn the nation-state into a human approximation of the superorganisms found in nature.

---

94   Tsukuba, "Kaisetsu" [Commentary], 430–31.
95   Migita, *Tennosei to Shinkaron*, 35.
96   Ibid. See the Introduction for a discussion of the significance of *Chūō Kōron* in the Meiji era.
97   Ibid., 44–45.

Though fellow members of the intelligentsia held positions that roughly corresponded to Oka's approach, popular appropriations in the "boom" period of Darwinism after the war did not seem to endorse this corporatist biology. Instead, diverse responses to evolution appeared which tended to celebrate not organic cohesion but individual endeavor.

Such anomic individualism was most apparent in the postwar "ideologies of striving and success" that we encountered earlier. The message of *risshin shusse*, "getting ahead in the world," that magazines and self-help manuals peddled to individuals flooding the urban centers in search of a more and more elusive success was almost always couched in terms "not of social harmony but of Darwinian struggle for survival."[98] The "money world"[99] that many felt they had now entered was indistinguishable from this all-against-all struggle. Indeed, the "social fevers" of *bunmei byō* that moral commentators lamented can simply be seen as the intense and occasionally frenzied reaction of newly untethered individuals to a highly competitive "material civilization" where success and survival seemed to depend on personal striving. Education fever, city fever, and, most obviously, the forms of enterprise fever were, at bottom, manifestations of makeshift laissez-faire social Darwinism that had its precedents earlier in Japanese history. "Rising in the world" had been a Neo-Confucian value espoused during the Tokugawa period, but it was only with the modernization program and introduction of *shinkaron* in the early Meiji period that *risshin shusse* became conceptualized as a struggle for material success. Part of this was the result, as Gluck explains, of the ambiguous manner in which slogans such as "rich nation, strong army" seemed to turn the pursuit of mammon into a virtue.[100]

Yet the way *shinkaron* was first appropriated after its introduction by Hilgendorf and Morse in the mid-1870s was an equally important factor. While stray passages from the *Origin of Species* and the *Descent of Man* had been translated here and there in combination with commentary by Huxley and others, the overwhelming majority of evolutionary writings available in the 1880s and 1890s were those of Herbert Spencer. Not only had thirty-two translations of his works appeared in Japan by 1900, but coinages of his such as "survival of the fittest" (*yūsho reppai*), "struggle for survival"

---

98 Gluck, *Japan's Modern Myths*, 206.
99 Ibid., 207.
100 Ibid., 209; Oka, "Generational Conflict after the Russo-Japanese War," 203.

(*seizon kyōsō*) and "social evolution" become the lexicon of a "social Dar-winian" *shinkaron* that, as we suggested earlier, was not necessarily aware of Darwin himself. In the early Meiji period, when this Spencerian *shinkaron* was being appropriated, people's interest in evolution "consisted in its social and political implications rather than in a biological theory."[101] The socio-political implications of Spencer's evolutionism were clear: although he es-poused his own theory of the "social organism," Spencer was a liberal who promoted natural rights and looked forward to a peaceful, industrial society that cherishes individualism. The kind of superorganism that Oka idealized for its perpetual war mobilization and its total subordination of individuals to the commonweal was explicitly dismissed by Spencer as a "militant stage" that must be overcome in the course of social evolution. It was this liberal outlook that led Katō Hiroyuki to complain in 1900 that while "Spencer re-alized that importance of the organismic nature of society, he made an obvi-ous mistake in considering the security and happiness of individuals as the ultimate ends."[102]

During the early Meiji period this Spencerian individualism was con-strained by the nationalist goals of the modernizing state. *Risshin shusse*, accordingly, was embedded within collectivist aspirations—either, as we mentioned earlier, in elevating the reputation of one's family or village, or in acquiring a government post.[103] After the war with Russia, however, "ris-ing in the world" came to be about individual ambition and was measured by the "attainment of wealth."[104] According to Gluck, by this juncture *risshin shusse*, which she calls "the Meiji doctrine of progress expressed on the level of the individual"[105] had become part of the common sense of Japanese, one of the unremarkable "meanings socially held in common"[106] and taken for granted as true and relevant. Though Spencer himself was becoming a for-gotten figure in the late Meiji period, the new, more content-rich and biolog-ically based *shinkaron* promoted by Oka—and which finally included full translations of Darwin's works—in the context of a "complicated" open so-ciety led many to reach for *risshin shusse* which "had become the common

---

101 Shimao, "Darwinism in Japan," 93.
102 Nagai, "Herbert Spencer in Early Meiji Japan."
103 Oka, "Generational Conflict after the Russo-Japanese War," 198.
104 Ibid.
105 Gluck, *Japan's Modern Myths*, 257.
106 Ibid., 253.

justification for all manner of individual striving."[107] The Darwin boom, to Oka's dismay, was helping revive the sort of anomic, disembedding individualism that his sociopolitical essays were meant to overcome.

As we saw in the last chapter, Oka was not at liberty to just simply reject this sort of social Darwinism that championed individual striving. His human-way was to be embraced not because egoistic self-interest was bad in some final, ontological sense but because it undermined the nomic cohesion of the nation which he thought should be conceived as a higher form of organic individuality "selfishly" struggling for survival. At times Oka even seemed to suggest, like Katō Hiroyuki had (Chapter 1), that the higher egoism of groups, nations, and races had its origins in the ad hoc unions that individual persons had formed to ensure their survival. However, in the end, as we will explore in the next chapter, Oka came to regard the persistence of lesser egoism within these larger sociopolitical entities as the etiology of decadence. The failure of these individuated "persons" to reintegrate once the nation or race had epigenetically differentiated was evidence that nomic instincts were absent. Along with a number of symptoms of physical weakness apparent in the urbanizing, industrializing society of early-twentieth-century Japan, individuals who lived free of regulating norms and conventions indicated the onset of degeneration.

Left-wing Misappropriation

As many Japanese concerned with *shakai mondai* (social issues) did at this time, Oka associated this disembedded individualism as much with socialism and related doctrines, as with unregulated capitalism. One reason for this was that, as Shimazu has explained, the socialists and anarchists at the forefront of the antiwar movement in 1904–5 had championed individualism—indeed, their message was pitched more to middle-class individualists than to laborers.[108] A related and yet deeper reason was simply that the wholly new socioeconomic order that socialism and anarchism imagined depended on the preexistence of "free-thinking" individuals. It was such individuals whose interests would be satisfied in a socialistic order—and, despite

---

107 Ibid., 257.
108 Shimazu, *Japanese Society at War*, 36.

a collectivist rhetoric similar in many ways to Oka's, it was their well-being, considered in aggregate, that would be the ultimate measure of success. This opened the possibility that self-interested individuals could simply contrive a vision of a new order and attempt to implement it—in single step. Like the other social fevers of the 1900s, revolutionary action threatened to overturn the existing norms and conventions in the name of satisfying unmet aspirations. It could thereby potentially bring about what Yamagata ominously labeled *shakaihakaishugi*—"social destructionism."[109]

Oka was especially eager to dissociate himself from socialism and anarchism because his superorganisms were in danger of being construed as blueprints for a socialist utopia. After all, the imitable features he ascribed to moss animal colonies read like the demands of a radical political agenda: full employment, joint ownership of property, absence of class and status distinctions, and perfect harmony.[110] In fact, with his suggestion that law, morality, and government had been rendered superfluous inside moss animal nations, Oka's "ideal group life," at times, seemed to approach closer to anarchist doctrine than socialist. Due to these similarities Oka, in "Ideal Group Life" made it explicit that he was not endorsing anything like a revolutionary doctrine: "[I]t is absolutely impossible for contemporary human beings to try in a single bound to imitate moss animal society."[111] As he explains, "having joint ownership of property, getting rid of differences in wealth and poverty, abolishing the class system, leveling social distinctions among the people, and eliminating self-regard while promoting fellowship and mutual aid, it is hardly possible to do these things today."[112] The status quo should be maintained because it had "its beginnings in some original necessity and then passed, along with accompanying social changes, through a fixed historical path to arrive at its present state."[113] Humans remain selfish creatures and until human nature is "recast" the best that can be hoped for is gradual reform.

Of course, Oka's differences with the left ran much deeper than views on the historical pace of change. As Chapter 4 laid out, the evolutionary realpolitik Oka articulated in "War and Peace" and "Mankind's Struggle for Exis-

---

109 Gluck, *Japan's Modern Myths*, 176.
110 Oka, "Minshu Kaizengaku no Jissai Kachi" [The actual value of the study of racial improvement], 67–69.
111 Ibid., 74.
112 Ibid.
113 Ibid.

tence" was intended, in part, as a sharp retort to the peace movement and its espousal of the brotherhood of man. For Oka, collectivism was synonymous with war mobilization and the basis of equity and harmony in the life of the group was the fact that the "same blood circulates within the entire nation."[114] Given, then, these stark and fundamental differences it may be asked why Oka had to expend any effort at all, in the end, to distance his evolutionism from the left. The answer appears to be that for the non-Christian left Oka's evolutionism became an indispensable device for undermining the official orthodoxy that was being constructed around the lineage of the imperial house. Just as fevered individualists used Darwinism after the war to justify a Spencerian type of rising in the world, so socialists and anarchists found in the common ancestry of all organic life a powerful critique of the emerging *kokutai* system and its belief in the emperor-centered historical view.

The self-described materialists among the activist staff at the Heimin Association were especially enthusiastic about Oka's *Lectures on Evolutionary Theory.* As was discussed in Chapter 4, it was the publishing company Heiminsha that not only stood at the forefront of the antiwar movement but, through its newspaper, *Heimin Shimbun,* published a translation of Tolstoy's "Bethink Yourselves!" during the early months of the conflict. Though many among the left-wing activist vanguard would have agreed with the religious message that Tolstoy imparted, the materialists, most of whom considered themselves atheists, sought a secular basis for their humanitarian vision of social evolution. For the founders of the Heimin Association, Kōtoku Shūsui and Sakai Toshihiko, and the editor of the Heimin newspaper, Ōsugi Sakae,[115] the outline of organic evolution in Oka's *Lectures on Evolutionary Theory* fit the bill. It was Ōsugi who, as we saw earlier, claimed that "an unknown, fantastically wondrous world"[116] had been opened up by Oka's text. Looking back, he recalls avidly reading and discussing Oka with his colleagues at Heiminsha: the book enabled them not only to know "what biology or the theory of evolution is" but "understand the truth of human society seen from biology or evolutionary theory."[117] Eventually Ōsugi would describe himself as the "one faithful pupil of the Professor [Oka]."[118]

---

114 Ibid., 70.
115 Migita, *Tennosei to Shinkaron,* 35–36.
116 Ibid., 35–36.
117 Ibid., 36.
118 Ibid., 65–66.

The importance of Oka's *shinkaron* to the Heimin leadership was on display in the second issue of their newspaper. This 31 January issue opened with an editorial, most likely written by Kōtoku Shūsui, that explicitly stated that "it is doubtful that socialism contradicts the theory of evolution of living things."[119] Later on, in the section on "Introducing New Publications," Sakai Toshihiko favorably reviewed *Lectures on Evolutionary Theory*, which had been published in the preceding weeks, excitedly claiming that "its 800 pages are so appealing that it can be read in just a day or two. We finished reading it in one day."[120] The advertising section of the newspaper also went out of its way to promote Oka's book, according *Lectures on Evolutionary Theory* a place of prominence next to Kōtoku's *The Quintessence of Socialism*.

It was after the war, however, that the influence of *Lectures on Evolutionary Theory* became especially pronounced. Though the Commoner Association had been forced to disband for a second and final time in 1905,[121] the core of its non-Christian leadership—prominent among whom were Sakai Toshihiko, Yamagawa Hitoshi, Kōtoku Shūsui, and Ōsugi Sakae—managed to stick together and under the auspices of the Yurakusha Company put out a series of general science books in 1907 and 1908 with Sakai acting as general editor. Entitled *Commoner Science (Heimin Kagaku)* and projecting six volumes in all, this series intended to make up for the lack of basic science education in the schools by "supplying natural science for the proletariat"[122] at a fraction of the cost of other commercially available science texts. Central to this project of "making the working class knowledgeable" was the theory of "the evolution of living things" which Sakai and the other writers hoped would "provide an easily understood antithesis to the emperor-centered historical view."[123] According to Migita, the compilers of these *Commoner Science* texts "faithfully took their direction from Oka Asajirō."[124]

The History of Human Events, the first volume in the Commoner Science series, and *All Things Are One Family*, the sixth volume, both illustrate how the increasingly anarchist-leaning left hoped to use Oka to subvert belief in the historical *kokutai*. Published in November 1907, just as the Darwin

119 Ibid., 63.
120 Ibid., 64.
121 Ibid., 35.
122 Ibid., 65.
123 Ibid.
124 Ibid.

boom was gathering strength, and written by Sakai, *The History of Human Events* takes a particularly audacious swipe at both religion and the emperor-centered historical view:

> That the ancestors of humans are monkeys, lampreys, and single-celled organisms has no connection with the value of today's human beings. That humans are special things—beings that god has created especially—is no reason that the value of humans increases. Along with birds, animals, grass and trees, beings without souls and that are not humans carry on [with life]. Along with gold, stone, wind and water, inorganic, nonliving, inanimate objects carry on. Though we take pride in alone standing on the top as miraculous, excellent humans, this does not mean our position is rising and our happiness increasing. The theories of human uniqueness, god-creation, and the miraculous are the same as silly class ideas such as the divine country is 2,600 years old and, out of childish pride, to be thought of as different than others—or that our lineage continued as a distinguished family for generations since the time of the goddess of the east being granted territory.[125]

Published seven months later, in July 1908, *All Things Are One Family* was even more explicit in its appropriation from Oka, as can be seen in how its author, Ōsugi Sakai, explicated its title: "*All Things Are One Family* which means everything that comes to be in this universe is a relative, a kinsman. That is to say, the gist of this book is that all things have a common ancestor: things born in the water, the sand, holes in the earth, in trees, in palaces, or that live in nests or build empires. They are all of one lineage, one clan."[126]

As it happened, the publication of this series coincided with events on the other side of the Pacific Ocean that would provoke a brief yet significant crackdown against literature promoting *shinkaron*. On the third of November 1907, the same month in which Sakai's *History of Human Events* was released, a group of expatriate left-wing activists posted handbills in San Francisco on the porch of the Japanese consulate and around the city attacking the emperor. The occasion was the emperor's birthday and the group in question had been personally organized by the central figure of Heiminsha,

---

125 Ibid., 66.

126 Ibid., 65–66. Though Ōsugi would publish his own Japanese translation of the *Origin of Species* in 1914, he would criticize Oka in a May 1917 *Chūō Kōron* article entitled "Arguments with Professor Oka's Biological View of Human Society." See Tsukuba, "Kaisetsu" [Commentary], 430–55.

Kōtoku Shūsui. Kōtoku had spent five months, from February to July 1905, in Sugamo Prison for violating the press laws in connection with his anti-war activities at Heiminsha, and in the aftermath of his release he decided to travel to San Francisco in order to "criticize freely the position of 'His Majesty' from [a] foreign land where the pernicious hand of 'His Majesty' cannot reach."[127] The roughly seven months that Kōtoku passed in the United States—from December 1905 to June 1906—in the company of anarchist activists from a variety of nations and Japanese expatriate members of the San Francisco branch of Heiminsha—which outlived the Tokyo office—had the effect of radicalizing both him and, by extension, the Japanese socialist movement. Abandoning the strategy of socialist participation in parliamentary politics and embracing anarchist "direct action" tactics such as a general strike, Kōtoku, before returning to Japan in summer 1906 to help start a newspaper for the revived Japanese Socialist Party, put special effort into leaving behind "a well-organized core of young Japanese radicals"[128] on the model of contemporary would-be Russian revolutionaries who were able to criticize the Tsarist regime from exile in Switzerland. Focusing on Iwasa Sakutarō and Takeuchi Tetsugorō, Kōtoku managed to inaugurate the Social Revolutionary Party of Oakland (Okurando no Shakai Kakumei Tou) just four days before his departure. It turned out to be these two individuals who were primarily responsible for the "Emperor's Birthday Incident" a year and a half later, boldly distributing an "Open Letter to Mutsuhito, the Emperor of Japan, from Anarchist Terrorists."[129]

The closing lines of this handbill convey why, as Itoya Toshio and Matsuo Takayoshi argue, it "gave the ruling class quite a shock"[130]: "Your Excellency Matsuhito, old friend! Poor old friend, Mutsuhito! Your time is just about up. The bomb is right in your surroundings, just about to blow up. Bye, your Excellency, old friend."[131] Yet it was not just the threat to assassinate the emperor but the rationale for doing so that was particularly inflammatory to the Home Ministry and other organs of the state. Killing the emperor would reveal that he was a mere man, an impure and imperfect human—indeed, extremely imperfect given that his ancestors had

---

127 Notehelfer, *Kōtoku Shusui*, 116.
128 Ibid., 132.
129 Ibid., 152.
130 Migita, *Tennosei to Shinkaron*, 68.
131 Notehelfer, *Kōtoku Shusui*, 152–53.

been, as the letter claimed, "evil" and immoral" enslavers of the Japanese people. The emperor was therefore neither divine nor inviolable. In fact, blowing him up would verify his animal nature, confirming that his ancestors were not gods but—and this blasphemy was so appalling that Japanese newspapermen in San Francisco were reluctant to report it to their home offices—"primates."[132]

According to Itoya Toshio this use of the common ancestry of humans and animals constituted the "first documented case since the beginning of the Meiji era" of exposing the emperor-centered historical view as a fraud.[133] When the handbill was smuggled immediately into Japan, the Home Ministry scrambled to confiscate and suppress copies of it.[134] Hara Kei, the head of the ministry, alerted embassies and consulates around the world and a concerted effort was launched to investigate the background of the incident. Because of his role in the founding of the Oakland Social Revolutionary Party and his contributions to the *Revolution*, the newspaper of this Oakland party, advocating direct action and the violent overthrow of the political order,[135] Kōtoku was suspected from the beginning of having had a hand in the contents of the letter to the emperor. Kōtoku had, in fact, carried a copy of Haeckel's *The Riddle of the Universe* (see Chapter 3) with him to Sugamo Prison and studied it assiduously along with Kropotkin's *Fields, Factories and Workshops*.[136] He had also been slated to write the fourth installment of the Commoner Science series, a volume whose proposed title was *The Morality of the Animal World*.[137] As a result of the Home Ministry investigation of the Emperor's Birthday Incident, not only was this upcoming volume canceled but *The History of Human Events* and *All Things Are One Family* came under sales prohibition. From this point onward elements within the Home and Justice Ministries would associate the theory of evolution with "dangerous thoughts" in opposition to the national body (*kokutai*) and its historical roots.[138] Within the Ministry of Education it became common wisdom that knowledge of "evolution breeds socialism."[139]

132 Migita, *Tennosei to Shinkaron*, 68.
133 Ibid.
134 Ibid.
135 Notehelfer, *Kōtoku Shusui*, 153–54.
136 Ibid., 112–13.
137 Migita, *Tennosei to Shinkaron*, 69.
138 Ibid., 76.
139 Ibid., 108.

Oka soon felt the reverberations of these controversies. About the same time that the Commoner Science series received its punishment, the Imperial Household Agency and the Office of the Deputy Inspector targeted *Lectures on Evolutionary Theory*. As with the problems Oka ran into with initial publication of this text in 1904, questions were raised about the danger it might pose to public morals—yet on this occasion, in 1908, at the height of the "Darwin boom," it was, according to Tsukuba Hisaharu and Nezu Masashi, very nearly prohibited from sales.[140] The Special Higher Police also began to keep tabs on Oka, calling on him on several occasions.[141] Though unsuccessful in banning his best-selling text, the Imperial Household Agency broadened its efforts against Oka in the coming years by pushing for his dismissal from the Tokyo Higher Normal School and the Ministry of Education's textbook compilation committee. A former pupil of Oka's, Inoue Kiyoshi, claimed that the bureaucrats in the imperial household were particularly upset that the promoter of a theory that insults the sacred image of the imperial family was training teachers at a national normal school. In Migita's estimation, it can be said that "the government, from the late Meiji to the beginning of Taisho, hated the spread of evolutionary theory to the general public due to contradictions with the emperor-centered historical view and that, within this context, it continued to subject Oka to various forms of meddling."[142]

This continued "meddling" was certainly incited by the simultaneity of the Darwin boom and the escalating radicalism of the Heiminsha materialists. Not only the raucous Red Flag Incident of 1908 but, most especially, the High Treason Incident and Trial of 1910–11 seemed to confirm the "social destructionism" intended by those who had blasphemed the emperor as nothing but a mortal and highly corrupt primate. Even after the execution of Kōtoku and eleven of his alleged coconspirators on the emperor's life, the association of *shinkaron* with anti-imperial radicalism was further cemented with Ōsugi Sakae's translation of Darwin's *Origin of Species* in 1914–15.[143] By the late 1910s a Marxist Boom began to take hold among educated youth who considered materialism and evolutionary theory as axiomatic

---

140 Ibid., 78.
141 Ibid., 110.
142 Ibid., 116.
143 Ibid., 70.

and looked to Oka as one of the primary sources of this materialist message. In his *Shinkaron and Tennosei*, Migita cites various examples of young men whose reading of Oka in their teens led them first to discover Darwin, Huxley, Haeckel, and finally, from this historical materialist basis, to an engagement with Marx. For these future critics and opponents of the political order Oka provided the rudiments of an "alternative map"[144] to the cosmology being inculcated by the state.

Migita and other scholars have portrayed this appropriation of Oka as evidence to support their contention that Oka's writings amounted to an artfully indirect code to attack the emperor-centered historical view. From Migita's perspective, evolutionary theory and *kokutai* orthodoxy were utterly irreconcilable, with no overlap between the two, and the eventual triumph of science and socialism, along with the technological necessities of national survival, dictated that evolutionism would inevitably shoulder "*kokutai* supremacism"[145] aside. Oka's "alternative map" was destined to become the only map, and the embrace of his *shinkaron* by the materialist left suggests that they were together in furthering the "universal trend"[146] of modern history.

However, as our next chapter will delineate, Oka distanced himself from the left. For him, socialism and anarchism were manifestations of individualism and indicators of decadence. Surely part of Oka's reaction to the left had to do with the sense of chaos and internal division that events such as the Ashio Coal Strike of 1907, the Red Flag Incident of 1908, and the High Treason Incident conveyed. Yet at a more basic level his metapolitics was carefully crafted to promote higher unity and not only was it unequivocally nationalistic but it had hoped to reform the existing order, not overturn it. And, perhaps more to the point, while Oka's materialism and rejection of egoistic laissez-faire conditions made him intellectually closer to the socialists, the ethical purport, the normative intent, of his evolutionism was closer to that of the reactionary statists in the government. The left may have been able to translate his materialism and collectivism into its own idiom, which became increasing Marxist over the coming years, but this does not mean that Oka in any way endorsed the overthrow of the imperial system. Oka's

---

144 Ibid., 42.
145 Ibid., 78.
146 Ibid., 18. See Chapter 3, note 273, for a discussion of Migita's scientism.

approach was, instead, to pry the *kokumin* away from belief in the divine origins of an immutable national body (*kokutai*). The late-nineteenth-century notion of the *kokutai* was, after all, constructed in part out of organic conceptions of the nation-state. The superorganism was a correlate of this organic conception, an invention of the "corporate biology"[147] that socio-politically concerned evolutionary morphologists, race hygienists, and eugenicists had devised to promote national cohesion in the 1880s and 1890s. Oka's implicit hope seems to have been that the concrete, consanguineous ties of the family-state could be reinterpreted according to the biological terms of his metapolitics. What disturbed him about the left is that its apparent indifference to the moral and geopolitical aspects of his message jeopardized the concrete qualities, the organic cohesion, that he believed to be essential for national survival. To Oka, working away in his modest lab, the radical transformation imagined by socialists, anarchists, and Marxists did not seem like the beginning of a new age. It looked like the onset of anomy.

COSMIZATION OF THE FAMILY-STATE

Oka's dissociation with the left and his affinity with the government's goals of securing "social foundations"[148] were not lost on establishment elements who recognized the critical importance of a scientific view of the world for modern Japan. Sharing the same reformist scientistic perspective that Oka started out with, highly placed members of the intellectual community, especially those connected with the government, sought to protect evolutionism by placing brackets around its more "dangerous" truths. The biological view of the *kokumin* and the common ancestry of humans and other animals would be treated as "esoteric" truths, reserved for the educated elites and made available to them as part of the knowledge of the natural world necessary for effectively running the nation-state from behind the screen. The family-state orthodoxy (*kokutairon*) meanwhile, would be countenanced as a unifying device for public consumption—an "exoteric" truth doled out to the hoi polloi who would dissolve into a mass of striving individuals if they knew the harsh biological facts of the human condition. As we have al-

---

147 Weindling, *Health, Race and German Politics*, 45.
148 Gluck, *Japan's Modern Myths*, 157.

ready intimated in the previous two chapters, this was not Oka's position. Not only would this misappropriation of evolutionary theory, like the fevers of individualism and political radicalism, convince him that his message needed to take on a more urgently cosmological cast, but it would set up the central conflict of his career by opening the door to an aggressive promotion of a fundamentalist version of the family-state orthodoxy. Called "reactionary Shinto ultranationalism" by Walter Skya, this late Meiji version of state Shinto would prove to be Oka's primary contender for control of the normative disposition of the *kokumin*.

Bracketed Biology

It was the evolution "in parenthesis" outlook that most likely accounts for the failure to ban Oka's *Lectures on Evolutionary Theory* and remove him from the Tokyo Higher Normal School. According to Migita, it also explains why Ōsugi's was the last text pertaining to evolutionary theory subject to sales prohibition under the Meiji constitutional order. In fact, Migita wonders whether it was actually banned at all in the end.[149] In his view, the nationalist imperative to promote science that began during the Bakumatsu period and was placed front and center during the *bunmei kaika* era of the 1870s resulted in a "dualistic policy"[150] that held not only through the Taisho and early Showa periods but into the phase of "national body supremacism"— what we will call, after Skya, radical Shinto ultranationalism—of the 1930s and 1940s. According to this self-enforced doublethink, the dissemination of information on the theory of evolution would be tolerated so long as it did not touch on the roots of the imperial family. This approach was devised to satisfy both Home and Justice Ministry bureaucrats who considered evolutionism dangerously subversive, and reformists who regarded knowledge of modern natural science to be indispensable to national survival. The problem of the contradiction between the emperor-centered historical view and the common ancestry of humans and animals would be placed in parenthesis and—many seemed to have hoped—simply ignored. The Home and Justice Ministries, for instance, came to tacitly permit the spread of evolu-

---

149 Migita, *Tennosei to Shinkaron*, 76–77.
150 Ibid., 80.

tionary biology through society and no educators were arrested for teaching evolution in schools.[151] The *kokumin* would learn modern science and only the favored few at the elite educational entry points—in particularly Todai and Kyodai—would be privy to the "radical knowledge"[152] that the origins of the imperial house were not divine but simian.

One of the prime proponents of this "in parenthesis" approach was the founder of Todai, Katō Hiroyuki, who, as we saw in Chapter 1, had since the early 1880s been, in the spirit of reformist statism, basing the *kokutai* on the theories of organic individuality from evolutionary morphology. In 1907, as the Darwin boom was gaining momentum and anarchists were plotting the "Emperor's Birthday Incident," Katō, in a book entitled *Our National Body [Kokutai] and Christianity*, attacked Japanese Christians for placing their loyalty to God above their loyalty to the emperor. In response to this book, prominent Christian intellectuals in Japan homed in on the glaring historical contradiction at the heart of Katō's own thought—namely the discrepancy between the founding of the *kokutai* and the evolutionary account of human origins. Ebina Danjō, the president of Doshisha University, mocked that "Katō, perhaps as one may have expected, has brought his materialist evolutionism and the national body [*kokutai*] into concord. This is something we very much want to hear about. As an evolutionist, Professor Katō does not just believe human evolution is based on the history of the ethnic nation [*minzoku*] but on the development of plants and animals. We want to hear how he is able to do research both in a scientific vein and on the theory of the national body founded on folk classics."[153] Similarly, a protestant teacher, Muko Gunji, pointedly asked: "The professor, a believer in the notion that natural laws alone rule the universe, also places his imperial majesty under the rule of natural laws. Yet we must query the professor: Is his the viewpoint that the ancestors of human beings are primates—or does the imperial majesty have a supernatural existence?"[154]

Forced into a corner, Katō replied the following year, 1908, with an awkward attempt to reconcile *shinkaron* and the *kokutai*. Included in his book *Critique of a Critique*, Katō posited a two-phased approach to history

151 Ibid., 81.
152 Ibid., 57.
153 Ibid., 55.
154 Ibid.

whereby the theory of evolution applied up until the moment when the ethnic nations (*minzoku*)—perhaps drawing on Haeckel's monophyletic account of human evolution from *The History of Creation*—separated from one another. After such racial separation occurred paternalism prevailed over the life of the national body. As he explains at length:

> Because I believe in the theory of evolution I am certain beyond doubt that humans came about due to evolution. I can't believe in theories such as the special creation of organisms. However, my theorizing about the national body [*kokutai*] does not at all discuss such things from before the appearance of humans. Such matters are not necessary with regard to the national body. Only what occurred in the world of humankind after the ethnic nations separated is discussed. And since the Japanese ethnic nation was created, the emperor, from the head family, has taken hold of the supreme power of government rule; and we subjects, from the branch family, have done our obedient duty under this reign.[155]

In Migita's estimation this relegation of the national body and the theory of evolution to "different phases"[156] constitutes a deliberate avoidance of the problem concerning which view of human origins is correct. The whole troublesome issue was placed "in parenthesis." Katō "does not write that the theory of evolution and such apply also to the roots of the imperial family. However, he also consistently avoids declaring that the theory of evolution cannot be applied to the imperial family. Because it discusses an era since the appearance of humans his own discourse of the national polity makes it not at all necessary to bring up the period 'before humans' as explained by the theory of animal evolution."[157] According to Migita, this manner of coping with this intractable problem was common to prewar evolutionists and biologists and accounts for the fact that "rare are the examples that clearly refer to the problem of the imperial house's lineage from an evolutionary standpoint."[158]

Migita attempts to lump Oka in with this approach, claiming that he used "skillful rhetoric that was just barely legal" to "deny the emperor-centered historical view."[159] However, the primary consequence of this "in pa-

---

155 Ibid., 56. Also see Katō, *Meisōteki Uchūkan "Waga Kokutai to Kirisuto-kyō" no Hihyō no Hihyō*, 264–65.
156 Ibid., 57.
157 Ibid., 56–57.
158 Ibid., 57.
159 Ibid., 57.

renthesis" strategy—that it opened the door to fundamentalism and other forms of superstition—was anathema to Oka. A vivid example of this can be seen in the evolving position of Inoue Tetsujirō who, as we explored in Chapter 1 and earlier in this chapter, had written a widely distributed commentary for the government on the Rescript of Education in 1891 that "fabricated the rudiments of the family-state ideology from Confucian analogies of ruler to father and Western organic theories of the state."[160] Inoue had construed the Rescript as inculcating a sense of public duty and willingness to sacrifice that would prepare the nation for inevitable future emergencies: "[I]f we do not unite the people, fortifications and warships will not suffice. If we do unite them, then even a million formidable foes will be unable to harm us."[161] He identified the *kokutai* from the Rescript with "collective patriotism" and, like Katō, he turned against Japanese Christians, accusing them of "nonnationalism" in order to help highlight what true nationalism (*kokkashugi*) was. Also, like Katō, Inoue, who had spent most of the 1880s in Germany, was an enthusiast for evolutionism, recommending the *Origin of Species* and the *Descent of Man* when asked to comment in a 1902 journal survey on "the greatest writings of the nineteenth century."[162] In 1889, when prospects of mixed residency with Westerners was being considered, Inoue warned against the idea because the latest scientific theories had shown that Japanese possessed a smaller cranial capacity.[163] For Migita, Inoue represents the epitome of the esoteric-exoteric dichotomy: "publically declaring the dignity of the *kokutai*" while dismissing the emperor-centered historical view to "companions at the imperial university" and "cockily gossiping about the imperial family."[164]

Yet Migita is too quick to dismiss Inoue's stance to a "strong elite consciousness" eager "to confirm its own superiority by making a display of the latest knowledge which the public did not know."[165] As we will see with Oka, Inoue's position evolved as he was confronted with the limited effectiveness of merely enunciating a national ethos. For instance, Inoue, in the early 1890s, seemed to believe that it was a "civilizational advantage" of the

160 Gluck, *Japan's Modern Myths*, 129.
161 Ibid., 130.
162 Migita, *Tennosei to Shinkaron*, 61.
163 Gluck, *Japan's Modern Myths*, 136.
164 Migita, *Tennosei to Shinkaron*, 61–62.
165 Ibid., 62.

Japanese that they were "free of any religious affiliation."[166] Japan alone among the nations of Asia and the West could "conduct a pure form of moral education"[167] and experience no impediments to absorbing the knowledge of scientific civilization. A decade and a half later Inoue still harbored disdain for religion, but now he also understood its utility for instilling the kind of national morality he had been hoping to promote. In 1907 he opined that "Shinto as a vulgar Shinto is mere superstition, but as ancestor worship [*sosen kyō*] of the Japanese, it possesses great power."[168] By 1911 he was referring to Shinto, despite its secular status under the Meiji Constitution, as akin to a "national religion." As he explained, "as a religion Shinto is primitive, but it is not merely a religion; in its relation to Japan's *kokutai* it is related to Japan's fate as a nation."[169]

Accommodation

While Katō and Inoue, coming out of the reformist statist tradition (see Chapter 1), seem to have entertained notions that the Shinto national body (*kokutai*) could serve as an acceptable public surrogate for the actual biological body of the nation, the logic they employed to bracket evolutionary truth was echoed by Shintoist and nativist fundamentalists. Unlike Katō and Inoue, these nativist scholars eyed evolutionary biology as a mortal threat that needed to be neutralized if not discredited. Their fear was that the theory of evolution would completely undermine the authority of *Nihonshoki* and *Kojiki* by calling into question the accuracy of the creation story which these seventh-century texts imparted. To preserve the status of Shinto and the "social foundations" that were sanctified on its basis, they sought to reconcile its cosmology with the scientific one of evolutionary theory.

Migita identifies two strategies devised to achieve this accommodation. The first assigns Shinto a metaphysical status that makes it the animating cosmic force underlying not only terrestrial evolution but the development of the entire universe. An article by Nakashima Kosei published after the Russo-Japanese War in an issue of the *Report of the National Association of*

---

166 Gluck, *Japan's Modern Myths*, 134.
167 Ibid.
168 Ibid., 142.
169 Ibid.

Shinto Priests elaborately describes "seven ages" over the course of which the two divine ancestors, Izangi-no-Mikoto and Izanami-no-Migoto, facilitated the birth of the universe and ushered along the development of a handful of species "into the millions of species we see today."[170] Thus, the "scientific theory of evolution" and the Shinto creation story "very much agree"[171] except that the direct ancestors of humans were not these organic creatures but the two creation deities: "[T]he human beings of the world are all descendants of these gods."[172] As with Katō's two phases argument the evolutionary development of life and the history of humankind are segregated from one another.

The second strategy of accommodation, one which Migita considers especially influential, also partitions the growth of the *kokutai* from that of nature as a whole. In this view, the unique qualities of the Yamato *minzoku* (Japanese ethnic nation) enabled it to transcend the struggle for existence and the evolutionary processes of the organic world. As Migita explains in some detail, the primary exponent of this approach was the "person of highest responsibility in the worlds of Shintoism and nativism."[173] Sasaki Takayuki (1830–1910), a privy councilor and onetime assistant to the Meiji emperor, he was also the president of the two academic institutions that served as the "headquarters of the worlds of nativism and Shintoism"[174]: Kokugakuin (National Studies) University and the Research Institution of the Department of Imperial Lectures. Sasaki took a keen interest in Oka's writings, thoroughly absorbing the contents of *Lectures on Evolutionary Theory* and, in response to Oka, published his own attempt to reconcile *shinkaron* and *kokutairon* in July 1907, the very same month "Ideal Group Life" appeared. Entitled "Our Empire as Seen by the Theory of Evolution," and appearing in the *Journal of the Academy of Classical Literature*, Sasaki's article maintains that "there seem to be many things the study of evolution just cannot explain" and presents itself as an exercise in "temporary"[175] disbelief in order to work out what the theory of the *kokutai* might look like if what evolution imparts is true. The result is a version of the two-phases argument which accepts that evolution and the strug-

---

170 Migita, *Tennosei to Shinkaron*, 49. See Nakashima, "Beyond the Shinto View," 23.
171 Ibid.
172 Ibid. See Nakashima, "Shintoism," 24–25.
173 Ibid., 53.
174 Ibid., 52.
175 Ibid., 50–51.

gle for existence occurs, but asserts that "our Yamato ethnic nation [*minzoku*] and our empire" has come to achieve such a decisive and final victory that it has come to "exist at a height that transcends the general world of living things where there is a ceaseless struggle for existence."[176] Paradoxically, Japan is the "summa cum laude in the survival of the fittest" and does not need to engage in "unjustifiable wars" and real maltreatment of "foreign races."[177]

Why "our country alone has developed into a stable and secure group" is, according to Sasaki, the fact that the sovereign emperor is the "common ancestor" of all subjects and the emperor and his subjects are "connected through a parent-child bond" that fosters "mutual familiarity, respect, reliance, and assistance."[178] Japan's superior standing is, in this way, founded on "loyalty and patriotism."[179] Japan is the "champion" among "the most evolved humans" because of "its ancestor-god"[180] which establishes unique sociopolitical foundations. As a result "the theory of evolution is not at all a hindrance"[181] and Sasaki concludes that "even if the theory of evolution is true, the national body [*kokutai*] is not shaken by it."[182]

Grafting the immutable *kokutai* onto the evolutionary process of universal organic development would, over the long haul, not prove a viable formula for the emerging Shintoist orthodoxy. Not only, as Migita suggests, did scientific knowledge continue to accumulate, but, as Walter Skya argues, the appeal of such an account of the national body would have limited appeal to a *kokumin* who had accepted the progress of civilization as commonsensical and unremarkable.[183] In particular, the reactionary historicism of this orthodoxy which depicted any change or deviance from original conditions as decadent was in direct conflict with the developmental historicism of both evolutionary theory and modern society. In the next chapter we will see that Oka's theory of decadence offered the orthodoxy a way out of this trap and that his regenerative vision may account, in part, for the transformation of Shinto ultranationalism from a reactionary to more future-oriented, developmental doctrine.

---

176 Ibid., 51. See Sasaki, "Shinkaron yori mitaru Waga Teikoku."
177 Ibid.
178 Ibid., 52.
179 Ibid.
180 Ibid.
181 Ibid.
182 Ibid., 53.
183 Gluck, *Japan's Modern Myths*, 254.

Absolutist Fundamentalism

In the short term, however, the attempt to partition *shinkaron* from the *kokutai* orthodoxy during the postwar years helped facilitate the rise to eminence of a fundamentalist version of this orthodoxy—what Walter Skya dubs reactionary Shinto ultranationalism. The exponent of this Shinto ultranationalism was Hozumi Yatsuka, the dean of the Todai Law School who, like Inoue Tetsujirō, spent the 1880s studying philosophy and constitutionalism in Germany. As we saw in Chapter 1, Hozumi had begun to formulate his version of the *kokutai* orthodoxy in the 1890s, asserting in 1892 that "ancestor worship [*sosen kyō*] is the source of public law" and in 1897 that it is "the foundation of Japan's distinctive *kokutai* and of its national morality."[184] However, according to Carol Gluck, it was not until after 1900, when the ideological emphasis shifted from building a sense of nation to shoring up the social foundations of the polity that Hozumi's invocations of the ancestrally based family state came to the fore. By the postwar period his reactionary Shinto ultranationalism was spearheading "the ideological offensive against social change"[185] that we discussed earlier in the chapter.

What distinguishes Hozumi's *kokutairon* from that of Katō—whom we saw also wanted to promote ancestral rites—was the thorough and unyielding aspiration to fully cosmicize the norms and conventions of the family-state. For Hozumi the family-state concept was not merely a form of patriarchal rule but of absolutist monarchy based genealogically and ethnically on blood. According to Skya, Hozumi "extended the concept of 'blood' to encircle the whole state, thus advocating the concept of the union of 'blood' and state' and of 'blood' and 'ethnicity.'"[186] Thus, in genealogical terms, the *kokutai* was a blood lineage, the imperial stem-line of the national body that extended back in an "unbroken line for ages eternal" to the divine progenitor. It is this sense in which, as Hozumi says, "Our race consists of blood relatives from the same womb."[187] In ethnic terms, the Japanese *minzoku* was an organic polity of such "blood relatives," a "family state" that "is a racial group."[188] And finally, in patriarchal terms, the members of the racial com-

---

184 Ibid., 186.
185 Ibid.
186 Skya, *Japan's Holy War*, 57.
187 Pyle, "Meiji Conservatism," 126.
188 Ibid.

munity of this nation-state, as branch lines of extended family, owe obedience to the family through the family head, the emperor: just as the "family is a small state," so is "the state a large family."[189] In this familial political order "the people were the emperor's children"[190] and *chūkō*, "loyalty and filial piety as one,"[191] became the paramount virtue. According to Skya the blood that bound the *kokutai* (national body), *minzoku* (ethnic or race nation), and *kazoku kokka* (family state) into an absolutist organic polity carried with it not only obvious biological significance but "a certain religiosity and mysticism."[192]

This religiosity of blood conditioned Hozumi's efforts to cosmicize the family state. In Hozumi's view such blood ties not only unified the *kokumin* but lent the political order in which they served the emperor an ontological heft—blood rendered it "natural." As Skya explains, "the group based on mutual blood relations was the only natural form of group solidarity and ... the formation of the state under the authority and spirit of the same progenitor was the only natural solidarity."[193] In ruling over the Japanese nation-state the emperor was manifesting the natural ontology and adhering to the "teachings of nature."[194] His blood relationship with the founder of the imperial lineage, Amaterasu Ōmikami, clothed him in an authority that was therefore absolute and inviolable. The emperor was "Amaterasu Ōmikami existing in the present"[195] and the nomos of the family state was identical with the cosmic order that the divine progenitor had brought into being.

For Hozumi the main threat to the family state was individualism, which had arisen because the other ethnic nations (*minzoku*) on the planet had surrendered their natural internal absolutism in favor of religious universalism. In his account of human history there was no common human race but a patchwork of segregated ethnicities each of which had grown up from a family to a village community and finally into a *völkisch* nation-state, something along the lines of a *Volksstaat*. Hozumi regarded the hierarchical and patriarchal internal relations of such racial states to be natural but only Ja-

---

189 Ibid.
190 Skya, *Japan's Holy War*, 65.
191 Ibid., 66.
192 Ibid., 57.
193 Ibid., 65.
194 Ibid.
195 Ibid., 56.

pan has preserved its naturalness and remained a true *kokuminzoku*, which was the term he coined for an ethnic or *völkisch* nation-state.[196] What corrupted the other *minzoku* (ethnicities) by convincing them to abandon their natural patriarchy was a conception of mankind as a single community. As Skya explains, a period of decline set in when certain individuals appeared who "concocted universal religions with their own internal systems of morality that applied to all individuals, ruler and subject alike, above and beyond the ethnic community. It was precisely at this point that we find the existence of the 'individual' for the first time."[197] In Hozumi's "ethnic theory of history,"[198] the emergence of individuals is, according to Skya, equivalent to the fall of man in the Christian cosmology.

The universal systems of world religions would inevitably usher in the fall of the "ethnic patriarchal state" because they "postulated the individual as a moral being with a raison d'être outside the *völkisch* state."[199] Providing "ontological grounds for the moral existence of the individual outside of the ethnic state or ethnic community" inevitably opened the door to "private morality" and, with it, the "inner freedom to defy authority."[200] Having acquired subjective freedom these real individuals would become aware "for the first time the distinction between state law [*kokuhō*] and religious doctrine [*kyōgi*]"[201] or between state law and morality. Nomos would be exposed as being not a manifestation of ultimate reality but a human construct. What Hozumi seems to have feared most of all is that individual autonomy would lead inexorably to the insight that the laws, norms, and conventions of the nation were invented and that individuals should be consulted in their creation. It was this that Hozumi believes he perceived happening in the dominance of Western political thought in the nineteenth century and, particularly, in the spread of contract theory of the state. Though like Katō, Inoue, and others, he lashed out frequently at the pernicious influence of Christianity, for him "the Enlightenment thought of Western liberal democracy was the ultimate ideological threat to the Japanese ethnic state."[202]

---

196 Ibid., 57.
197 Ibid., 72.
198 Ibid.
199 Ibid., 74.
200 Ibid., 72.
201 Ibid., 72.
202 Ibid., 76.

The notion that "society is made up of self-supporting individuals" who were brought together on a contractual basis would result in an internal struggle for survival that would destroy the ethnic nation-state. For Hozumi, Japan was engaged in a "holy war" against not only the individualist idea but with the "Enlightenment" and modern "Western civilization"[203] that portrayed nomoi as the invention of autonomous, self-aware individuals.

To preserve its *völkisch* arrangements against this threat Japanese needed not only to understand that their nomos "does not rest on a contract among equals"[204] but to learn how to embody what Hozumi called *kōdōshin*. Hozumi coined this term to refer to "the desire for two or more independent elements to become one" and, by his account, the ideal person was one who aspired to submerge themselves completely into the organic totality of society. Through this total assimilation, which was the "purpose of all ethics and morality,"[205] society and its component members would achieve a condition of *gōdō seizon*—a fused or amalgamated existence. According to Skya, "society was thus composed of the existence of merged individuals. The individual, in other words, was an element, or *bunshi*, of society. The individual thus became an irreducible constituent of a complete entity called society."[206]

To actualize *kōdōshin* into such a concrete group, imperial subjects were to practice ancestral rites. In 1897 Hozumi began his central ideological text *Kokumin Kyōiku: Aikokushin* (National education: Patriotism) with the assertion that "the foundation of our nation's unique *kokutai* and national morality is ancestor worship."[207] Paying homage to the ancestors is essential because doing so reaffirms that the binding laws, conventions, and norms are a natural inheritance, not products of mutable, individual artifice. Ancestor worship acknowledges that laws are the "word of Amaterasu Ōmikami,"[208] an extension of her will, and thus it guarantees not only "the unity of state law and religious doctrine" but that "the individual as an independent moral being does not come into existence."[209] Invoking the "authority of the ancestors" will reveal that the "blood relationship" between members of the fam-

---

203 Ibid.
204 Ibid.
205 Ibid., 69.
206 Ibid.
207 Ibid., 54.
208 Ibid., 71.
209 Ibid., 73.

ily state "cannot be severed and joined, or continued and discontinued according to advantages and disadvantages."[210] Rather "this bond is eternal,... this bond is rock solid."[211] The laws, conventions, and norms emanate from a natural ontology, a cosmos and what we call individuals have no choice but to submerge themselves utterly into the collective life that represents their embodiment—and do so with *chūkō*, complete loyalty and filial piety.

As the next chapter will reveal, Oka, too, associated the emergence of individualism with the decay of the ethnic state. Individuals who locate their "raison d'être" outside the realm of the organic polity and devise private moralities based on principles of humanitarian universalism usher in, for both Hozumi and Oka, ethnic disintegration and signal the onset of historical decline. Both also strove to restore the "blood community" of the nation-state by solidifying its nomic foundations in ultimate reality—rendering them "natural" and thereby impervious to the preferences of individual invention. In both cases, the individual would, in this way, be reduced to an element, a *bunshi*, of the social whole—a component and utterly subordinate cell of the composite organic group.

Both intellectuals were responding to the anomy of the late Meiji period—the sense of incipient normlessness and the perception of disintegrating social cohesion that accompanied urbanization, industrialization, the breakup of village life and the awakening of the masses to their "inner freedom to defy authority."[212] It is on the basis of this commonality that I am arguing that Oka's metapolitics aspired to reform the Meiji order, not overturn it. Yet, as it would turn out, it was the fundamentalist imperatives built into Hozumi's version of the blood community that would prove as worrisome to Oka as the decadent individualism and radical ideologies of the postwar and incite him to draw out the generative aspect of his scientistic organicism. The most profound of these imperative concerned the temporal dimension: Hozumi's fundamentalist belief that the present emperor was the reincarnation of the Sun Goddess meant that worship of him returned the blood community to the pristine circumstances of the primordial Japanese ethnic state. As the next chapter will explore, Oka's emphasis on the life cycle of superorganisms in his rendering of the blood community was,

210 Ibid., 76.
211 Ibid.
212 Ibid., 72.

in large part, a response to the static and emphatically reactionary quality of Hozumi's conception. Ultimately, Oka would provide a path to returning to a more cohesive and organic past without abandoning future development.

However, Oka's most immediate and pressing problem with the fundamentalist orthodoxy that Hozumi and his allies began to sponsor in the years after the war with Russia was the means it employed to cosmicize itself. Hozumi's consanguineous national polity—his patriarchal construction of the family state and *minzoku*—was a blood community of worshipers. Unlike the technologically able, scientifically educated members of Oka's blood community—who would build up nomic instincts by practicing race-specific altruism—the *bunshi* that comprised the amalgamated existence imagined in Hozumi's ethnic state were enjoined to pray to the apotheosized paterfamilias. As a result, an extensive program was soon launched to promote worship and focus the *kokumin* on the living god in the imperial palace. Not science but superstition would inform the collective life of the *kokumin*.

Oka's recommendation in "Ideal Group Life" that images of moss animals should be raised in the public spaces where religious statues now stand was a veiled response to the spread of state Shinto in the aftermath of the war. Though Oka specially singled out "statues of sect founders and the Buddha,"[213] these were safe, surrogate targets, selected to dodge scrutiny from state censors while making insinuations about the real threat: the state's concerted attempt during the postwar years to bring the imperial cult, as imagined by Hozumi, into the lives of the people. This aspiration was perhaps nowhere more apparent than in the efforts from 1906 onward to nationalize, regularize and consolidate the folk-oriented "people's shrines" [*minsha*] which were "centered in local hamlets, villages, towns and city neighborhoods"[214] across the nation. These nearly 200,000 people's or civic shrines had been part of elaborate plans in the early years of the Restoration to establish a standard, nationwide liturgy based on "a national calendar of rites centering on the nation and the imperial house."[215] However, during the middle years of the Meiji period, government support for Shinto waned: funding for people's shrines was cut off and their priests ceased to

---

213 Oka, "Risōteki Dantai Seikatsu" [Ideal group life], 71.
214 Fridell, "A Fresh Look at State Shinto," 559.
215 Hardacre, *Shinto and the State*, 101.

be government officials.[216] Even the more highly ranked imperial and national shrines which remained active participants in the national liturgical program throughout the Meiji period, were threatened in 1887 with having their state funding eventually removed. Not until the surge of patriotic support for Shinto that came with the Sino-Japanese War (1894–95) did priests at the people's shrines have their official status restored. In the aftermath of the war with Russia a new, aggressive attempt was made to impose a national liturgy by merging the people's shrines. According to Helen Hardacre, "to raise the status and social prominence of shrines in the train of heightened patriotism after the Russo-Japanese War … the state embarked upon a campaign to have not more than one shrine per village (*isson issha*), thereby aligning civil administrative districts with shrine territories, creating a parallel ritual and administrative hierarchy."[217]

Though the creation of this hierarchy met with resistance—in part due to the decrease in shrines "from 200,000 to 120,000" by 1914[218]—and was never completely successful, this administrative effort to reverse "millennia of local autonomy and uncoordinated shrine rites" was "revolutionary."[219] Its ambition consisted in nothing less than having "the liturgy of all the shrines of the nation … orchestrated according to single plan, penetrating all areas and all levels of society."[220] In Hardacre's account, the Grand Shrine of Ise, where the ancestral *kami* of the imperial family (Amaterasu Ōmikami, the Sun Goddess) was enshrined, functioned in an absolutist manner, employing its liturgical power to reach down into local areas:

> Through … various rites, the emperor's religious authority was based on the unity of his person with Amaterasu, the apical ancestress of the imperial house. The idea that all other deities were putatively descended from her had a parallel in the notion that all the Japanese people were ultimately descended from the imperial house. Similarly, all deities being ultimately linked to Amaterasu, all shrines were ultimately subordinate to Ise. Thus Ise was the apex of a pyramidal hierarchy of shrines, their rites should conform to imperial rites conducted both at Ise and in the palace. In the person of the

---

216 Fridell, "The Establishment of Shrine Shinto in Meiji Japan," 160.
217 Hardacre, *Shinto and the State*, 98.
218 Shimazono, "State Shinto in the Lives of the People," 118.
219 Hardacre, *Shinto and the State*, 102.
220 Ibid.

emperor was bound up the unity of the nation and its people and myriad deities. This unity was symbolized in local society by shrines and shrine rites.[221]

In both helping to cast the "emperor unambiguously in the role of head priest of the nation"[222] and orchestrating the shrine mergers the Home Ministry hoped to "integrate shrines into social life more thoroughly than before"[223] and thereby imbue the nomos of the nation with the cosmic significance of the *kokutai*. The Boshin Rescript that the ministry had the emperor issue in 1908 called not only for "all classes of Our people to act in unison"[224] but for the shrines to be "utilized in promoting the unification and administration of the country."[225] Accordingly, "it became a matter of national policy to integrate the shrines with such bureaucratically inspired movements as national youth groups, women's groups, and army reserve units."[226]

As Gluck, Hardacre, and Shimazu all point out, this integration was not merely a top-down, unidirectional affair. Instead it involved willing collaboration and even inspired initiative by those who perceived opportunities for local interests in accessing the liturgical power in the state. This can be seen especially in how the *chihō jichi seido* (local self-government system) and the *chihō dantai* (voluntary local organizations) became ideological agents after the Russo-Japanese War, furthering the Home Ministry's nomic and administrative agenda. During the war both had displayed exemplary service to the nation, evincing the spirit of *Kyokoku itchi* (national unity) in which, as a top ministry bureaucrat remembered, "everyone in the country worked in complete unity."[227] For this reason the local organizations became not only the primary device for the local improvement that the Home Ministry launched in 1909, but a conduit for *shakai kyōiku* or social education through which the government could "influence sections of the population who were otherwise out of range of such state institutions as the schools and the army."[228] Likewise, the system of local self-government was turned to in order to maintain the "social harmony" of ancestral village life.

---

221 Ibid.
222 Ibid.
223 Ibid.
224 Lu, *Japan*, 603.
225 Hardacre, *Shinto and the State*, 38.
226 Ibid.
227 Gluck, *Japan's Modern Myths*, 194.
228 Ibid., 200–201.

Conceived along the lines of *Selbstverwaltung*[229] under the influence Rudolf von Gneist and Albert Mosse in the 1880s, this system of local self-administration was intended as a "safely apolitical means of national integration"[230] that "tied the *chihō* as closely as possible to the center" while denying them "any semblance of political autonomy."[231]

With the financial difficulties and "social destructionism" that arrived after the war not only was even more stress placed on "selfless self-governance" but "*jichi* was now extended to include moral exhortation."[232] The chief Home Ministry ideologue spoke of "the mores of the country" being "restored"[233] through *jichi*. Eventually it came to be regarded as an administrative equivalent to the national body espoused by state Shinto: "the *kokutai* of local government."[234] As Gluck explains, "just as *kokutai* signified the ideological essence of the nation, *jichi* stood as a public sign of the countryside."[235]

Competing Cosmologies: Textbooks and Education

The primary institution, however, through which the moral-religious imperatives of the state impacted the lives of average Japanese was the one in which Oka was directly invested: education. Scholars can debate about the degree of adherence of shrine Shinto to state directives—and while local organizations and local self-government were certainly open to religious messages, the so-called "*kokutai* of local self-government" cannot be said to constitute the community of worshipers that Hozumi envisioned. In contrast, the national education system did increasingly become a venue for liturgical inculcation during the late Meiji years. For Oka it was above all this aspect of the government response to the general nomic crisis that turned into a crisis in its own right—one that forced him to match the Shinto cosmization of norms and conventions with an historicist presentation of his evolutionism.

---

229 Ibid., 192.
230 Ibid.
231 Ibid., 193.
232 Ibid.
233 Ibid.
234 Ibid., 197.
235 Ibid.

State Shinto insinuated itself into the public school system via the Imperial Rescript on Education. As was discussed earlier in the chapter, the Rescript had been promulgated in 1890 in order to allay concerns in various quarters during the late 1880s that Japan was lacking the "spirit nation-mindedness" and the "socio-moral bonds"[236]—that is the ethical life needed to bolster the anticipated constitutional order and ensure survival in the competitive international arena. Offered as a new "civic creed" in keeping with "the familiar code of customary social morality,"[237] the Rescript was enshrined in the schools in a manner that gave state Shinto a firm foothold. "Revered as holy writ" copies of the Rescript came to form, along with the official photo of the Meiji emperor which had been distributed to all the schools over the course of the 1880s, "a liturgical set."[238] According to Hardacre, "the scroll on which the rescript was written and the photograph had to be housed in some portion of the school not used for any other purpose. Sometimes a special room was constructed and a special night guard hired to protect them in case of fire or other emergency. They were placed in a shrinelike box, and offerings set before them. When opening the box, one had to bow low enough to place the hands on the knees, an obvious borrowing from shrine etiquette."[239] From early in the 1890s Home Ministry directives were distributed by shrine priests stipulating not only rules for this careful handling but the manner and timing of ceremonial readings. Readings were conducted on three of the imperial holidays established in the early years of the Meiji period, and

> for a school's first reading of the Rescript the scroll had to be paraded to the school by teachers, pupils, local notables, the mayor, the post office chief, local people in government, and the area's oldest residents. A sacred space was prepared for the reading with fresh gravel and hung with red, white, and blue curtains. An offering of rice cakes was presented to the scroll as if it were a deity. The school principal assumed the priestly role, donning white gloves to intone the text.[240]

---

236 Ibid., 110, 120.
237 Ibid., 127.
238 Hardacre, *Shinto and the State*, 108.
239 Ibid.
240 Ibid., 108–9.

While local officials eager to co-opt state authority for their own purposes may have added their own embellishments, this basic ceremonial form of school rites was established across the country in the 1890s. As Gluck portrays it,

[S]choolchildren heard the principal intone the Rescript on each national holiday, each school ceremony, and at special monthly convocations held expressly for the purpose. In the lower three grades the children repeated the words after the teacher in *shūshin* [ethics] class; in fourth grade and above they were expected to recite it from memory. The ceremonial recitation of the Rescript, like the Pledge of Allegiance to the flag in the United States, became an emblematic moment in school ritual. It was associated with the principal and the emperor—that is, with both local and national authority—and with obedient demeanor and solemn sanctity.[241]

The seriousness with which this sanctification was regarded is indicated by instances in which principals took their own lives after mispronouncing a single syllable from the text of the Rescript.[242]

In the final years of the Meiji period, a moment of nomic crisis we are describing in this chapter, the bonds between Shinto and the schools further consolidated. Shrines for *kami, kamidana,* could be found at 70 percent of the nation's schools and many such schools supplemented the Rescript and the imperial portrait with special shrines for talisman from the Ise Grand Shrine which housed Amaterasu Ōmikami.[243] Some local principals even used their authority to greatly increase the number of shrine festivals, thereby multiplying the ritual occasions upon which the emperor was invoked as a manifest deity. By 1911 the Ministry of Education was instructing schools to include shrine visits in the academic calendar.[244] "Monthly shrine visits and monthly shrine cleaning by pupils," which included formal offerings at shrine alters that were mostly overseen by priests, became integral to the educational routine. Perhaps the greatest influence was the growing presence of this Shinto clergy in the classroom as instructors. According to Hardacre, "priests who held the rank of *kundō* (second form the lowest) and higher were automatically qualified as primary school teachers" and

241 Gluck, *Japan's Modern Myths*, 148–49.
242 Hardacre, *Shinto and the State*, 109.
243 Ibid.
244 Gluck, *Japan's Modern Myths*, 141.

many priests of civic shrines, who were in need of "by-employment of some kind"[245] took up the opportunity. In this manner, Shinto, though still considered "nonreligious rites of state," had begun to infuse its cosmology into the life experiences of the population and define its normative disposition.

As a professor at the nation's top normal school, Oka warned that this creeping Shintoist infiltration was "something which those engaged in education must think about very deeply."[246] In May 1911, the same year the Ministry of Education began to order schools to make shrine visits, Oka gave an address which three months later appeared under the title "Education and Superstition" in the expanded second edition of *Evolution and Human Life*. The eighth and final section of this lecture-cum-essay was labeled "A Caveat for Education" and it focused directly on this issue of school excursions: "According to newspaper reports, it seems that in our nation of late the practice of visiting shrines and temples has been adopted as a means of education. Often there appear stories about the principals at elementary schools in some villages leading all the students to the village shrine, making offerings and then returning, or stories of the student group at a certain school visiting some temple. I think there is an issue here about which educators should be very cautious."[247]

What has Oka worried is that students who have been exposed to shrines and temples in this manner will not learn the habit of "avoiding superstition."[248] While he admits that "visiting temples and shrines is an old custom in our nation" and even educated people, such as Oka and his audience, tend to "pay reverence when going to a place where are shrines and temples," he reminds his listeners that "the origins of shrines and temples involve written oracles" from "the uncivilized days long ago" and that, therefore, from the standpoint of "today's knowledge we are satisfied that we have clearly no choice but to regard them as products of superstition."[249] Making "school pupils" go and "worship gods and Buddhas" is likely to instill in them "something like hesitation about rejecting this sort of superstition as superstition."[250] Even "if one can remove those aspects of contemporary re-

245 Hardacre, *Shinto and the State*, 109.
246 Oka, "Kyōiku to Meishin" [Education and superstition], 127.
247 Ibid., 126.
248 Ibid.
249 Ibid.
250 Ibid.

ligion which are classified as superstition and then lead the people to revere the remaining parts"—something which, from his metapolitical perspective, "is, in truth, acceptable"—the residue of reverence for gods and Buddhas might "unconsciously transmit and spread superstition."[251] If this were to happen, "the harm done would far outnumber the benefits gained"[252] because the scientific basis of education would be fatally undermined.

In this same final section of his Hibiya library speech of May 1911—"Education and Superstition"—Oka is equally critical of contemporary attempts to restore nomic bonds through religion. "It is doubtful whether encouraging the worship of gods and Buddhas from the onset of education would bring about the improvement of the world's manners and customs."[253] Even when religious practices become popular, such as going on "pilgrimages," which entail "beating drums, uttering holy invocations" and holding parades, "it cannot really be thought that the customs of the world become commendable."[254] While Oka concedes that "it might be a good thing to preserve customs from long ago such as prefectural governors in the costume of Shinto priests visiting shrines and presenting a Chinese chest covered with gold brocade against a red field" or "processions through the streets featuring court nobles, court musicians with court dress, children in damask brocade loose *suikan* blouses with their hair hanging down the back, and high priests in purple robes," he believes that "planning to prevent a moral setback by means of these customs is inappropriate for contemporary times."[255]

Why the dangers of "allaying the decline in public morals"[256] by means of traditional culture and religion became an especially personal issue for Oka—one that impelled him to reconstitute the cosmic parameters of his scientism—was due to his experiences on the Ministry of Education's textbook committee from 1904 until 1918. Though participation on this committee was part of his job at the Tokyo Higher Normal School, and were duties which he shared with at least two other faculty members, Oka seems to have regarded his position on the committee as a unique opportunity to realize the goal that motivated his essays and books: disseminating knowledge of

---

251 Ibid., 127.
252 Ibid., 126.
253 Ibid., 127.
254 Ibid.
255 Ibid.
256 Ibid.

science among the general public.[257] It cannot be emphasized enough that over the long term, Oka was extremely successful in meeting this goal: his work as an educator, researcher, and popularizer contributed profoundly to elevating the prestige of biology and influence not only in Japan but in East Asia.[258] As we have intimated several times already, the corporatist imperatives of his scientism did not diminish his achievements as a genuine scientist and science promoter. Unfortunately, as Migita has established, this accomplishment did not begin to register until the 1920s after he had quit the curriculum committee out of frustration and as his literary, scholarly, and educational career was winding down. In the short term—that is, during the late Meiji period and for most of the Taisho period—Oka's efforts were thwarted. In no area did he experience greater frustration and dismay than in his activities on the textbook curriculum committee.

Although Oka's selection to this committee at its inception in July 1904 occurred just six months after his best-selling *Lectures on Evolutionary Theory* had been published, his inclusion was, in the opinion of Migita, due to his critical approach to education and not his growing fame and authority as an expert on evolutionary biology.[259] Since the early Meiji period there had been an ongoing debate within the Ministry of Education about whether the emphasis of the school curriculum should be on instilling ethics or imparting knowledge about the world and developing practical skills. During the 1870s, under the influence of the Charter Oath, which had called for "seeking knowledge throughout the world," education policy adopted a progressive orientation of "reformist civil bureaucrats," focusing on the "useful knowledge and skills"[260] of modern civilization to the neglect of morality and native customs. By the end of the decade this exclusively pragmatic approach provoked a conservative reaction with the result that the new guidelines for elementary education drawn up in 1880 and 1881 made *shūshin* (ethics instruction) the first priority among school subjects.[261] While the culmination of this stress on "moral education" was, as we have already

---

257 Migita, *Tennosei to Shinkaron*, 108.
258 See especially Li, "Lu Xun and Oka Asajirō." Though it never mentions Oka, James Pusey thoroughly delineates the reliance of Lu Xun on the same Haeckelian version of evolutionism that we are arguing Oka espoused. See Pusey, *Lu Xun and Evolution*, 37–65.
259 Migita, *Tennosei to Shinkaron*, 106–7.
260 Gluck, *Japan's Modern Myths*, 104–5.
261 Ibid., 108.

described, the Imperial Rescript on Education, faithfully inculcating "the Way" of this document among the *kokumin* presented a whole new set of difficulties. Not only were classroom instructors often untrained and ideologically unreliable but the textbooks that private publishers began to produce in large quantities were of questionable quality.[262] After the Ministry of Education struggled unsuccessfully to curtail this problem by establishing a process by which ethics textbooks would be examined and approved, the Diet ordered the ministry to compile its own official textbooks in 1897. Before the committee, which was chaired by Katō Hiroyuki, could compile ethics texts for all elementary grades, it was decided in 1902 that all elementary textbooks would be produced by the government. The first such textbooks came out in 1903.[263]

In keeping with the progressive spirit of the 1903 ethics textbook—which emphasized "vocational ethics" and downplayed patriotism and loyalty[264]—the committee that Oka joined the following year was assigned the task of devising an official "Ordinary Elementary School Science Book" for use in the nation's classrooms.[265] Oka was an obvious choice for this committee not only due to his reformist educational philosophy, which he articulated in a 1901 book entitled *Education and Natural History*,[266] but because he had already produced four biology textbooks for use in the nation's schools: *Modern Textbook of Biology* (1896), *Modern Textbook on Physiology* (1898), *Modern Textbook of Zoology* (1899), and *Short Lecture on Zoology* (1902). According to Migita, Oka "took charge of the part of the curriculum connected with biology" in this proposed textbook project and saw his work as a "golden opportunity" to "introduce the theory of organic evolution into the compulsory school curriculum."[267]

The stakes involved with this particular textbook could not have been higher for someone whose raison d'être was to instill knowledge of natural science and evolutionary biology in the general public. Though by 1906 an extraordinary 98 percent of school-age children were enrolled in the nation's

---

262 Fridell, "Government Ethics Textbooks in Late Meiji Japan," 825.
263 Ibid., 826; Gluck, *Japan's Modern Myths*, 147.
264 Fridell, "Government Ethics Textbooks in Late Meiji Japan," 826.
265 Migita, *Tennosei to Shinkaron*, 106–7.
266 Ibid., 107.
267 Ibid., 108.

schools,[268] only a small minority progressed beyond elementary school. For instance, Migita claims that in 1910 Japan had a total of 6,861,000 students in ordinary elementary schools but a mere 154,000 in junior and senior high schools as well as normal schools.[269] The numbers decreased even more steeply for higher education with only 5,000 students enrolled in the two imperial universities at Tokyo and Kyoto in 1906. The conclusion was obvious for Oka: if evolutionary theory was to become a fixture in Japanese life, it would have to be included in the elementary school curriculum. While from the 1890s natural science subjects had been offered above the level of elementary schools,[270] so far elementary textbooks had only a crude lesson on "science materials" in the Japanese-language reader.[271] With proposals to expand compulsory education to eight years—realized in 1908—and the inclusion of science subjects in the fifth and eighth grades a "golden opportunity" did, indeed, present itself.[272]

The complete absence of any mention of the theory of evolution not only in the Ministry of Education's first official science textbook, which finally appeared in April 1911, but in its subsequent 1918 revision, triggered, I want to argue, a seismic shift in Oka's approach. Though Oka struggled for a total of fourteen years to have materials on evolutionary theory included in the Ministry's official science textbook for elementary schools, it was clearly during the years leading up to the 1911 text—the same years of nomic crisis after the Russo-Japanese War—that this shift took place. In fact, "Ideal Group Life," the 1907 article that we cited at the start of this chapter marks Oka's mounting awareness that the "nonreligious" religion that the government was in the process of inventing had begun to erect formidable obstacles to the dissemination of *shinkaron*.

Oka's response to these ideological barriers was twofold. On the one hand, as we will explore in the next chapter, he comicized his *shinkaron* into a theory of decadence. On the other hand, he intensified his criticism of "superstition"—his code word for state Shinto—so that it became, for a time, not only bolder and less indirect, but, in an essay entitled "Bite of the Sleep-

268 Gluck, *Japan's Modern Myths*, 164.
269 Migita, *Tennosei to Shinkaron*, 103.
270 Ibid., 102.
271 Ibid., 105.
272 Ibid., 106.

ing Dog,"[273] briefly approached lèse-majesté. Writing in the prestigious New Year's issue of *Chūō Kōron* in 1913, Oka, in a manner that carefully omitted mention of the country to which he was referring, described a "powerful tyranny" which "borrows the gods that ordinary people had come to worship in the past" in order to enforce a compulsory faith."[274] Indoctrination occurs under this regime through the school system where children are "made to bow before an oil painting, sing hymns, and stand respectfully while reading a sutra" and "the history of country is also arranged to favorably amplify the compelled faith."[275] While "priests and scholars who follow the commands of authority and convey compulsory faith" in this order are allowed to "express themselves loudly, true thinkers have no recourse aside from the protection of silence."[276] The result of this reign of superstition is dire for the nation in question: "research into natural developments is looked down upon in education and therefore research in this field does not advance."[277] Surrounded on "all four sides" by competitors who "enthusiastically develop themselves," the nation falls hopelessly behind and gradually begins to slide "on a downward slope because of the compulsion of this absolutely fixed faith and the artificial cessation of progress in the world of ideas."[278]

According to Migita, the issue of *Chūō Kōron* that carried "Bite of the Sleeping Dog" was subject to sales prohibition, which was not enforced until 20,000 copies had been circulated. However, it remains unclear whether this measure was provoked by Oka's article or, as was officially claimed, an offending piece by Aoyagi Yumi entitled "The Corruption of Manners and Customs."[279] Whichever the case, it is not difficult to discern why Oka's "boldly irreverent expression,"[280] as Fukuhara Rintarō has described "Bite of the Sleeping Dog," might have alarmed the authorities: not only does it suggest that the emperor-centered historical view was a myth constructed

---

273 The title of Oka's article is "Sawaranu kami ni tatari," which is a play on a well-known proverb, "Sawaranu kami ni tatarinashi." Because the original proverb means something to the effect of "Let sleeping dogs lie," I have rendered Oka's version as "Bite of the sleeping dog." However, a literal reading of the proverb would be "Gods who are not touched (or meddled with) do not curse." The "dog" in question is, in other words, a god or gods (*kami*), something highly relevant to the context of this essay.

274 Migita, *Tennosei to Shinkaron*, 111.

275 Ibid., 112.

276 Ibid.

277 Ibid.

278 Ibid., 113.

279 Ibid., 115. For the edition in which Aoyagi and Oka's articles appear, see *Chūō Kōron* 28, no. 1 (1913).

280 Ibid., 114.

out of "old stories" and "fanciful legends"[281]; it also alludes to the process by which superstition had come to suppress evolutionary science in the official elementary school textbook of 1911. The turning point where textbooks in general were concerned appears to have been the appointment of Komatsubara Eitarō as Minister of Education in 1908 by Prime Minister Katsura. Engrossed with *kokumin dōtoku* (national morality) and the dangers of literature which "corrupted morals and incited the 'spirit of speculation,'"[282] Komatsubara established what was considered a blue chip committee to "rectify and review elementary school ethics, history and language texts,"[283] as well as any other textbook materials he personally decided needed scrutiny. The purport of this "rectification" campaign can be gleaned from the chairman he selected to head the revision of ethics textbooks: Hozumi Yatsuka.[284] Reversing the reformist outlook of the 1903 ethics texts, Hozumi saturated the texts with the truisms of family state orthodoxy, evidently with a mind of actualizing his vision of Japan as a blood community of worshipers that we discussed above. As Wilbur M. Fridell summarizes, such rectified instruction came to stress in the 1911 ethics textbooks the apotheosis of the emperor and his lineage, the "super family of the nation," and "absolute lord-loyalty"[285] to the emperor-led state. Not only was the "doctrine of political absolutism" to be granted the "final sanctions of religious belief,"[286] but Shinto mythology was actually presented—much as Oka suggested it was in "Bite of the Sleeping Dog"—as "believable historical fact."[287]

In such an atmosphere evolutionary theory, which had come to be associated with anarchism after the Emperor's Birthday Incident, stood little chance of reaching the impressionable ears of schoolchildren. Yet the sharpness of Oka's response in 1913—a year and a half after evolutionism was excluded from elementary school texts—should not lead us to conclude that he had joined in any way with the political opposition or abandoned his metapolitics. Migita suggests that Oka "gave up" after "Bite of the Sleeping Dog," by which he seems to imply that up until this time Oka's writings had in-

---

281 Ibid., 111–12.
282 Gluck, *Japan's Modern Myths*, 171.
283 Fridell, "Government Ethics Textbooks in Late Meiji Japan," 826.
284 Ibid.
285 Ibid., 824.
286 Holtom, *The Political Philosophy of Modern Shinto*, 236.
287 Fridell, "Government Ethics Textbooks in Late Meiji Japan," 832.

tended to actively subvert the official orthodoxy. But it is precisely here that Migita gets it wrong. Certainly Oka privately rejected the emperor-centered historical view—and certainly he would have preferred a thoroughly secular political order for Japan. Nonetheless, his stance was reformist, not revolutionary, and that this continued to be the case even after January 1913 is illustrated by his actions. Far from surrendering to superstition Oka continued to produce both classroom textbooks—*An Outline of Intermediate Education in Natural History, Woman's Science Textbook of Physiology and Hygiene,* and *Woman's Science Textbook of Animals,* all in 1914—and popular works on biology and evolutionary theory—most notably *Seibutsugaku Kōwa* (Lectures on biology) of 1916[288]—throughout the 1910s. His essay writing also did not tail off, with anthologies of his lectures and pieces from journals and magazines appearing in 1914 (*Jinrui no Kako Genzai oyobi Mirai* [Past, present and future of mankind]), 1921 (*Hammon to Jiyū* [Anguish and freedom]), and 1926 (*Saru no Mure Kara Kyōwakoku made* [From monkey herd to the republic]).[289] Perhaps most significantly of all, he remained on the textbook committee fighting for a place for evolutionary biology in the curriculum, until 1918 when the second version of the elementary school science textbook came out and, once again, excluded any mention of evolution. Migita portrays Oka as quitting the committee out of frustration but it is also clear from his being made a member of the Imperial Academy in 1925 that he didn't leave on bad terms with the government. The connection Oka apparently formed around the time of his retirement with Emperor Hirohito, a subject we will return to in the epilogue—also indicates that wariness of the "sleeping dog" of imperial-centered superstition did not bring his designs to metapolitically reform the so-called "emperor system" to a halt.

Oka, in fact, argued at more than one juncture for the utility of superstition in politics. For instance, earlier in the same 1911 Hibiya Library lecture, "Education and Superstition," in which he warned educators that exposing school children to Shinto rituals might compromise their critical faculties, he conceded that "ruling over the people through superstition is not necessarily blameworthy."[290] Careful to distinguish such an arrangement from the "the nation's present-day constitutional government," Oka described

288 Watanabe, *The Japanese and Western Science,* 86.
289 Oka, *Jinrui no kako genzai oyobi mirai;* Oka, *Hanmon to Jiyu;* Oka, *Saru no Mura kara Kyowakoku made.*
290 Oka, "Kyōiku to Meishin" [Education and superstition], 124.

the premodern polity as one in which "the sovereign was believed to be the representative of god" and, therefore, "the sovereign's will was god's will" and constitutes "something that should be obeyed absolutely."[291] Such a "device," as Oka called it, was "extremely convenient" and if "it is carried out thoroughly, rule can be sustained for a long time."[292] For those ruled over such an order can prove highly beneficial: "so long as the sovereign pampers the people without being too lawless, they will gladly be ruled over for a long while and perhaps be able to enjoy safety for generations, praising the blessings of peace."[293]

Where this device of "ruling over the people" became "extremely harmful"[294] were circumstances in which the country in question faced outside competition. When "nation has no superior in the world it is appropriate just to rule well and provide for the happiness of the people, employing superstition to achieve this goal."[295] Yet "it becomes difficult to maintain superstitions as they existed in the past when the world moves on, traffic opens up, and popular ideas come to be widespread."[296] Oka believes that the "great efforts to maintain superstitions, doing such things as exercising authority, employing Buddhist priests or handing down orders to educators" will stifle skepticism and suppress "the heart of research in the people."[297] Such adherence to superstition will become an "obstacle to the progress of scientific knowledge" and "inevitably retard the advance of civilization."[298] This lack of progress is something modern Japan cannot afford in the cutthroat international system of the new imperialism: "seeing that there are many nations on earth and that each extends its power, engaging in intense competition, a nation cannot be free of anxiety by merely setting the internal peace and security of the nation as the only goal. Certainly we must progress just so as not to be defeated by others."[299]

A *minzoku* that it scientifically aware and technologically adept—Oka reiterates some version of this formula for national progress and survival in

---

291 Ibid.
292 Ibid.
293 Ibid.
294 Ibid., 125.
295 Ibid., 124–25.
296 Ibid., 124.
297 Ibid.
298 Ibid.
299 Oka, *Shinka to Jinsei*, 125.

nearly every essay in *Evolution and Human Life*. However, only in his "Education and Superstition" lecture is he perfectly explicit about his model for a techno-scientific ethnic nation-state: his contemporary Germany. In fact, extolling an idealized version of Wilhelmine Germany—and doing so in terms reminiscent of tracts produced by Haeckel's Monist League—was integral in this Hibiya Library speech to his warnings about the fatal liabilities of official superstitions. The logic of this lecture turned on Japan's failure to attain the basic aim of education: "to cultivate upcoming generations of a nation's people ... to do just what it takes to stand up in the arena of competition among the nations of the world and thrive on their own."[300] To illustrate the hollowness of Japan's conceit that it possesses first-rank status among the nations of the world due to its victories over Qing China and imperial Russia, Oka points to the prevalence of superstitions and the crudeness of the nation's technological products. Yet the fundamental shortcoming was in science education, as exemplified by the grossly inadequate scientific textbook for elementary schools that Oka himself had just assisted in compiling. It is in this area which he draws his unfavorable comparison with Germany. In contrast to Japan's "second or third rank"[301] achievements, Germany has streaked ahead and is presently winning the global "war of peace" in the indispensable realms of technology and commerce due to its domestic promotion of scientific knowledge. Germany's "superiority" is even admitted to by its main competitor, England, a country that Oka is quick to point out is itself "far superior to our own nation."[302]

What the Germans have gotten right, in Oka's estimation, is the intrinsic connection between general science education, pure research, and technological applications. By cultivating what he calls "the spirit of science"—by which Oka means "investigating the true nature of things on one's own" and seeking "explanations from reality"[303]—through the education system, Germany, Oka suggests, has been successful in "arousing the heart of research."[304] Research in this case signifies "pure research" which is performed without consideration for future technological applications—but which, counterintuitively, makes such applications possible. For Oka, "the original great dis-

---

300 Ibid., 117.
301 Ibid., 118.
302 Ibid., 119.
303 Ibid., 120.
304 Ibid., 121.

coveries of science, such as electricity and x-rays, were reached only as a result of pure research which did not take into consideration their applications. Research that aims from the beginning at its application never ranks with great discoveries" because "trying to apply science right away is like omitting the foundation and basement and attempting to construct the second floor alone—it is absolutely impossible."[305] Once these foundations in pure science have been laid, however, they serve "as a forerunner for the progress of applied science."[306] It is this "reasoning" that the Germans evince they are "clearly aware" by "making efforts to advance science in both its pure and applied forms."[307] In Oka's estimation, "the newly established Kaiser Wilhelm Institute for the Encouragement of Science and other organizations like it" typify the German approach: they "aim at advancing scientific research without any necessary connection to present-day applications"[308] yet still result in medical and technological achievements unmatched anywhere else on the planet.

For Oka, the success of this German model does not rest on training a population of professional scientists. Rather, as explained about a year before the "Education and Superstition" lecture, "the number of people doing research in pure science is not more than a few" and "because there are not many people suited for science" only a "few specialty scholars"[309] will actually emerge. The role of the common run of people will be to help implement the new technology that materializes from the foundations laid by these researchers. In other words, just as the population supports pure research due to its first rate science education, so is it also prepared to make use of the applications that inevitably result from such research. It is for this reason that even German-made toys on display on the Ginza are superior to "the domestically manufactured scientific instruments in schools, which tend to break immediately."[310] Ultimately, German excellence depends on the scientific sophistication of the average worker: things like these German products cannot be made at all if it has not happened that scientific knowledge has spread to workers." These workers "actually understand the

---

305 Ibid.
306 Ibid.
307 Ibid.
308 Ibid.
309 Oka, "Minzoku no Hatten to Rika" [Science and the development of the race-nation], 116.
310 Oka, "Kyōiku to Meishin" [Education and superstition], 119.

logic" of these products and, as a result, "do not merely imitate the outward appearance."[311]

In his *Tennosei to Shinkaron*, Migita attributes the conflict of Oka's evolutionism with Shinto orthodoxy to there being "no overlap"[312] between naturalistic descent, as described by evolutionary theory, and the emperor-centered historical view. However, from Oka's point of view, the basic "incompatibility of science and superstition"[313] ultimately rests not on this theoretical question of origins but, rather, on the practical question of technological prowess. "We cannot try to combine science and superstition in the same brain" because "a brain fit for science is unfit for superstition, and a brain fit for superstition is unfit for science."[314] As far as Oka could tell from his position at the Tokyo Higher Normal School and on the Ministry of Education's textbook compilation committee, the "brains unfit for science" among the future workers of the Japanese ethnic nation were gaining the upper hand: "the position of our nation with respect to scientific learning and its application is far inferior in comparison to other first-rank nations. If we do not put a great deal of effort into this in the future we will not at all be able to rank with these other nations and take a stand in the arena of competition."[315] Compared to Germany, in fact, the situation is "quite extreme"[316] and Oka claims to be, as a result, "at the height of despair."[317]

TOWARD GENERATIVE SCIENTISM

Oka's despair at the prevalence and seeming ascendancy of superstition is much like Haeckel's clash with ultramontane Catholicism. In both cases the reaction not only directly threatened science education but undermined an accommodationist stance that sought to reform the traditional nomos by degrees, not abruptly overthrow it. However, in Oka's case, the response was more like Haeckel's protégés than that of Haeckel himself. As we have seen, Oka's reaction to the nomic crisis after the Russo-Japanese War had a great

---

311 Ibid.
312 Migita, *Tennosei to Shinkaron*, 14.
313 Oka, "Kyōiku to Meishin" [Education and superstition], 122.
314 Ibid.
315 Ibid., 121.
316 Ibid., 123.
317 Ibid., 121.

deal in common with that of the reactionary statists. Each in its own way prescribed shoring up the nomic disposition of the people in order to preserve the organic and concrete consanguineous bonds of the nation. Both positions deplored social "fevers" that exacerbated unfettered individuals and related ideologies such as laissez-faire social Darwinism, socialism, and anarchism, all of which seemed to undermine nomic cohesion. Oka's evolutionism relied on the atemporal organicism of interdependence and seemed to offer this as a modern, scientific basis—a metapolitics—upon which to reform traditional norms and conventions. However, the emergence of state Shinto as an aggressive force designed to counter the same anomy that Oka hoped to turn back brought evolutionism and orthodoxy into direct conflict. Especially as Shinto began to successfully invade the sanctum of public education and inject superstition into the curriculum Oka was forced to resort to measures, beyond reformist metapolitics, that would match and perhaps turn the tables on Hozumi's reactionary Shintoist "blood community of worshipers."

Though, as we saw above Oka came close to directly attacking the reign of superstition in 1913, his primary gambit, one we will argue proved highly successful in the long term, was to historicize his organicism. This move can be seen in both the Hibiya Library lecture and another talk that Oka gave in Shizuoka a year before which was given the title "Science and the Development of the Ethnic Nation" in the second edition of *Evolution and Human Life*. As we have already seen "to cultivate upcoming generations" for autarkic competition is the stated aim of education in Oka's "Education and Superstition" lecture.[318] Conversely, continuing to govern through the "superstitions of old" will prove "a great disadvantage for the future of the nation."[319] The "Science and the Development of the Ethnic Nation" lecture is even more emphatic in its future orientation, ending with a warning that "if the kind of person who has an interest in science, though not the confidence to master science in a special area, and who always lends support to the planning of scientific advancement, does not greatly increase from here on, I think the future fate of our nation cannot be one of long-term prosperity."[320]

---

318 Ibid., 117.
319 Ibid., 125.
320 Ibid., 116.

More than just averring to the folly of emperor worship through his critique of superstition, it is this invocation of future historical development that will comprise Oka's response to the liturgical cosmization of Hozumi's family state. In the Shizuoka lecture ongoing appropriation of ever-advancing "new civilized knowledge" is the essential activity of modern nation-states, and accordingly, Oka places future generations of technologically adept workers, who are versed in this new civilized knowledge, at the center of Japan's continued survival, growth, and expansion. This participatory vision of ethnic nationalism is in stark contrast to Hozumi's absolutist national body (*kokutai*) which not only rejected imperialism—because empire would pollute the blood community—but reduced the *kokumin* to dutiful and docile children of the sacrosanct emperor-father. As Walter Skya argues, Hozumi's reactionary answer to the crisis of cohesion after the Russo-Japanese War—what we have called a nomic crisis—was always going to prove inadequate because the subjectivity that the war had helped arouse would never accept a return to old regime arrangements. Skya describes how alternate ideologies that did take subjectivity into account ultimately forced Hozumi's "reactionary Shinto ultranationalism" to transform into a "radical Shinto ultranationalism" that posited the participation of the awakened masses in national political projects. Like socialism, anarchism, and, especially, Minobe Tatsukichi's organ theory, which promoted party politics, Oka's vision of a superorganic nation-state of technologically adept worker cells who, by practicing an instinct-engendering human-way, would achieve an organic cohesion that was more congruent with the lives, experiences, and aspirations of members of an industrializing, urbanizing, and increasingly cosmopolitan nation than Hozumi's absolutism or the performance of arcane rituals.

Yet the advantage Oka's metapolitics had over these alternate ideologies is that it also spoke to the longings for community that the emerging Shinto orthodoxy was attempting to co-opt. As we have seen, Oka, like Hozumi and other government intellectuals who wanted to keep evolution in parenthesis, regarded the postwar turbulence as a nomic crisis that could be answered by instilling a moral disposition into the population, one that would render the nation a concrete, organic body with the same cohesion and shared inner purpose as a family or a village. Though his goal was to engender instincts, not promote ritual obedience, this similarity of approach allowed Oka to meet the orthodoxy, in a sense, on its own ground and offer more compelling ontological underpinnings to the norms, conventions, and laws that bound the nation together into a whole. To achieve this, Oka seems to have realized the polemical insufficiency of a metapolitics that relied merely on the example of the organicism of interdependence found in nature to scientistically reform the polity. His experiences during the "Darwin boom" and with the Shintoist reaction to modern anomy had revealed to him something his colleagues in Germany had also discovered: that for evolutionary biology to hold its own and not be sidelined by competing ideologies or suppressed by a religious revival it had to emphasize the temporal dimension of its organicism. The reformist scientism of his wartime and early postwar writings would have to be supplemented by a scientism that, like the scientism of Haeckel and his followers, drew on the epigenetic process of growth: the nation would not just exhibit the structure of an organism but develop through life-cycle stages which would measure health, establish purpose and generate values. It was this generative scientism that presented an alternative to the ontology offered by religion: just as images of gods and Buddhas were to be supplanted by representations of the super-organismic moss animal, so too would the reactionary vision of Hozumi's family state be replaced by a dynamic developmental process that infused not only the genealogy of the nation but its binding norms and conventions with cosmic significance. The nomos of the human-way would be cosmicized by identifying it with national destiny.

As the next chapter will reveal, Oka avoided the heretical implications of his generative scientism by offering it as a theory of degeneration. The nomic crisis described in this chapter will be seen as a sign of senility and, in particular, the rise of individualism will be portrayed as indicative of a modern life gone awry. By intimating that the moment of healthy, organic cohesion lay in a past that correct hygiene might, at least, partially retrieve, Oka was not only offering the orthodoxy a metapolitical ontology in which it could place its own genealogical conception of the "national body" but opening the way to imaging a new kind of human being through the techniques of eugenics and racial hygiene. In the end we will argue that Oka's *shinkaron* makes available a palingenetic ontology that envisions the regeneration of the nation through the programmatic modernist initiatives of such "new civilized knowledge."

CHAPTER 7

DECADENCE AND DESTINY

In the 1910 New Year's issue of Meiji Japan's premiere intellectual journal, *Chūō Kōron*, Oka showcased his answer not only to the postwar nomic crisis but to the reactionary measures undertaken by the state to reverse that crisis and restore traditional, organic relationships between members of body politic. Traveling under the portentous title "The Future of Humankind," Oka's lengthy article expanded his organicist evolutionism into an historicist vision of cosmic development that aspired to outdo Shinto fundamentalism in providing ontological foundations for a communitarian nomos. Acknowledging in its opening paragraph that "to expound on the limitless future is not easy" and that "even many weather forecasts based on science do not come true," the article, nevertheless, argued against the common wisdom that it takes a "more than human" prophet to foretell the future. Wasn't the public, after all, anticipating that very spring the appearance of Halley's Comet in the skies above Japan? Astronomers, Oka pointed out, had been able to predict the coming of the comet according to a particular method: "measuring heavenly bodies in bygone days, searching for laws that guide such movements, applying these laws to the future, and making predictions." This same method, he contended, could be employed to predict the future of humankind: "examining past change in the world of living things, measuring the laws that govern the rise and decline of each species and applying these laws to the human case." While prognosticating the exact timing of future events with mathematical precision was not possible, an understanding of the laws of natural change would yield a

reliable estimate of the "direction of development" and the "final destination" of the human species.[1]

The evolutionary laws Oka consulted did not predict a progressive future
for humankind. Instead, Oka conjured for his increasingly sophisticated
late Meiji readership what seemed to be a tragic vision of the future: decline
and extinction, not prosperity and progress, were in the offing for the various "species" that comprised humankind. Oka's "The Future of Humankind," in fact, articulated a theory of degeneration, one that extrapolated on
Haeckel's recapitulationist paradigm (see Chapter 2) in a manner similar to
his contemporaries in Europe (see Chapter 3). Working in a period known
to historians of science as the eclipse of Darwinism, Oka devised his own
account of degeneration by drawing on a non-Darwinian theory of evolution known as orthogenesis. Based on the analogy of evolution with embryological development that both the *Naturalphilosophen* and Haeckel had espoused, orthogenesis provided not only an evolutionary but an historical
law by which Oka could predict the direction and eventual destination of
human life. According to this doctrine, degeneration and death were the inevitable outcomes of biological growth at all levels of individuality: just as
individual organisms were predestined to go through stages of growth, maturity, senescence, and eventual death, so too were species, peoples, and,
most importantly for Oka, races and nations destined to evolve through life
cycles toward their own eventual extinction.[2]

Although, as we will see, Oka employed this organicist life-cycle analogy to indict the modern mode of life in postwar Japan as having entered a
stage of overdeveloped dissolution that he diagnosed as senescence, I will
argue here that his theory of degeneration, in fact, presents a palingenetic
vision of national development that, in the long term, proved to be more
credible than the reactionary Shinto orthodoxy in establishing the ontological foundations for nomic cohesion. As will be illustrated, not only by the
content of this New Year's article but, most especially, by his endorsement,
shortly thereafter, of racial hygiene, Oka's account of national degeneration
pointed inexorably toward regeneration, a return to earlier phases in the life

---

1   Asajirō Oka, "Jinrui no shōrai" [The future of humankind], in *Shinka to Jinsei* [Evolution and human life]
    (Tokyo: Yūseidō Shuppan, 1968), 204–5.

2   Apparently unaware of the doctrine of orthogenesis and its impact on evolutionary science, Watanabe
    Masao attributes Oka's pessimism to his temperament and the influence of Buddhism on Japanese cul-
    ture. See Watanabe, *The Japanese and Western Science*, 90–98.

cycle when hygienic integration was still intact and growth into a healthily differentiated modern mode of existence was still possible. Whereas Hozumi's reactionary Shintoism provided a purely static vision of the nation, one in which all change was portrayed as decay, Oka, in contrast, placed the nation along a life-cycle continuum that embraced development and sought to overcome decline not by retreating to an immutable past but by recapturing and starting anew from an earlier phase of healthy integration.

As with the emerging orthodoxy, a primary target of Oka's mature *shinkaron* was individualism—which he portrayed as a form of egoism and therefore a primary source of group-destroying anomy. Oka, also like promoters of Shinto fundamentalism, attempted to reverse this anomy by establishing an ontological basis for nomic cohesion. Yet, as I will argue, not only did his future-oriented *shinkaron* contribute a narrative of national destiny more congruent with the urbanizing, industrializing, and specializing world of the *minzoku*. The scientism it made available also served simultaneously as a source of value and a means of transformation. It is due to this duel capacity that I have attached the term "generative scientism" to Oka's evolutionism. It is the comicizing life-cycle narrative of growth, maturity, senescence, and death that performs two concurrent operations: generating values by measuring health in terms of maturation into an optimal state of integrated differentiation—unity-in-difference—and elucidating the workings of the growth process in a manner that facilitates eugenic restoration. In other words, the cosmological incontestability associated with religion and the "transparency of the real" required for technological manipulation were embedded together in Oka's temporal organicism. The degenerate anomy of egoism will be overcome and the true concrete community revived through the embodiment of value-generating, cosmically grounded nomic instincts in the rejuvenated superindividuality of the ethnic nation.

At the end of this chapter, and more extensively in the epilogue, we will suggest that the technologically transformative, value-positing, futural orientation of Oka's generative scientism meant that it would eventually contribute to the renovation of the orthodoxy it was intended to counter. Though the reactionary version of the *kokutai* orthodoxy, Hozumi's family-state made significant inroads at the end of the Meiji period and the early years of Taisho, Oka's organicist evolutionism looked ahead to an alternate, healthy modern lifestyle in a way that such reactionary Shintoism did not. Restoring the certainty of something like a sacred canopy but not rejecting progress and development, Oka's generative scientism qualifies as an early Japanese form of programmatic modernism. A vision of national-biological reconstruction equipped with both meaning-generating ultimate ends and techniques for transformation, Oka's organicist, developmental program would, a decade after "The Future of Humankind," come to occupy a place alongside the orthodoxy once the Great War in Europe had established once and for all the indispensability of science and technology for national survival. Toward the close of this study we will explore whether this semiofficial condition of coexistence might in part account for the transformation of the latter into a more programmatic doctrine that, in the end, was less familialist and more totalitarian in its outlook.

1. Orthogenetic Overdevelopment

It was from his training in evolutionary science—which we described in Chapter 2—that Oka derived the historical law that enabled him to foresee the "final destination" of humankind and call for regenerative measures that would delay the decline of the Japanese *minzoku*. The future "direction of development" of humanity—and, most critically, that of its constituent ethnic nations—could be predicted because its trajectory adhered to the law of evolution that was at the basis of all life. However, we should be careful, once again, to distinguish evolution as Oka understood it from Darwinism. Darwin, in fact, conceived of naturalistic descent with modification as a haphazard, branching process that did not at all lend itself to the sort of prognostication that preoccupied Oka. Oka's *shinkaron*, in contrast, was shaped by organicist evolutionary theories from a largely non-Darwinian basis that advanced a developmental vision of evolution according to an analogy with individual growth.[3] The notion that the future of species, nations, and races would unfold as phases of a foreseeable life cycle rested on this analogy—an analogy in the form of a metaphysical conceit that, despite its prescientific origins, had insinuated itself at the very heart of the scientific circles where Oka received his graduate training.

In Chapter 2 we explained how this organicist growth analogy was the central feature of the research paradigm in Rudolf Leuckart's laboratory at

---

3   Bowler, *The Non-Darwinian Revolution*, 28–30, 51–52; Weindling, *Health, Race and German Politics*, 36–48.

Leipzig University where Oka studied in the early 1890s. Devised by Ernst Haeckel, the Jena University zoologist who was primarily responsible for interpreting Darwin to the late-nineteenth-century global audience, this paradigm, known as evolutionary morphology, construed the developmental, life-cycle analogy from the early, pre-Darwinian "idealist morphology" as the central principle of evolution—what he called "biogenetic law." According to this law, the life-cycle stages an individual organism passes through from conception up to mature adulthood (ontology) merely repeat the evolutionary history of its species back to the beginning of life on earth (phylogeny).[4] By implication, this law, which Haeckel famously summarized as "ontogeny recapitulates phylogeny," could also be read in the opposite direction: the life history of a species can be said to unfold in adherence to the same phases of birth, growth, maturity, senescence, and death experienced by individual organisms. Species, in short, are destined to progress through the phases and transitions of an individual life in a sort of biographical story arc. The certainty of biogenetic law allowed evolutionists such as Oka not only to use the evidence of embryology to look back and try to fill in gaps in the paleontological record, but also to anticipate future evolutionary developments.

Inherent in this life-cyclical view of evolution founded on biogenetic law was another non-Darwinian presupposition: that of a hierarchy of organic individuality. Ultimately, the idea of recapitulation at the heart of biogenetic law made sense because evolutionary morphologists assumed that particular organisms and the species to which they belonged were similar phenomena: they were both "unities of life," parallel instances of living nature realizing an innate tendency to form itself into organic wholes through an epigenetic process of differentiation and reintegration. Whether individual persons or species construed as individuals, these self-contained organisms might be thought of as selves or even as personalities or egos. For Haeckel this essential quality of life extended to every level of living nature. His evolutionary morphology envisioned the world of living things structured as successively more and more complex and inclusive echelons of organic individuality. As we saw in Chapters 2 and 3, Haeckel, in such worldwide best sellers as *The Wonders of Life* (1904), simplified this hierarchy to cells, per-

---

4   Gould, *Ontogeny and Phylogeny*, 76–85; Bowler, *The Non-Darwinian Revolution*, 76–90.

sons (individuals as we usually think of them), and colonies in such a way that persons consisted of higher unities of cells (cell-states) and colonies as yet higher unities of persons (superorganisms or corms). All three levels constituted sentient, ego-possessing organisms in their own right, with the highest level, the superorganism, being how Haeckel portrayed the lives of gregarious creatures.

In the best-selling book that established his reputation among the Japanese public, *Lectures on Evolutionary Theory* (*Shinkaron no Kōza*), Oka presents biogenetic law as *the* law of evolution.[5] This should come as no surprise as it was the research program of evolutionary morphology that enabled Oka to perform physiological and embryological analyses on *kanten kokemushi* (moss animals), the species of freshwater bryozoan that inhabited the ponds in and around Tokyo Imperial University. As we have seen throughout this study, it was the collective existence displayed by these moss animals—which Oka depicted in terms of biogenetic law and its hierarchy of organic individuality—that came to serve as the metapolitical model, the "ideal group life," according to which he hoped the Japanese nation-state would eventually conform. While these hopes for the instinctual, nomic cohesion of the "human-way" seemed to have been momentarily realized under the conditions of the Russo-Japanese War, the war's aftermath, as we described in the last chapter, seemed to unleash "social fevers" that threatened subversion, dissolution, and anomy. Alarmed by these developments, the Home and Education Ministries adopted aggressive initiatives to shore up the social foundations by promoting a Shinto-infused nation-creed focused on the sacredness and historical centrality of the imperial house. By 1910 Oka found his efforts to promote his nation-as-superorganism account derived from biogenetic law undermined and marginalized: not only did individualist ideologies of political radicalism and self-interested striving rejected his corporatist Darwinism but the Education Ministry committee on which he had served for over five years was about to issue an official science textbook that excluded any mention of the theory of evolution.

Oka responded to this crisis within a crisis by turning, in the "The Future of Humankind," to the theory of orthogenesis. It was this theory in particular that translated seamlessly into an historical law and allowed Oka to

---

5 Oka, "Kyōiku to Meishin" [Education and superstition], 122–23.

predict the decline and extinction of humankind. However, construing evolution as orthogenesis did not at all represent a break with Haeckel's evolutionary morphology. Rather, orthogenesis extrapolated on biogenetic law, taking its central developmental analogy with individual growth and transforming it into a force within a species, one that causes it to evolve in a fixed direction through the life-cycle phases of birth, growth, maturity, senility, and death. Because this innate evolutionary drive was nonadaptive, much more emphasis was placed on the end stages of the life cycle: how senility and extinction occurred in formerly thriving species now needed explaining. The answer that espousers of orthogenesis came up with involved what they called the overdevelopment of once beneficial traits. As we will see it was this notion that emerged as the central feature of Oka's theory of decadence.

Overdevelopment, like orthogenesis itself, presupposed Haeckel's research paradigm of evolutionary morphology. As was established in Chapter 2, this paradigm featured not only biogenetic law, but a non-Darwinian mechanism as the primary agent of evolutionary change: Lamarckism. In Haeckel's account, once an organism "recapitulated"—that is, once it reached maturity by epigenetically developing through the evolutionary stages its ancestors had experienced—it then had the potential to add on new characteristics through its own behavior. Habitual action would cause an organism to "acquire characteristics" that could be passed on to the next generation of offspring. Such offspring would exhibit this new characteristic as the final stage of their own growth into maturity before they too added novel, yet inheritable characteristics via the Lamarckian mechanism.[6]

Sometimes called "use-inheritance," Lamarckism, in conjunction with biogenetic law, became the basis of many of the non-Darwinian theories that challenged the priority of natural selection around the turn of the century—the period of so-called non-Darwinian revolution. Indeed, the scientists who formulated the doctrine of orthogenesis can be thought of as Lamarckians with a background in evolutionary morphology. This was true not only of Theodor Eimer (1843–1898), the German zoologist who coined the term orthogenesis and in the 1890s explained the theory to the world in his *On Orthogenesis and the Impotence of Natural Selection in Species-Forma-*

---

6   Bowler, *The Non-Darwinian Revolution*, 84–85.

tion (1898), but of Alpheus Hyatt (1838–1902), the widely influential Massachusetts Institute of Technology paleontologist who was most active in synthesizing orthogenesis and Lamarckism into a theory of degeneration through overdevelopment. Hyatt argued that "adaptive trends established by the Lamarckian effect almost always carried beyond the point of maximal utility and drove the species inexorably toward 'racial senility' and death."[7] In other words, progressive traits developed through use-inheritance would inevitably take on a momentum of their own, becoming an increasingly nonadaptive liability. Such liability marked the onset of decadence—for from the moment the traits overdeveloped the species would begin to down cycle, becoming "senile" and finally going extinct.

In its full-blown version, orthogenesis imagined forces from within species driving this process along a predetermined trajectory. Evolution was conceived as "consistently directed along a single path,"[8] while the orthogenetic drive within it caused species to trace a parabolic arc which, in most versions of the theory, paralleled the life cycle of an individual organism through stages of growth, senility, and death or extinction. The overdeveloped traits that evolved through the Lamarckian mechanism acted as the agent of this orthogenetic drive. At first these traits had been of great benefit to the species in question, enabling them not only to grow into maturity but to thrive and even dominate. Yet, inevitability, their very success turned into a disadvantage: the cunning of evolution, through an elemental inner process, encouraged the traits to become fatally exaggerated, thereby initiating the downward trajectory toward extinction. Either the species in question would become easy prey for hitherto inferior competitors and be annihilated, or else their overdevelopment would make them so dysfunctional that they simply died out.[9] Whichever the case, for adherents to the orthogenetic doctrine such as Eimer, Hyatt, and, as we will see, their fellow Lamarckian colleague Oka Asajirō, the appearance of such overdeveloped traits indicated that the unseen force within evolution was pushing a species inexorably through the declining stages of the biogenetic life cycle.

---

7   Bowler, *Evolution*, 247–50.
8   Bowler, *The Eclipse of Darwinism*, 7.
9   Bowler, *Evolution*, 141–81.

2. Downfall of the Dinosaurs

Oka may have been compelled to embrace the doctrine of orthogenesis, especially Hyatt's version of it, because the notion of overdevelopment was being applied to his subfield in zoology. Certain varieties of the aquatic invertebrates he was researching, bryozoan or moss animals, displayed a self-destructive tendency to elaborate their shells well past the point of utility. While the shells of these particular bryozoan species had initially served as a supporting structure for the colony, they had, over generations, become so onerous that they increasingly cut these minute members of the colony off from their surrounding environment. Haeckel himself had addressed this problem, but it was W. D. Lang, a paleontologist at the British Museum, who offered the accepted explanation—namely that a self-generated orthogenetic compulsion to excrete calcium carbonate accounted for both the initial beneficial emergence of the shells and their eventual deleterious overdevelopment. In other words, the shells evolved not due to adaptation to the environment via natural selection, but as the result of an in-built, nonadaptive urge to produce calcium carbonate. The rise and fall of these species of bryozoans through the stages of the life cycle was predetermined by this inner evolutionary force.[10]

In "The Future of Humankind," Oka was particularly interested in a certain variety of species that had been brought low by this process of orthogenesis: "animals that occupied a preeminent position akin to today's human beings and that, for a time, did not have any competitors to challenge them."[11] In Oka's portrayal, the tragic fate of these once dominant creatures offered another stark illustration of the inner workings of evolution: their rise and fall limned a parabolic arc through which all such species must pass during their evolutionary life cycle. Yet, as the quote suggests, such species also served as something more: a precedent for the human predicament and, as such, a scientistic index against which human affairs could be interpreted. For Oka the tragic decline of these once dominant creatures, our precursors in preeminence, presented a glimpse of human destiny. Not only was theirs a story which humankind was fated to endure, but the onset of human deca-

---

10 Lang's research was not published until 1921. See Bowler, *The Eclipse of Darwinism*, 165–67.
11 Oka, "Jinrui no shōrai" [The Future of Humankind], 208–9.

dence could be read in the tell-tale signs of overdevelopment made available through the fossil record they left behind.

Among these once dominant precursors, Oka held special fascination for the almost unimaginable "vitality and strength attained by species of lizards in the Mesozoic era." He marveled at the Alantosaurus, a dinosaur whose fossils had recently been excavated in North America and which, at almost thirty meters in length, was "bigger than the largest whale of the present day." Equally astounding to Oka were whalelike aquatic lizards such as the "Plesiosaurus and Ichyosaurus" and the airborne pteranodon that sported a wingspan over six meters and was "three times the size of today's largest flying bird, the South American Condor." These dinosaur species were "entirely alone in walking the earth, swimming in the seas and soaring through the air so that no other creature should equal them even to the least extent."[12]

The great mammals of the Tertiary period provided their own vivid examples of single species habitat dominance. During this time there walked the earth, for instance, a variety of elephant called Deinotherium that featured a gargantuan skull, a species of saber-toothed tiger known as the Machiaradus whose "tusks were nearly as big as daggers," and a type of deer whose antlers spanned almost four meters. As with the dinosaurs of Mesozoic times, these beasts were so overwhelmingly powerful that "not even in a dream" was it possible that one can imagine them being vanquished. They reigned supreme without evolutionary challengers.[13]

Explaining why these "great lizards of the Mesozoic era" and "terrifying beasts of the Tertiary period" came suddenly to represent "figures of utter defeat" for subsequent epochs involved debunking the standard view of their decline and extinction. In Oka's estimation, his contemporary paleontologists and biologists were greatly mistaken in assuming that "superior animals appeared" and then defeated previously dominant creatures. This interpretation made little sense because it would have been nearly impossible "for a species from among those who, up until now, had been inferior suddenly and rapidly to acquire power, surpass those who had hitherto been absolutely superior and cause their prompt annihilation." A better explanation, according to Oka, was that the dominant species were weakened

---

12 Ibid., 209.
13 Ibid., 209–10.

due to a cause "from within those species of animals themselves." This "inner cause of their decline works itself out and they come to incline toward their fate: all at once they are brought low by those who until now occupied an inferior position."[14]

Though Oka evidently did not want to unduly complicate matters for his lay audience by introducing scientific jargon, this internal cause of inevitable self-destruction was clearly none other than the orthogenetic drive behind evolution itself—the drive that, like its antecedent biogenetic law, made both species and individuals develop through stages of growth, maturity, senility, and death. In the case of dominant species this drive was manifested in the overdevelopment of traits. Specifically, "the cause that works from within is, in a manner of speaking, identical to what made a species in the beginning, and allowed it to defeat all of its opponents and attain a superior position." According to Oka, the "examples from the study of fossils have revealed" that "the same characteristics" which allow species to "overcome other animals and attain a supreme position soon bring disaster." Impelled by the inner workings of evolution, once advantageous characteristics first acquired through Lamarckian use-inheritance become a liability. If these "liabilities exceed a fixed degree" the traits in question cause the species to be annihilated in the struggle for existence by their erstwhile inferiors.[15]

For the dinosaurs of the Mesozoic era it was, Oka suggested, their great size and strength that, paradoxically, did them in. While he conceded that "size and strength are certainly conducive to defeating others in the struggle for existence" these advantageous traits also could burden an animal. These burdens included: "needing great quantities of food in daily life, requiring many months and years to mature, needing a long breeding period and lacking quickness in work." At a certain point these disadvantages added up and the dinosaurs were vanquished. Likewise, the ferocious tigers and elephants of the Tertiary period developed "large and sharp horns and tusks" that "were undoubtedly extremely advantageous for defeating enemies." Yet, in the end, the singular overdevelopment of such successful traits was also what undermined these dominant creatures: "A skull and jaw bone supporting these horns and tusks, muscles for putting them to practical use, blood

14   Ibid., 210–11.
15   Ibid., 212–14.

vessels to replenish these muscles—all of these together must develop. Consequently, if horns and tusks alone grow large, the burden on the animal becomes heavy and when this too exceeds a certain point it becomes unsuitable for the struggle for existence."[16]

According to Oka, it was the moment of victory over other creatures that marked the onset of overdevelopment and the beginning of decline. This occurred because members of the triumphant species now turned on one another, employing the same traits used to gain mastery over the rest of the animal kingdom. As Oka describes the logic at work: "Species that conquer the world through muscular strength later on complete within their own species through muscular strength. Species that occupy a superior position due to their tusks later on fight with others of their own species using tusks. Consequently, more and more it is the case that if their bodies are not large and their tusks not strong they cannot survive. In this way, traits used by species to prevail over others are in a state where they can limitlessly develop without end."[17] Such negative competition was ultimately what determines which traits will overdevelop. Once this process starts it cannot easily be reversed. As we will see, slowing or resetting this process to an earlier, healthier moment of growth will turn out to be Oka's response to what looks like inevitable decline.

3. The Triumph of Brains and Hands

Oka's anthropological account of the rise and fall of humankind traced a similar trajectory. Beneficial traits emerged and provided the creatures that eventually evolved into human beings such an absolute advantage that they came to reign supreme on earth. Nevertheless, in the end, the internal mechanism of evolution would turn these assets into liabilities—they were destined to overdevelop and result in members of the species setting upon each other and falling prey to erstwhile weaker competitors. This internal strife was especially fatal in the case of humans because, unlike their dinosaur and great mammal precursors in habitat dominance, human beings were gregarious creatures for whom the struggle for existence took place at the group

16 Ibid., 212.
17 Ibid., 213.

level. Once this group ceased to function like a single organism it would begin to cycle into decline and eventual extinction.

Oka attributed the "present-day superior position" of human groups to the emergence of two uniquely sophisticated faculties, brains and hands. These traits not only provided the human equivalent of the moss animal collective with distinct edge over competitors, but they explained the transition from ape to human. Indeed, "The Future of Humankind" offers a sketch of human evolution in which the brains and hands of apes developed in tandem until full humanity was achieved. True to his non-Darwinian predilections, Oka imagined this evolution to be a Lamarckian process emphasizing habitual action—in this case the use of tools. According to Oka, "perhaps tens of millions or hundreds of millions of years ago, there was among the apes one type that moved from an arboreal existence to life lived on the ground, supporting their bodies on their hind quarters alone and walking upright. The erect posture of this ape freed up the front legs which then could be employed to manipulate simple tools, or pick up stones and throw them at others, or break off branches and fashion them into sticks to protect against enemies. Or else they set up some stones and broke them so that they could use the resulting sharp edges as swords or axes."[18]

The making and manipulation of tools began the evolution of ape into man. In fashioning "simple instruments" the fingers inherited from apes became more and more sophisticated. This, in turn, meant the hands could produce more refined tools, such as arrows, until, finally, humans were able to create fire for themselves and use that fire to make earthenware or cast weapons out of iron and bronze. In this way humans became the "animals that use technology"[19] and they employed this technological prowess to eliminate "not only those they already had to fear as enemies, but every beast that had caused them harm." In the end, the human species "gradually bred and spread out over the entire world, until we finally progressed to the present circumstances wherein, if we speak of warfare, we only mean warfare between human species."[20]

This technological triumph was, by Oka's reckoning, also an intellectual one: along with the hands the brain developed as well. Though it acquired the

18 Ibid., 207.
19 Ibid., 206.
20 Ibid., 208.

ability "to make estimates" and to "invent things," what most distinguished the brain, in Oka's view, was its capacity for language. Along with their aptitude for technology, humans were also "the animal that uses language." As Oka explains, "ordinarily language is considered to be something spoken with the mouth, but, in reality, the mouth is needed merely as an organ to give voice to language and, in truth, the organ we use is the brain. Thus, it is always preferable to say that we are speaking with our brains." As with the implement-wielding hands, the larger linguistically oriented human brain enabled humans to organize their societies, better analyze their world and, thereby, overcome "various other creatures" to attain their "present-day superior position."[21]

The Lamarckian element in the development of brains and hands was unmistakable. Hands evolved in tandem with the implements they devised. Likewise, the brain evolved in tandem with the hands in a Lamarckian feedback process. "As a general rule, whichever tool is in use, at the same time the hands are being employed so is the brain and in the making of implements the brain is used still more. In making and using tools devised by the brain, the hand gradually becomes skilled and, over time, gains the ability to do elaborate work. Due to the experience of manipulating the hands, the brain develops further and becomes better able to think. The hand and brain assist one another and together they gradually develop."[22] For Oka the development of these interrelated attributes did not occur "in a sudden single step" but, in keeping with the central life-cycle analogy, "through a sequence of necessary steps" that resulted from a gradual "piling up of experiences."[23] The hands and the brain were, in other words, characteristics acquired through habitual action. A Lamarckian, and not a Darwinian, process was primarily at work.

The brains and hands that Lamarckism produced were viewed by Oka, initially at least, as specialized attributes that contributed to the health and power of the higher organic individuality of the human group. While humans may have come down from the trees and stood upright, they still relied on gregarious, group-oriented instincts for survival. Not only did individual humans subsume their self-interested, lesser egos to the greater good of the group, but the human struggle for existence took place at that group

---

21   Ibid., 207.
22   Ibid., 206.
23   Ibid., 206–7.

level. The group was an individual with an ego and interests of its own and, just like the moss animal, its evolutionary health was measured by its ability to unite itself internally for competition with other social organisms. The implements employed by developing hands and the language made use of by the increasingly sophisticated brains yielded, respectively, technology and abstract ideas, both of which fortified the superorganism. In the case of technology, it translated into group power through outward force projection: the manufacture of more and more sophisticated armaments that allowed human groups to vanquish competing species and, later, one another. Abstract ideas, meanwhile, not only made modern science possible—which in turn rendered human weaponry increasingly lethal—but they enabled human superorganisms to consolidate themselves through laws, morality, state institutions and communications. As Oka pointed out repeatedly in his writings in language that appeared to draw on the account of human evolution from Haeckel's *The Wonders of Life* (see Chapter 3), the evolutionary winners among humans were the "civilized" human species that have organized themselves through their advanced technological and mental capacities to triumph over weaker, less rigorously collectivized "barbarians."

4. HUMAN DEGENERACY

For Oka and many of his contemporaries victory in the Russo-Japanese War seemed not only to confirm such "civilized" status for Japan, but to represent a moment when the longed-for *Kyokoku itchi* (national unity) of the *minzoku* had finally been realized.[24] Yet, as the last chapter explored, this sense of national integration was deceptive: the society that had rallied behind the war effort now revealed its conflicted nature.[25] Not only did the awakened subjectivity of individualism begin to manifest as anomic social fevers and acts of political subversion, but the stifling reactionary response to this dissolution threatened to exacerbate it through a nationwide inculcation of anachronistic superstitions. In response, Oka's postwar writings were infused with a sense of peril that Japan was losing the nomic solidarity it had seemingly actualized during the war. As we have seen, the essays he began to contribute to

---

24 Shimazu, *Japanese Society at War*, 19.
25 Ibid., 17–54; Gluck, *Japan's Modern Myths*, 157–212; Skya, *Japan's Holy War*, 154–55; Oka, "Generational Conflict after the Russo-Japanese War."

leading journals were written to educate the public about Japan's evolutionary situation in the hopes of convincing individuals to subsume their lesser selves to the greater good of the *minzoku*. Myopic self-interest and the evolutionarily deleterious social divisions it wrought increasingly became Oka's preoccupation until, in "The Future of Humankind," he began to describe what he perceived as rampant egoism as itself an expression of the inner logic of evolution.[26] Oka now argued that the brains and hands that had secured human success had overdeveloped. Not only was this causing the superorganism of the ethnic nation to disintegrate, but it was part of an inevitable process: the tragic life-cycle trajectory that all dominant species are destined to follow.

Oka did not attempt to explain how overdeveloped brains and hands translated into ego overdevelopment. Instead he focused on what he took to be the excesses of contemporary material civilization and treated these as vivid signs of impending decline. Thus, the accoutrements and novelties of the late Meiji period came to serve as indicators that the evolutionary era of sociopolitical solidarity was drawing to a close. Looking at the world around him Oka did not see progress but incipient degeneration—the material accomplishments and new social arrangements were signs that the lesser egoism of individuals was undermining the greater egoism of the nation. They marked the ominous transition toward inevitable decline and extinction.

The prime indicator of this transition was the money economy—or "money world."[27] For Oka laissez-faire capitalism represented the onset of this degenerate phase of evolution, one in which individuals within each *minzoku* engaged in negative competition against one another. In his view "humankind survives by forming societies: combining strength together and helping one another are important above all else. Yet this fellowship grows more and more faint when public consciousness degenerates in conjunction with life problems" brought about when competition between individuals so intensifies that one can do nothing but "calculate and plan from the vantage point of one's gains and losses." Once the pursuit of "egoistic

---

26 A transformation during these postwar years seems to have occurred in the concept of *risshin shusse* (getting ahead in the world), which had been associated with Darwinism from the early Meiji period, from stressing success for one's group to success for one's self, often through the acquisition of wealth. Oka's evolutionism can be seen as attempt to provide correct scientific grounds for the intense efforts by opinion leaders and government agents to reconstruct national unity and curb free-wheeling individualism. See Oka, "Generational Conflict after the Russo-Japanese War," 197–203; Gluck, *Japan's Modern Myths*, 204–12.

27 Gluck, *Japan's Modern Myths*, 207.

self-interestedness" becomes the overriding concern "the very fragile instinct for cooperation and consensus" loses efficacy and the superorganism of the people begins to disintegrate.[28] The money economy of capitalism and the enfeebling conveniences it concocts come to count, as Oka saw it, as sure signs of the *minzoku*'s incipient degeneration.

How capitalism was weakening the collective life of the nation interested Oka more than the manner in which overdeveloped brains and hands fabricated the money economy. We can glean from his passing remarks that somehow the technological and linguistic advantages that brains and hands afforded certain humans resulted in the appearance of private property and "at the same time a system of lending and collecting interest." From these developments a society emerged that was disastrously divided against itself into competing classes, one in which "value is attached to money alone."[29] While it is commonly presumed that social Darwinists of this period regarded such circumstances as evidence that the "struggle for existence" was functioning properly, Oka saw it as just the opposite: "with humankind the workings of natural selection are suspended after money—along with other things that can be exchanged—came into circulation." What private property did was set up a more intense, yet false and evolutionary disadvantageous, struggle for existence "in which the standard that determines winners and losers is not necessarily superiority of body and spirit."[30] Where the struggle for existence during the period of human ascendancy selected for individual specimens who contributed to the commonweal with strong bodies and a public-spirited mental makeup, the new, ersatz fittest of Oka's late Meiji modernity were either simply crafty self-promoters or sickly hangers-on, subsisting off of inherited wealth.

Thus, the petty egomania of the market place simultaneously fragmented and weakened the organically cohesive original *minzoku*. Unable to gather together its collective will, the superorganism was fated to fall easy prey to hitherto inferior competitors and eventually die out. In order to capture how palpably ominous this transition to degeneration was for Oka from his scholarly nook at Tokyo's Higher Normal School, it will be useful to analyze his account of this process of fragmentation and enfeeblement into two components. First,

---

28 Oka, "Jinrui no shōrai" [The future of humankind], 227.
29 Ibid., 214–15.
30 Ibid., 219.

we will explain how the false selection based on money and private property was, in his view, destroying the physical health of the race-nation. Then, secondly, we will address its degenerative impact on socially binding morality.

a. Physical Degeneration

For Oka the material civilization of the present age had resulted in human life becoming "estranged from the conditions of nature." No longer hardened by the competition with other human groups, individuals lived in pursuit of the technological conveniences and luxuries that money could buy. "Using machines for everything," the "resistance of the body to nature decreases and it becomes emasculated." The very technology that enabled humankind to light the night, cook its food, clothe itself and keep warm in winter and cool in summer—that is, innovations such as electric lights, coal fires, ice machines, electric fans, and the like—had so weakened the human body that "even if exposed to small degrees of cold it falls ill right away." Oka claimed there were "already examples of Westerners who are in danger of catching cold when not wearing socks" and that eating boiled food over generations has decreased "the ability to bite into tough objects" with the result that "compared to savages, civilized people have generally weak teeth."[31]

This growing enfeeblement led to an even greater dependence on technological products in order to maintain the health of human beings. Oka, who was famous among his students for the spare, technologically minimalist laboratory he kept,[32] cited objects as wide-ranging as "gloves, ear protectors, respirators, goggles," and "mood pills" as examples of the kinds of things that "when even one of these is lacking illness befalls right away."[33] Just as mammoth tusks and saber-toothed tiger fangs necessitated costly and evolutionary deleterious adjustments in other areas, a similar logic, according to Oka, prevailed with regard to modern technological comforts: "the numerous things needed to sustain life become extremely large, and, to that extent, the cost of life goes up, the degree of problems increases and still more effort is required for the struggle for existence."[34]

31 Ibid., 219.
32 Tsukuba, "Kaisetsu" [Commentary], 437–39.
33 Oka, "Jinrui no shōrai" [The future of humankind], 217.
34 Ibid.

Of these elaborate processes now needed to sustain life, Oka recognized the internationalization and industrialization of food production to be particularly dangerous. "When the world remained closed off, farm products passed directly into the hands of consumers" and so "food and drinks were not artificially mixed." Yet now, with a global economy, the manufacturing industry required not only manufacturing food products in "great quantities in a single place" but adding in preservatives while these products are temporarily placed in storage and mixing products together to "obtain extravagant profits." In Oka's view, that it was "already popular to do such things as add salicylic acid to alcohol, mix granules into sugar and flour, and put saccharine into sho-sake" did not bode well for humankind: "over a long period of time" these practices would "harm the body little by little."[35]

A more immediate threat, however, to human physical health was the very technological landscape that the overdeveloped brains and hands of laissez faire capitalism had created. The world of industrial processes, of machines and gadgets and mass entertainments, was not only weakening the body—it was also exacting a psychic cost that was driving humans to various self-destructive vices.

This physical cost was most obviously apparent with the advance of the manufacturing industry. As work became more "specialized according to the division of labor," the "actions of the body also come to be inclined in a single direction." As a consequence "those whose work consists in using the ears, use the ears alone to an excessive degree. Those whose work involves using the eyes make use of the eyes to an excessive degree." With many workers also finding themselves doing such things as "breathing cotton fibers all year around or smelling the smoke of hydrochloric acid," the outcome was that "each job comes to have a particular disease associated with it," a fact that was particularly devastating in the eyes of a Lamarckian such as Oka who believed acquired traits would be handed down across generations. He thus concluded that under such conditions "the body gradually worsens" and "to the extent that the countryside declines and the cities grow the range of this harm widens."[36]

---

35 Ibid.
36 Ibid., 223–24.

However, the harm engendered by industrialism did not by any means cease at the factory doors. In Oka's view, just living with technology weakened humans, for the hubbub of modern urban life was forcing the individual to react to his environment with a constancy and to a degree never required of our more healthy ancestors. While primitive humans had to deal with an exacting struggle for survival, they did so "unconsciously"—it was just a fact of existence. In contrast, technologically pampered, ego-inflated, physically feeble modern humans were confronted with circumstances which were paradoxically less challenging, but more taxing: a false struggle for more and more which was typified by the clatter and tumult of big city life.

All of this ego-driven turbulence manifested itself in an overload on the nervous system. As Oka would have it, "the instruments human beings make are for convenience or recreation, but in either case they are things that just stimulate the nerves with great intensity." When "we ride electric cars and steam trains," a "clamorous sound passes through the auditory nerves and strongly stimulates the brain's center." Though we may become less aware of this clamor as we acclimate to the urban landscape, the stimulation "caused to the ear, nerves and brain" lingers on without decreasing. The same effect was brought on by viewing motion pictures: while moviegoers may have thought they were merely experiencing a "movement of images," the stimulation of the "retina, optic nerve and brain" with "alterations of light and darkness" was occurring at a "rate of more than ten times per second."[37] Like the riding of public transportation or, indeed, the operating factory machinery, attending the cinema overstimulated the brain and the senses that serve it.

This overstimulation had a deleterious impact on the health of the whole nervous system. Not only did "the nerves gradually weaken" but "such action brings on oversensitivity" and, eventually "an onset of morbidity" and acute anxiety. Oka imagined modern humans to have become, as a result, skittish, apprehensive creatures for whom "small and trivial things cause extreme worry and concern," prone to passing fancies of the moment and in desperate need of escape from their worries so that "the least adversity leads immediately to disappointment and discouragement or desperation." In his view, the tendency, as degeneration deepens, would be for more and more

---

37 Ibid., 217.

people to fall prey to final despair or to find deliverance from anxiety in a variety of socially destructive vices. "According to statistics, the number of mentally ill people, suicides, and criminals increases every year. In the future, in accordance with the increase of such cases, we must be even more ready for the enormity of these developments."[38]

Those who did not end up in mental hospitals, morgues or prison houses would tend to take refuge in drugs and, in particular, alcohol. Oka even claimed that "savages," upon "coming into contact with civilized people," soon demanded "alcohol and tobacco first and foremost" in order to relieve the psychic "pressure brought on by the use of machinery." For the civilized urbanites that resorted to these vices under this same unrelenting pressure the consequences of using these "poisonous substances" could not have been more dire: "toxicosis," "deliriums of fear and trembling," and dimming eyesight. Worst of all, was, in his estimation, the harm that would come to "the constitution of descendants" of these tipplers: "[A]ccording to medical statistics, people who are mentally ill, imbecilic, and abnormal almost all had parents who were drinkers."[39]

b. Moral Degeneration

Yet as bad as this money and ego-inspired era of the machine had been for humankind's intergenerational physical makeup, the harm it was doing to morality was much more dire. As we discussed extensively in Part II, "Metapolitics," Oka's stress on the moral and mental faculties over the physical resulted from his estimation that it was between collectives, among, that is, racialist superorganisms, where the human struggle for existence properly took place. The weakness of individual bodies was only a concern insofar as it was dangerous for the superorganism of the *minzoku* to have weak cells. If particular people were unhealthy, they could always be cast off—just as any complex organism sheds unnecessary cells. Morality, in contrast, was conceived by the Lamarckian Oka as the active force that unified the people-cells as a whole into a higher organic self: practicing altruistic, public-spirited moral habits would literally serve to engrain the "nomic" instincts

---

38 Ibid., 217–18.
39 Ibid., 222.

needed for cooperation and consensus. The failure of morality—or ethical life—would therefore be catastrophic: it would signal the disintegration of the superorganism, the onset of its decline. But it is just this failure that Oka was portending.

While the remote cause of this tragic downturn was the overdevelopment of brains and hands, the visible trigger was widening discontent with the sociopolitical order and the authority that supported it. The dexterous hands and big brains that fashioned technological wonders for an economy based on private property had also produced envious have-nots.[40] According to Oka, as the "rich got richer" and the "poor poorer, it came about that within a single society there were a small number of extremely wealthy people living and playing in extreme luxury alongside numberless extremely impoverished people who lacked, no matter how hard they toiled, even basic food and clothing." Seduced by the lure of "the splendorous lives of the rich," the poor were beginning to believe they too could live extravagantly if only they acquired enough capital. Thus, it happened that "value is attached to money alone" and determination and success came to be measured solely as "the ability to save money." Though the whole society urged the young to work and save no matter the hardship, the reality was that "all of the strivers cannot possibly hope to succeed" and "these masses will continue to compete intensely for an indefinite time and, finally, while in pain, their lives will end."[41]

Discontent began to appear as the have-nots started to wise up to their situation. Big brains and improved education had given them "the capacity to judge and discriminate all by one's own power" and, as a result, they became acutely "aware at times that there are unreasonable institutions in society." Unlike the "eras of ignorant savages and semicivilization" in which the common people lacked subjective freedom and did not question socioeconomic disparities, remaining content if they were safe and sound, today's educated masses, according to Oka, "want to know the reason for all things." In the face of great wealth "there is an intense feeling of wrongdoing and, as a result, discontent arises at the difficulty of putting up with being placed in a disadvantaged position."[42]

40 In a recent essay, Sanuki Masakazu explains how class conflict became a central preoccupation of Oka's later writings. See Sanuki, "Kindai nihon ni okeru kyowashugi."

41 Oka, "Jinrui no shōrai" [The future of humankind], 215.

42 Ibid., 218.

Ultimately this acute discontent would translate into class resentment and political subversion. Lacking opportunities, the common people would begin to target the privileged few, among whom Oka seems to count himself a member: they "do not have any idea that we suffer every day to have clothes to wear and food to eat, and they, who certainly have less physical and mental capacity than we do, wonder why we occupy a superior position in society" and "for what reason they should respect those who are dishonest and greedy." Finally, the situation would reach a crisis moment as the already technologically exhausted "nerves approach a point of oversensitivity due to excess stimuli" and the masses decide they "are not able to endure it any longer." Malcontent political movements such as "nihilism, anarchism, and socialism" would arise. "Gangs appear one after another and are so bold as to carry out barbarous acts out of excess of resentment. Even today such things as assassinations and insurrections often occur—and without a doubt they will happen still more often in the future."[43]

Compounding this social disintegration were the haves whose growing skepticism and cynicism matched the discontent of these have-nots. Their allegedly greater brain power enabled them to understand that humankind had entered a period when "the morality of the past must be changed and examined from its foundations." Like the underprivileged masses they too saw a world in which "the good perish and the bad thrive"—in which "families that have accumulated virtues over time suddenly go extinct, while those who have accumulated wickedness instead are rewarded." Based on this, many "with even just a little learning" came to question "whether there is such a things as morality." Perhaps most ominous of all for Oka was the majority who, under the pressures of the market place, had taken this disaffection "one step further": "[I]n the actual conduct of their lives they easily make light of morality. They calculate from their interests and, on the basis of the struggle for existence, they respect morality when it benefits them to adhere to morals, and they discard morality without looking back when it benefits them to violate morals." This cynical expediency was making it impossible to develop a shared general ethic that reached into all areas of life and united a human community. "Once public sentiment reaches this level, morality, of course, can no longer hold any in-

---

43 Ibid., 218–19.

tegrity for people." Finally, morality would come to seem "to be like an antique known in a past era."[44]

The collapse of morality under the weight of discontent and cynicism was rendering the social organism unable to cohere. Indeed, what Oka was describing was a condition of total anomy: a complete loss of faith in norms, conventions, and laws. Let loose in a socioeconomic order that did not demand they reintegrate their differentiated interests for the sake of the common good, oversized brains were employing their capacity to recognize the constructed nature of nomos to reject morality itself. Lacking a self-regulating *Sittlichkeit*, egoist individualism was running rampant, accelerating even further capitalism's ersatz struggle of existence and heightening the physically and psychologically debilitating clamor of the technological urban landscape. Just as overdeveloped tusks of the mammoth marked its decline toward extinction, the nomic chaos and political subversion spurred on by the "money world" signaled the degeneration of the biological entity that has reigned supreme over the earth—the superorganisms of human *minzoku*.

5. SYPHILIZATION

For Oka the anomy of contemporary life found its ultimate physical expression in the inability and unwillingness to procreate. The stresses, frustrations and debilitating comforts of life in the present day had begun to badly warp human sexuality. Severed from nature by technology and spurred endlessly onward by the capitalist order to covet what they could not possess, humans were forced to think not of the greater biological unit to which they belonged—whether it be the family or the *minzoku*—but of their own carnal desires, even when doing so risked disease and possible death.

This sexual irresponsibility was unleashed by the money economy—an economy which was making it increasingly difficult to marry. According to Oka, "as living expenses rise, marrying and supporting a family becomes less and less easy. Because one cannot marry until suitable assets have been built up, it naturally comes about that people marry late. The number of people who are not allowed to marry till middle age grows." This postponement of marriage, however, did not postpone carnal interest along with it: "[S]ex-

---

44 Ibid., 224–25.

ual desire among humans in a natural state is a most powerful force. At such times of life when youth burns it is hardly the case that it must be able to be controlled coldly by reason." The result was that "youth pursues its satisfactions through some other means" and "intimate moral habits cannot help but be thrown gradually into disorder."[45]

This "disorder" in "intimate moral habits" was Oka's delicate way of suggesting an onset of sexual licentiousness. Young men who were forced into an extended bachelorhood "leading single lives from the beginning," and young women "who lead unavoidably single lives due to the absence of partners to marry" were both, due to their nearly irrepressible instincts, naturally prone to promiscuity. In the case of women, there was the further temptation, under the pressure of the money economy, to exploit "the anatomy of their bodies" when "they run up against life problems" or "they lack the money needed to fulfill their vanity." Thus, "it easily comes about that in gradations" a significant number of young women "decide to sell their bodies to supplement this lack of money"—and Oka even alluded to terrible cases where there are "coeds secretly working in order to obtain their tuition fees."[46]

The direct consequence of this widespread sexual immorality and disorder was the infection of the body politic with illnesses transmitted by promiscuous behavior. "If the world becomes this way, syphilis, gonorrhea, soft chancre and other venereal diseases spread right away and there is no known way to stop them." Oka regarded syphilis as particularly lethal: not only did it "horribly weaken the body" but it attacked the nervous system, eventually causing the onset of excruciating mental illness for two or three years "from which the victim will certainly die." Worst of all, because it was sexually transmitted, "syphilis is passed along to descendants" and "the general health of successive generations weakens." Inserting an untranslated English phrase into his text, Oka predicted that the final outcome of this moral pandemic would be that "Civilization becomes syphilization."[47]

Yet an even greater threat than so-called "syphilization" to the survival of the racial superorganism was the declining birthrate. In Oka's view, egoism, late marriage, carnal license and the obsession with money all added up

---

45 Ibid., 220–21.
46 Ibid., 221.
47 Ibid., 221–22.

to a distortion of goals once people got around to tying the knot. "The reasons are no longer those of the past: creating an honorable family and bearing and raising up healthy, successful individuals." Both men and women were, instead, interested in acquiring wealth through marriage: "men plan to marry the daughter of a rich person and gain a hand to rise up in the world" and "women too try to marry rich, living luxuriously without worrying about the problems of life."[48]

The "problems" which women were least keen to bother themselves about were pregnancy and child-rearing. According to Oka, women nowadays "hate pregnancy, the result of natural marriage, and they consider every method to try to avoid it."[49] In one sense this avoidance was understandable, for Oka himself explains at length how being "estranged from the conditions of nature" has brought about a situation in which women had become dependent on midwives, nurses, and obstetricians. Unlike "primitives of Africa and Australia" who, in their primordial health, were still quickly able to give birth on the move, alone "in the bushes" on the side of the road, before "scampering" to catch up with the tribe, modern women, weakened by the often elaborate conveniences of the modern world, tended more and more to suffer through "hard labor."[50] However, for Oka these intense birth pangs only served to further encourage the growing tendency of married people to "avoid the trouble of child-rearing while seeking sexual satisfaction inside and outside the home." Even when they did bother to give birth the women in these selfish marriages looked to "leave the upbringing to assistants" in order to preserve "their own happiness." As a result, the capacity of such mothers "to secrete milk degenerates" and "in the West there is already year by year growth in the number of women who cannot produce milk though they have given birth."[51]

The steep drop in the birthrate that follows from this decline in the institution of marriage was perhaps the ultimate indicator that degeneration of the species was already underway.[52] The concrete biological unit in which humans manage to survive, the ethnic superorganism, would quite liter-

---

48 Ibid., 222.
49 Ibid., 222.
50 Ibid., 216–17.
51 Ibid., 222.
52 On the subject of fertility in early-twentieth-century Japan, see Otsubo, "Engendering Eugenics"; Otsubo, "The Female Body and Eugenic Thought in Meiji Japan"; Driscoll, "Seeds and (Nest) Eggs of Empire."

ally not be able to perpetuate itself once its constituent "cells," the individuals that make it up, fail to reproduce. The moral and physical weakening brought on by capitalist egoism—which itself was a function of overdeveloped brains and hands—was culminating in the slow death of the collective over generations.

6. Battle of the Invalids

Oka summarized his account of humankind's destiny of degeneration as follows:

> [Human groups] triumphed in the beginning over other animals through the power of their brains and hands and thereby occupying an absolutely superior position. But, in the future, as a result of the advanced operations of such brains and hands, differences in wealth and poverty will become stark, life problems increase, the body degenerate, nerves grow oversensitive, feelings of doubt and dissatisfaction advance, mere self-interest will gain in popularity, and the capacity to cooperate and achieve consensus becomes an impossibility. Even in the case of humankind, the same traits which in the beginning were most favorable in the struggle for existence and developed without limit, they, in the end, caused calamity.[53]

Significantly, Oka looked to conditions in his contemporary West for portents that decline and extinction were indeed inevitable. This not only revealed how closely attuned he was to the European discourse on decadence which, from the time Oka was student in Leipzig, had been documenting the indicators of degeneration, but it is consistent with the doctrine of orthogenesis: Western leadership in evolutionary progress also meant Western leadership in evolutionary decline—the biological entities which these nations represent were simply ahead of Japan in the universal life-cycle process of birth, growth, maturity, senescence, and death. Throughout "The Future of Humankind" the examples that Oka drew on to illustrate the downward trajectory Japan had begun to follow were almost all taken from Europe and the United States. It was Westerners who were so weakened that

---

53 Oka, "Jinrui no shōrai" [The future of humankind], 229.

they take ill if they forget to wear socks.[54] It was at the University of Berlin where venereal diseases had become so prevalent that "special lectures" had to be given to warn students of the long-term health risks. It was in France where women's breasts had begun to dry up and the birthrate had become so low "there is a fear that national power is weakening" and measures were being taken to prevent the trend.[55] It was "among the civilized countries of the West" that the biopolitically corrosive movements of "nihilism, anarchism, and socialism" had infected the people.[56] And, of course, it was to the English language that the polyglot Oka turned for the phrase that encapsulated this advancing decay: Civilization becomes syphilization.

Oka had this allegedly more advanced decadence of the West in mind when he offered his advice concerning the practical measures that Japan, a nation keenly aware of its late-developing, "followership" status, should take in the face of this inevitable and tragic trend.[57] For him "today's humans are in a condition like that at the start of an incurable illness, and each ethnic nation, though its condition is still not serious, should be compared to an ill person whose complete recovery is beyond hope." However, unlike individual persons who can "discard other matters and peacefully rest," the racial superorganism of the *minzoku* cannot afford such luxury: "[E]ach ethnic nation which occupies the earth's surface is at daggers with the others and because, when there is even a slight opening, it expects it will be laid low, it cannot solely be devoted to nursing its illness." Instead, the *minzoku* must understand that "wars in the future will be like a battle between invalids" and that "those with inferior war preparations" or "in whom illness has advanced the quickest will be gradually vanquished by their adversaries" and annihilated first.[58]

Even though Oka saw it as a necessity to "always be superior to other ethnic nations in both these areas"—that is martial prowess and moral health— he seemed to take it for granted that the state was devoted to "strengthening military preparations." Thus, it was "humankind's incurably sick moral decadence" as evinced in the West that preoccupied him most. In Oka's view the palliative for this moral sickness, this pathological anomy, needed to be fo-

---

54 Ibid., 216.
55 Ibid., 222.
56 Ibid., 218.
57 Pyle, "Advantages of Followership."
58 Oka, "Jinrui no shōrai" [The future of humankind], 230.

cused on Japan preserving the "capacity to cooperate and achieve consensus" as long as possible.[59] The Japanese had to remember their ethnic nation was a biological entity, an organism in its own right, and that without the ability to unify its individuals, the organism would grow decadent and die. While Western countries had already begun to disintegrate due to a combination of the kind of rampant egoism and physical enfeeblement described above—again, both brought on by overdeveloped hands and brains—follower Japan had to seek its own advantage in global competition by finding a way to regenerate itself or at the very least check the incurable illness of modern life.

What Oka's experiences since the war with Russia had taught him was that it was impossible to achieve this end by simply devising a secular, scientifically based version of traditional morality that would reform the nation-state. Despite the applicability of its evolutionary realpolitik to Japan's circumstances, the metapolitics of the "human-way" had depended on a society and an educational apparatus that was receptive to the organicist vision that he packaged along with his promotion of evolutionary theory. As we have seen though, the "overdeveloped" brains and hands of late Meiji Japan responded, at least initially, to the message of Oka's evolutionism according to their own lights. Subjectively free strivers, who were leaving behind the traditional life of villages and towns for the atomized existence of metropolitan industrial centers, construed it as an alternative ideology that facilitated their supposedly fevered ambitions to "rise in the world." Political radicals, disgusted by the exploitation and suppression of the seemingly retrogressive imperial order, looked to Oka's evolution as a materialist account of universal progress that could permanently delegitimize the "primate" emperor and his oligarchic puppet masters. Meanwhile, reformist statists, though they recognized the scientific possibilities of evolutionism, believed it should remain an esoteric truth—a body of dangerously potent knowledge which was to be parenthetically confined to the educated elite and kept from the unpredictable multitudes who were better off with the exoteric account of imperial divinity. Finally, reactionary statists regarded evolutionism as a source of heresy, subversion and social dissolution—a counter-narrative that they sought to suppress through limited press censorship and widespread fundamentalist indoctrination, especially in schools.

---

59 Ibid., 229–30.

In short, the "complicated society" that Gluck describes—which includes the money economy, industrialism and the technological conveniences that came with them—had produced a fragmented nation comprised of confused radicals, aloof technocrats, empowered reactionaries, and, above all, volatile masses of greedy, discontented, and constitutionally weak egoists. While Oka still held out belief that implementation of the Golden Rule, via the "human-way," would cause "the degeneration of morality and the corruption of public consciousness" to "instantly dissipate," thereby turning the world, right away, into "a Buddhist paradise," he no longer thought such implementation possible. The capitalist rat race had made the costs of altruism for the individual too high, reaching the point where "it cannot possibly be hoped that all of the individuals inside a given race-nation will practice these teachings" of sages such Confucius, Buddha and Jesus.[60] The lesser egoism of striving, agitated individuals rendered any morality, even one based on evolutionary science, impotent to protect and promote the greater egoism of the ethnic nation.

Oka made it clear that democracy also provided no real answers to the problem of nomic cohesion. While he admitted that, theoretically, the Japanese Diet could promote social cohesion in the way its members were "accepted and elected by many people," in reality, it had become a vehicle for egoism and greed. With the "prevalence of self-interestedness" those with an eye for profits had put their names forth, embarked on campaigns that "noisily urge on the voters" and even resorted to violence in the attempt to "have their opponents rejected." Likewise, though the United States possessed "an ideal of government whereby the politics are republican" and "there are no differences between individuals, rich and poor, high and low" due to a constitution that has "given equal rights to all," the actual process left voters frustrated and discontented. "If we were to imagine ourselves coming to reside in New York City, the political rights that we were in reality to possess would merely be the right to be able to freely make one choice among two possibilities: selecting candidates that we do not like or abstaining from voting." The cynicism that is thus promoted only made it increasingly difficult to undertake "activities that require cooperation and consensus."[61]

---

60 Ibid., 231.
61 Ibid., 228. It is passages such as this one that had led me to disagree with Sanuki Masakazu and Migita Hiroki, who prefer to see Oka as a defender of liberal democracy. In my view, Oka recognized the need

7. Generative Scientism:
Maximizing the Minzoku as a Religio-Eugenic Quest

If a secular, altruistic morality that gestured to religious tradition could not slow inevitable disintegration and decline and if, in addition, democracy only exacerbated egoism and discontent, then what would work to keep the spirit of "cooperation and consensus" alive? According to Oka, with "no basic remedy" available, "there is no way other than to seek out alternative measures" especially those "already being taken today in various civilized nations."[62]

The alternative measures Oka put forth did not merely involve policy initiatives—most of which, we will see, entailed state intervention—but a programmatic modernist vision of national regeneration through racial hygiene and eugenics. Oka's version of this restoration, which we saw in Chapter 3 had precedents among his cohort in Europe, is integral to what we mean by generative scientism. This term, as we explained in Chapter 3, refers to the dual aspect of the historicist-organicist account of the nation as a living being cycling through epigenetic growth stages: this process not only exposes natural causality in a manner that renders life transparent to technological manipulation but establishes, at the same time, an ontological developmental order into which values and norms have been cosmically embedded. In other words, generative scientism envisions the simultaneous valuation and transformation of human life. In Oka's case, this means that the superorganism of the *minzoku* will realize its optimal condition of vitality through interventions made possible and given purpose by the developmental order delineated by evolutionary science. Health and power—both of which are defined by the complete hygienic integration of specialized individual parts—will be achieved, via this generative scientism, in the dual sense of indicating both the prime stage of organic maturation and the means to perpetuate that stage. Staving off senility—that is, organic disintegration—and retaining the vigor and strength of the ethnic nation's "early adulthood" will become the ultimate value—and restoring such youthful health and power will be the raison d'être of his biopolitical technology. As we will suggest, this palinge-

---

for a unifying orthodoxy and sought to underwrite it with his evolutionism. Though he hoped to mitigate superstition, the organicist assumptions of evolutionary morphology made him an advocate of statism—even if the state were centered on the imperial cult—not liberal democracy. See Sanuki, "Kindai nihon ni okeru kyowashugi"; Migita, "Meijiki Chishikijin ni okeru seibutsu shinkaron no hayari saikou."

62 Oka, "Jinrui no shōrai" [The future of humankind], 231.

netic regeneration of an earlier moment of maximum vitality will eventually become the basis of an accommodation between Oka's "progressive" evolutionism and the reactionary orthodoxy of the family-state.

In chapters four and five we saw what such healthy integration looked like for Oka and the power he attributed to it. His evolutionary realpolitik imagined an atemporal organicism in which all members of the superorganism were instilled with an anomy-proof human-way that instinctually bound their interests to the higher individuality of the nation. After the war with Russia, however, Oka had to recognize that the nation had overspecialized: its individual members had overdeveloped and their egoism was pulling the nation apart—as evidenced by the corrosive anomy of the feverish laissez-faire economic order. More powerful and invasive measures would be required to reverse this decadence and return to the earlier stage of healthy, presenescent maturation when the organically unifying instincts were intact. The eugenic measures that Oka has in mind are introduced at the end of "The Future of Humankind" but they are only fully described in light of their programmatic modernist purport in a follow-up essay from 1911: "The Actual Value of the Study of Racial Improvement." Together, these two essays reveal how Oka's organicist vision lays down a program of modernist rejuvenation that will be the lasting legacy of *Evolution and Human Life*.

In "The Future of Humankind" Oka introduces eugenics as part of an array of interventionist measures adopted to reverse the degenerative effects of anomic egoism. This degeneracy, as we have seen, was already in evidence in the West, presumably because of the advanced degree of capitalist egoism and social fragmentation there. To check the accumulation of wealth and the increase in class divisions Oka suggested that measures such as "trustbusting" and "progressive inheritance laws" might be tried. At the other end of the societal spectrum, he mentioned "methods of relief" that will quiet the discontent and agitation of the have-nots. These included "orphanages, reformatories, charities, associations for sheltering released prisoners, depots for cheap food distribution, free hostels for travelers, funds for worker retirement homes, relief agencies for the impoverished among other means of lending assistance."[63]

---

63 Ibid., 231.

Though these were unremarkable initiatives—indicative of the Bismarckian welfare state that he had seen firsthand as a graduate student—Oka likened them explicitly to "surgical medical procedures."[64] Eugenics was, in fact, cleverly introduced as the extension of these procedures, part of the regimen designed to treat the degeneration of the national body. What particularly interests Oka at this juncture is a program of negative eugenics: the "compulsory prohibition of procreation for those with hereditary diseases."[65] Such prohibition was, according to Oka, "actually occurring in certain of the states of the United States of America."[66] As he did in his wartime speech "Evolutionary Theory and Hygiene," Oka was quick to answer those who might "argue against this on the basis of human rights and so on."[67] Such humanitarian concerns were, in his view, "meandering."[68] Objecting to race improvement was "the same as hesitating to amputate the diseased section of a gangrenous toe when rot has begun to set in for the sake of the rights of body cells."[69]

While "The Future of Humankind" admitted its proposals were "unavoidably makeshift" and would "not cure the cause of the disease but only address the symptoms," the historicist reasoning behind such extreme "surgical medical procedures" became even more explicitly the basis of a programmatic vision of eugenic regeneration in the follow-up essay of 1911, "The Actual Value of the Study of Racial Improvement." Sharing the goal of the earlier essay to "strive gradually to promote and, as much as possible, not abandon the spirit of cooperation and consensus,"[70] this later effort, published in the journal *Human Nature* in August 1911, unambiguously assigns supreme value to bodily health as measured in futural terms—as a rejuvenation that will secure the destiny of the nation. The fate of "future generations" will be invoked repeatedly to authorize and legitimize measures to transform human nature. A developmental cosmology featuring the process of organic growth at the macro level will serve to create healthy humans who embody a new table of ultimate values to compete with religion.

---

64 Ibid.
65 Ibid., 231–32.
66 Ibid.
67 Ibid.
68 Ibid.
69 Ibid.
70 Ibid., 231–32.

Oka conjures this healthy future destiny by reminding his readers of the threat of present-day decadence. For him "the really urgent business of to-day" consists in "investigating hereditary development among humans and other animals and preventing the degeneration of one's own race on the basis of such results."[71] The primary reason such preemptive measures are so vital has to do with the pressures of evolutionary realpolitik that we delineated in Chapter 4: "[T]o stand up as an independent people in the future arena of international competition one must strive to prevent with great dispatch the degeneration of our race and to hold one's ground unyieldingly in circumstances where other races are superior."[72] However, just as important as the external geopolitical realities of the New Imperialism were the troubling signs of internal decay which, as we have seen, he spoke of in "The Future of Humankind": "in each country the problem of degeneration is avidly discussed among scholars" and "according to statistics in recent years the number of suicides, criminals and mentally ill persons have increased year by year in various civilized nations."[73] In Oka's estimation, "it seems that the average condition of human beings is certainly degenerating."[74]

Oka derives his regenerative vision of the nation as the obverse side of this universal degeneration. Beginning from the same geopolitical concerns about national fate, his generative scientism comes to attach supreme worth to health: "seeing that humans create societies, form nations and many of these stand in opposition to one another, excellence in mind and body is important above all else. Even if they are superior in other areas, those whose condition of mental and physical health is inferior in comparison to members of other nations have no chance of occupying an advantageous position in the arena of future international competition. Therefore, the most important issue for nations and races is the state of its mental and physical health."[75] The "actual value" from the title of his essay follows directly from this apotheosis of health: "the study of racial improvement" acquires value to the extent that it restores and maximizes the mental and physical health of the nation. "Racial improvement"—which is, again, his composite term for eugenics and racial hygiene—is therefore not like doctrines which are

71   Oka, "Minshu Kaizengaku no Jissai Kachi" [The actual value of the study of racial improvement], 202–3.
72   Ibid., 202.
73   Ibid., 201–2.
74   Ibid., 202.
75   Ibid., 199.

"well thought out" but have "really no value whatsoever" because they "cannot be actualized." Instead, the study of racial improvement "can be put into practice."[76] On this basis it represents initiatives that "should have a tremendous impact on the future of our ethnic nation [*minzoku*]."[77]

What Oka envisions is nothing less than a comprehensive "plan" designed "to apply the logic of the biological sciences to human society."[78] Carefully distinguishing this plan from the "old theory of race improvement" in the early Meiji period, which wrongheadedly proposed importing Caucasians "from abroad to create a mixed race,"[79] Oka, expanding on what he said in "The Future of Humankind," describes racial improvement as a program devised to apply biological knowledge and actualize potential through the control of reproduction: "[T]his theory of racial improvement is based on the idea that only those people, from among ordinary humans, who are recognized as being most suitable for producing the next generation of *kokumin* by virtue of their excellence in both mind and body are allowed to reproduce; those who it is thought will doubtlessly leave behind inferior offspring by virtue of their own inferiority in mind and spirit are not allowed to breed; in this manner the human race will come to improve year by year."[80] To clarify what he is proposing, Oka likens "racial improvement" to the artificial "breeding and cultivation of plants and animals" which "in a comparatively short number of months and years obtains surprising results."[81] He specifically cites the example of a contemporary biologist in California named Burbank "who improved many plants by unnatural means and even began to produce cacti that do not have needles."[82] According to Oka the study of racial improvement rests on the same reasoning "because species, whether they are plants or animals, are certainly able to improve in this way if, within each generation, [healthy] seeds are selected and only these are allowed to reproduce. Of course, human beings, as a kind of animal, can also be expected to improve by this method."[83]

---

76 Ibid., 202.
77 Ibid., 198.
78 Ibid.
79 Ibid.
80 Ibid.
81 Ibid.
82 Ibid.
83 Ibid., 198–99.

Oka imagines "the planning of racial improvement"[84] to entail programs of both negative and positive eugenics. Negative eugenics will be applied to "those who have diseases which it has been determined will certainly spread to offspring."[85] Not only does Oka insist that these individuals "must be strictly prevented from reproducing" but, he argues, "even if the disease itself is not handed down, if a disposition to easily contract such a disease is inherited, such offspring will often catch the disease" and, "as a consequence this too is the same as passing along the disease."[86] He thus concludes that "when sowing the seeds of fruit trees, one burns up all those seeds which have been found to have contracted a disease. This method is the most thorough. If even among human beings this method was practiced, perhaps it would be possible to wipe out a large part of human disease in a few generations. Therefore, it is necessary to control the reproduction of those we determine will pass down some disease or deformity of the mind or body after researching whether they have this inclination."[87]

In "The Actual Value of the Study of Racial Improvement" Oka urges that such a program of negative eugenics is among the "methods which should be able to be implemented" without delay. As he explains, "the reasoning which is based on the study of racial improvement is extremely clear. There is no doubt at all that the mind and the body of the nation's people both ought to gradually improve together if an appropriate theory has been devised and generally put into practice. There are today some methods which should be able to be implemented right away. Already at present various laws have been established in many of the states in the United States of America and there are limits on the reproduction of people with hereditary diseases. For instance, those who have come down with a mental illness are prohibited from marrying for three years even if they have completely recovered; one is not allowed to marry if there is not certification from a physician; and those with such things as epilepsy and alcoholism are also not allowed to marry. Many such regulations have been established. These kinds of regulations can be put into practice right away even if we do not especially alter today's social organization and political arrangements."[88]

---

84 Ibid., 199.
85 Ibid.
86 Ibid., 199–200.
87 Ibid., 200.
88 Ibid., 200.

Oka is somewhat more vague and tentative when it comes to implementing a positive eugenics program. Though he mentions the prospect "to gradually raise the average condition of both the people's body and mind," his focus is on "extraordinary geniuses who appear with extreme rarity—a single one showing up for every 100,000 or one million people."[89] By thoroughly investigating "the circumstances and causes under which a genius appears" one can "plan to provide a conducive environment and allow this great ability to exhibit itself for the sake of the entire nation."[90] However, Oka concludes that for the time being "nothing can be done" to create such superior beings "but wait for research into hereditary development."[91]

Along with frequent suggestions about the need for new sociopolitical arrangements, Oka's repeated emphasis on the as-of-yet inconclusive state of research into heredity exposes the tentativeness of his positive eugenics for what it is: an intimation of what it would really mean to implement and actualize a theory development that rendered the workings of heredity utterly transparent. Such complete access to natural processes would not only "raise the average condition of individuals" and foster geniuses but, more significantly, reconstitute the totality of life within the ethnic nation—and do so in a manner so radical that Oka would not dare to articulate his vision explicitly. The closest he comes is a passage toward the end of "The Actual Value of the Study of Racial Improvement" in which he argues that the "remarkable results" that "should certainly arise" if a final theory of heredity were put into practice and "actualized" would be severely curtailed "while the social system and human nature remain as they are today."[92] Even the benefits of negative eugenics, such as "restrictions connected with marriage," will come to naught unless Japanese are "prepared to transform human nature drastically and, for the sake of the next generation of *kokumin*, offer something as a sacrifice."[93]

Though Oka was noncommittal about the mechanism that would bring about this drastic transformation, the framework of organicist evolutionism within which it would be realized remained constant. As we described at length in Part I and again in this chapter, Oka carried out his research, wrote

---

89 Ibid.
90 Ibid.
91 Ibid.
92 Ibid., 202.
93 Ibid.

his textbooks, and presented his popular writings in an era during which Darwinian selectionism was contested by alternative theories of evolution. Dubbed "the eclipse of Darwinism" by P. J. Bowler, the two decades on either side of the turn of the century witnessed a proliferation of pre- and non-Darwinian theories. In "The Future of Humankind" we saw that the version of *shinkaron* that Oka came to espouse was, despite announcing itself as Darwinian, an amalgam of Lamarckian use-inheritance, Haeckel's recapitulationist hierarchy of organic individuality, and the theory of orthogenesis which extrapolated on Haeckel's recaptilationism or biogenetic law. Accepting this largely non-Darwinian framework based in evolutionary morphology did not, however, prevent Oka from recognizing and explicating other mechanisms. In particular, Oka, like Darwin and Haeckel before him, combined Lamarckism and natural selection together in his account of evolutionary transmutation. This nondogmatic approach was important because it made Oka receptive to the spread of Mendelian ideas in the early twentieth century which would eventually end the eclipse of Darwinism by confirming selectionism and result in a "modern synthesis" in scientific circles in the 1930s.[94] While Oka remained a Lamarckian, both the new editions of *Lectures on Evolutionary Theory* and the new popular primers that he published in the first years of the Taisho era included introductions to Mendelian theories of heredity.[95] Already at the time "The Actual Value of the Study of Racial Improvement" appeared in 1911, Oka was clearly aware that the question of heredity was still in need of being definitively sorted out.

Oka never doubted that such sorting out would occur. He also never seemed to have questioned what the ultimate result would be: a complete transparency of the heredity mechanism that would facilitate a possible total transformation of the future life of the ethnic nation. What troubled him, however, was the prospect that such regenerative mechanisms might be identified but not taken up and thoroughly implemented in Japan. In the last chapter we described how the nomic crisis in the period after the Russo-Japanese War exposed the impotence of "metapolitical" reformist scientism: Oka had previously hoped the nomos-constructing human-way could reform the ethnic nation, but anomic "civilization sickness" and the orthodox

---

94 Bowler, *The Eclipse of Darwinism*, 216–17.
95 Watanabe, *The Japanese and Western Science*, 86; Sanuki, "Kindai nihon ni okeru kyowashugi."

reaction to it indicated that this soft organicist evolutionism would be ignored, misunderstood or repressed in the dissonance of contending voices. In "The Actual Value of the Study of Racial Improvement," it is eugenics and racial hygiene that he worries that the anomic society will now misconstrue. This essay, in fact, opens with a long discussion of how the late Meiji predisposition for fads threatens the implementation of a program of racial improvement. Noting how in recent years both eugenics in England and racial hygiene in Germany have risen to prominence as academic fields of study and are now being "noisily advocated" and "popularly advanced,"[96] Oka anticipates "the time will probably arrive within two or three years when the study of racial improvement will suddenly be advocated even in our nation and you will certainly see one or two essays connected with this field of study in whichever magazine you open."[97] No doubt thinking of the "Darwin boom" in Japan which was just then petering out, Oka's concern is that "based on past examples" such a theory from the West will be treated like "a striped pattern which is the rage today in Tokyo" and "in a few months" reaches "remote areas to become the rage there." After first "taking the world by storm," it will be "forgotten" and in the end there will be "no memory of it"[98]—"the entirety of the theory is discarded and ignored."[99] The reason Oka emphasizes the "actual value" of the theory is so it will not be merely blindly followed by "those who lack a critical eye" and then cast aside like just another fad "without plumbing its true value."[100] For him, racial improvement, like evolution itself, is not akin to other theories that have little practical application but, as we noted earlier, one "which should have a tremendous influence on the future of our ethnic nation."[101]

The threat to racial improvement that ultimately preoccupies Oka in this essay is the one which concerned him so greatly during the war with Russia: humanitarianism. In particular, he finds it "highly regrettable" that those whose job it will be to implement these improvement measures, the "physicians," continue to misapprehend their "benevolent calling."[102] "Advances in

---

96 Oka, "Minshu Kaizengaku no Jissai Kachi" [The actual value of the study of racial improvement], 197.
97 Ibid.
98 Ibid.
99 Ibid.
100 Ibid.
101 Ibid., 198.
102 Ibid., 201.

the medical arts" are increasingly bringing about "such things as people in-born with an extremely weak constitution being saved or being allowed to survive, reproduce, and then, in turn, being allowed to leave behind weak children."[103] Recalling perhaps his earlier exhortations to the altruism of the human-way, Oka admits that "charity is, of course, a good thing" but pity can become pernicious if it means we "save mentally handicapped peo-ple who are unfit for social existence, allow them to reproduce and, further-more, let them hand down handicapped people."[104] "The next generation of *kokumin*" will not call these actions "benevolent."[105] Instead, suffering "tre-mendous inconveniences due to the existence of such handicapped people" future generations will most likely "curse the cruel mercy of the previous generation."[106] In the end, the "the next generation of citizens will see the burden on each individual grow heavier and might idolize those who have not advanced the medical arts."[107]

This emphatic and, indeed, contemptuous rejection of the supposed "cruel mercy" of humanitarianism is more than an example of elimination-ist reasoning. Invoking the vitality of future generations as an ultimate mea-sure of value, Oka reveals what it means to interpret the fate of the nation from "the standpoint of the study of racial improvement."[108] Though "racial improvement" is at the stage of "only precisely investigating hereditary de-velopment through experimental observations and statistics" and "the find-ings we are able to put into practice right away are extremely few,"[109] the his-toricist schema of his organicist evolutionism has already established that the future development of the community as a totality must override any consideration for its constituent parts. In particular, nonintegrating, un-supportive elements within the national body of future generations are re-garded not only as expendable but causal agents in the historical process of degeneration. Correcting this untoward historical trend and returning the *minzoku* to its original life trajectory of healthy development constitutes what Oka intends when he speaks of the "urgent business" of racial improve-

---

103 Ibid.
104 Ibid.
105 Ibid.
106 Ibid.
107 Ibid.
108 Ibid.
109 Ibid.

ment. In "The Actual Value of the Study of Racial Improvement" this restoration to health will be accomplished by weeding out weak individuals and
waiting for the biological sciences to elucidate the mechanism necessary to
positively engineer an improved human stock. In "The Future of Humankind," as we saw, such hygienic restoration involves stemming or reversing
an unraveling process of senescence which Oka identified broadly with the
individualistic modern life of industrializing and urbanizing late Meiji Japan. Together these two essays use the prospect of decline and extinction to
delineate a regenerative vision according to which the lesser individuality of
persons will be reintegrated—that is, subordinated and even "sacrificed"—
to the higher individuality of the ethnic nation-state. As in the case of so
many other early-twentieth-century historicisms, Oka's *shinkaron*, with its
schemes to restore wayward individuals to the organic unity of the commonweal, takes upon itself "the whole weight of responsibility for the superindividual life to come."[110]

As a whole, the essays that comprise *Evolution and Human Life* announce
a scientifically grounded regenerative program that will rejuvenate the organic cohesion needed for national survival. While Oka recognized that
competing *minzoku* represented the ultimate threat to Japan, his primary
focus was on strengthening and invigorating the nation internally. His approach, as we have explored, relied on promoting modern science not just to
raise up a technologically adept population primed for international competition, but to transform human nature in line with the collective end
of national prowess. In the earlier essays that make up the anthology the
hope was that this transformation would occur through a Lamarckian process based on education in the biological sciences: members of the *minzoku*
would come to understand the virtues of the human-way and practice race-
specific altruism that would inculcate organically binding nomic instincts.
However, coinciding with the fundamentalist reaction to postwar anomy,
the rejection of the Ministry of Education of any mention of evolutionary
theory in its textbooks forced Oka to radicalize his *shinkaron* beyond a mere
program of reform. Instead of merely emphasizing the interrelatedness of elements toward a common goal, Oka's organicism came to stress the temporal process of development: rejuvenating the cohesion of the nation would

---

110 Koestler, *Darkness at Noon*, 100.

be achieved by reversing the degenerative process of disaggregation into atomized parts and embedding the life of the *kokumin* back within the regenerative process of integrating growth. Explicit in both his theory of degeneration and his promotion of racial improvement was an understanding that
the unity necessary for national survival would only be secured through
technological intervention in the historical process of development.

Yet it is the message implicit in Oka's invocation of the grand trajectory
of evolutionary development that is of the greatest significance in *Evolution
and Human Life*. On top of the ability to engineer human nature, what Oka's
regenerative program posited was a new horizon of meaning within which
new values could be established. The introduction to this book began with
a pivotal passage from Oka's essay "Ideal Group Life" in which he mused
on the superior benefits that would result from replacing religious statues
with representations of the superorganismic existence of moss animal colonies. It was about the time Oka wrote this essay that he began to understand that the soft organicism of his reform scientism would not be sufficient: like the religious statues erected in the public square, evolutionism
would have to impart a cosmological vision that attached significance to human life in a modern idiom if it were to resonate with the population at large.
Thus, while Oka failed to get evolutionism into school textbooks—something which would have been the equivalent of moss animal statues in the
public square—he achieved this cosmological aim with his theory of degeneration and his proposals for racial improvement: individual lives were to be
granted meaning through the perpetuation of the national superorganism
into the future, a survival which would take place against the backdrop of a
developmental ontology of cosmic proportions. Via this ontology, evolution
could, like religion, cosmicize the norms, conventions, and laws of the nation. The anomy of contemporary life could be overcome by granting to individual participation in the extant nomos a new purpose that was validated
by the cosmological pattern of evolutionary development.

Expressed in his orthogenetic theory of degeneration and related eugenic
program of racial improvement, the regenerative vision of national destiny
in Oka's best-selling *Evolution and Human Life* speaks to the popular appeal
of programmatic modernist diagnosis in the final years of the Meiji period.
As we have seen earlier, Roger Griffin expanded the notion of modernism

to include systematic, sociopolitical initiatives in "Europeanized societies"[111] to revitalize a decayed nomic order. This programmatic modernism came to construct modern existence as decadent and began to envision an alternative modern life style that would supersede this decadence by rejuvenating an earlier state of coherence, purpose and health in a new, future-orientated manner. Though there had been forewarnings of a cultural crisis in the 1880s and, as we described in the last chapter, fears of *bunmei-byō* from the 1890s onward, it was Oka's *shinkaron* that introduced such a modernist program to the Japanese public. Along with enthusiasm for scientific knowledge, the wide popularity of his writings suggests a receptivity in Japan to what Griffin calls the dialectic between current decadence and future health. The nomic crisis of modern life was coming to be understood as evidence of degeneration and not only did Oka's generative scientism help articulate this consensus but it supplied hygiene-enhancing eugenic techniques that would cure the sickness of civilization and revitalize the nation.

For Roger Griffin such programmatic modernism also helps explain the success of a related vitalization movement, namely fascism, "a revolutionary species of political modernism originating in the early twentieth century whose mission is to combat the allegedly degenerative forces of contemporary history (decadence) by bringing about an alternative modernity and temporality (a 'new order' and a 'new era') based on the rebirth, or palingenesis, of the nation."[112] According to Griffin, the realization of a "totalizing vision of national or ethnic rebirth" will "overcome the decadence that has destroyed a sense of communal belonging and drained modernity of meaning and transcendence" and "usher in a new era of cultural homogeneity and health."[113] The specific vision of the nation-state that Griffin attributes to these revolutionary political modernists seems especially apropos to our analysis of Oka's generative scientist *shinkaron*: "Fascists conceive the nation as an organism shaped by historic, cultural, and in some cases, ethnic and hereditary factors, a mythic construct incompatible with liberal, conservative, and communist theories of society. The health of this organism they see undermined as much by the principles of institutional and cultural pluralism, individualism, and globalized consumerism promoted by liberal-

---

111 Griffin, *Modernism and Fascism*, 116.
112 Ibid., 181.
113 Ibid., 182.

ism as by the global regime of social justice and human equality identified by socialism in theory as the ultimate goal of history, or by the conservative defence of 'tradition.'"[114]

Despite these rather stark similarities, Oka's *shinkaron* was, as we stated in the introduction, neither fascist nor protofascist. Not only do his politics appear to be closer to the statism of Minobe Tatsukichi but, as we have discussed in the first two parts of this study, his preference was for reform, not revolution. His metapolitics grounded itself in a reformist scientism that hoped to educate the national entity, through the organicist humanway, into becoming a technologically sophisticated, hygienic superorganism. However, this nonfascist orientation is not the whole story, for, as we have delineated, the widespread perception of anomy, the rise of reactionary Shinto ultranationalism in response to it, and his own failure to convince the Ministry of Education to include evolution in its official textbooks inspired Oka to expand his *shinkaron* into a form of programmatic modernism along the lines of the eugenics and racial hygiene movements described in Chapter 3. While not fascist itself, this generative scientism, as we have called it, did contribute to attempts to formulate a fascist ideology in later decades. As Griffin portrays it, such a revitalizationist ideology is not a logical system but comes together through a process of syncretism, attempting to synthesize disparate and even contradictory elements to forge a new "mazeway" that will become the basis of "the founding principles and constitutive values needed for a new world to be constructed."[115] In the epilogue we will argue that Oka's organicist programmatic modernism was integral to the syncretic processes of forming Japanese fascism, not only providing a modern dynamic within which revived aspects of traditional culture could be situated, rendering them relevant and congruent with the lives of imperial subjects, but provoking Shinto fundamentalists, who it turns out were keenly attentive to evolutionary theory, to revise their orthodoxy as a developmentalist-organicist vision of the *kokutai* "blood community." In the end, as we will suggest, this new mazeway seems never to have come together— mainly because the synthesis of two of its primary elements, evolutionary science and the *kokutai*, remained unfinished.

---

114 Ibid., 181.
115 Ibid., 117.

EPILOGUE

EVOLUTION AND
THE NATIONAL BODY:
AN UNFINISHED SYNTHESIS

A time that tries to suppress and bypass science with ideological beliefs will be
retarded in the progress of the world. We have no choice but to be enveloped by
things like the theory of evolution.

THE SHOWA EMPEROR, 1935[1]

In *Japan's Modern Myths*, Carol Gluck writes of the incongruence of Meiji
orthodoxy with Japanese society over the course of the early twentieth century. According to her, the late Meiji period was the crucible in which this
orthodoxy was forged and by 1915 a "naturalization of meaning" had occurred whereby "socially created symbols" had been "transformed by time
and circumstantial ubiquity into the ideological equivalent of natural
monuments."[2] In Chapter 6 we referred to this process as cosmization, and
Gluck claims that its sustained attempts to instill a "sense of nation" and
project a vision of social order resulted in a "rendition of modernity" that,
"too entrenched to be easily outdone," remained, "until 1945, the authoritative one."[3] Though "new concerns were generally met with reformulations
of ideological material that had come into currency in the late Meiji period,
and wholly new elements were rare,"[4] the orthodoxy suffered from a basic
dissonance with the social experience of the *kokumin* (people):

---

1   Migita, *Tennosei to Shinkaron*, 152.
2   Gluck, *Japan's Modern Myths*, 253.
3   Ibid., 39–40.
4   Ibid., 36.

Compared to the views of the nation and even to those of politics, late Meiji views of society were less congruent from the first. This was in part a result of timing. For when the ideological elite raised their voices in concern over a "complicated society," it was in response to social change that they felt had somehow got ahead of them. The social and economic consequences of "civilization," which became increasingly manifest in the decade between the two Meiji wars, presented the ideologues with a twentieth-century project that was already under way when—with apparent surprise and no little chagrin—they began to respond to it. In this case the late Meiji figures appeared to be running after reality, constructing their versions of society on the heels of social change. Often the result was a gap between the situation they described— or, typically, the ills they diagnosed—and the prescriptions they offered to remedy them. Appearing after the social phenomena that provoked them, late Meiji views of society sometimes seemed perceptibly behind the times.[5]

As we have seen, the prescriptions that were offered involved reviving the supposedly organic relations of the past to counter socioeconomic change: the "agrarian myth" was "reinvigorated," village life "apotheosized," and above all, the traditional extended family projected on to the ethnic nation so that the imperial stem line and its divine ancestors came to wield consanguineous, parental authority over present-day subjects. Over time, as "the discrepancy between the official social myths and an urbanizing, industrializing society with an increasingly vulnerable agricultural sector only widened," it happened that "experience disconfirmed"[6] these constructions and the orthodoxy became "anachronism outpaced."[7] Yet, as Gluck explains, "the more experience gave them the lie, the more they were scrubbed and polished and enshrined"[8] and she depicts the ideological efforts from the beginning of Taisho to the end of the Second World War as cyclical dogmatic attempts to fit this reactionary vision of modern life to an increasingly fluid and elusive social reality.

Gluck's nuanced presentation of the functioning of Meiji orthodoxy can help us to understand how—less fearful of the future and more comfortable with change—the scientistic, programmatic modernism of Oka's *Evolution*

---

5   Ibid., 265.
6   Ibid., 266.
7   Ibid., 40.
8   Ibid., 266.

and Human Life could offer a vision of modern existence more congruent with the experience and sensibility of an urbanizing, industrializing nation in which customary norms and conventions seemed to be in peril. In Gluck's account the overt messages of the Japanese orthodoxy were grounded in less explicit, routinized assumptions—ones that were more firmly established aspects of the nomic background and, therefore, simply taken for granted and left unstated. Thus, beneath the ideological landscape defined by such surface features as the emperor, the *kokutai* (national body), the empire, patriotism, and the idealized relations of customary village and family life, lay a substrate of common sense perceptions that had over time become axiomatic. Gluck especially emphasizes the unquestioned collective referents, the "meanings socially held in common"[9] that since the beginning of the Meiji period had "by virtue of a half-century of unstressed but constant re-iteration" become "as natural to vast numbers of Japanese as they once had been to the learned few.[10] Among such commonsense generalities she lists "the nineteenth-century myths of progress, the Meiji dogmas of civilization, the political doctrines of constitutionalism, the social morality of success, the national and ethnic sense of being 'we, Japanese.'"[11] Gluck depicts these commonsense fixtures as the implicit part of ideological discourse, the dependent clauses that frame basic issue and thereby establish the common ground upon which issues are engaged.

Further down, beneath the level of these unstressed commonsense constructs, sits, according to Gluck, an even more elemental substrate where deep social meanings "unspoken, even unthought" are "enacted in social behavior."[12] "Embedded in social practice that makes the spoken language of ideology intelligible,"[13] this layer corresponds to the "groundless grounds" explored by later Wittgenstein and early Heidegger: the unarticulated, pretheoretical fundament of skillful coping where norms and conventions possess the certainty of natural facts—where nomos takes on an ontological heft equivalent to cosmic truth.[14] While Gluck mentions notions

---

9 Ibid., 253.
10 Ibid., 257.
11 Ibid.
12 Ibid., 260–61.
13 Ibid., 258.
14 In *On Certainty*, Wittgenstein offers that "at the foundation of well-founded belief lies belief that is not founded" and that "the end [to giving grounds] is not an ungrounded proposition: it is an ungrounded way of acting." Wittgenstein, *On Certainty*, 17, 33. For a discussion of "groundless grounds" and a cri-

of Confucian self-improvement and the distinctions between bureaucrats (*kan*) and common folk (*min*) as examples of this deepest substrate, it is, for our purposes, what she suggests about the ingrained propensity to rely on customary ethics in favor of legalities and to cherish community as a paramount value that is of interest. In her view, "the preference for morality and mores over law as the guarantees of civic order emerged against the background of the communitarian ethos that was the most familiar and practiced socio-moral form of the majority of the Japanese."[15] It was, in other words, this deep-seated ethos that infused norms and conventions and consecrated them with the "moral power of social sanction."[16] Such power was so fundamental to the normative disposition of Japanese that the two upper strata were circumscribed by concern with community and custom.

For Oka's metapolitics the challenge was to convert the strata of this cultural-ideological edifice to the corporatist biology he had brought back from his studies in Germany. The prospects for quick and easy success in this endeavor must have seemed quite promising to him. The collective life of moss animals, which he took as a moral-political exemplar, correlated neatly with this deepest substrate we have just described: not only did the structure of the superorganism correspond with the communitarian ethos but the instinctual altruism of their members reflected the preference for morals and mores before laws. If the soft organicism of interdependence seemed a good fit at this deepest level, the evolutionary morphology it was based on seemed ideal for the middle, commonsensical level of ideological construction. After all, the most prominent of the collective referents that had been established since the early Meiji period involved civilization and progress. As Gluck points out, the phrase "as civilization advances [*bunmei no shinpo to tomo ni*]"[17] had become, by the late Meiji period, an unremarkable and self-evident framing device for discussion and, as an internationally respected research scientist, Oka clearly felt that he could better delineate what constituted true progress and civilization. His cutting-edge evolutionary perspec-

---

tique of scientism, see Braver, *Groundless Grounds*. In my view, what Oka and other proponents of eugenics were trying to achieve was equivalent to the quest of logical positivists of the same generation: replace the nomic grounding of background practices described by Wittgenstein, Heidegger, and Berger with logical and scientistically transparent foundations.

15 Ibid.

16 Ibid., 259–60.

17 Ibid., 254.

tive could also be brought to bear not only in separating *risshin shusse* (rising in the world) from a spurious social Darwinism—which, as we saw in Chapters 4 and 5, was, in Oka's estimation, better suited to lone predators than gregarious human groups—but in offering a scientific rationale to constitutionalism and the commonplace trope of *wagakuni*, our nation.

It was, curiously, on the ideological surface, the most overt level or "middle of the message" where Oka's reformist scientism seemed least likely to succeed. Aside from selfless patriotism and the trumpeting of empire, both of which, as we saw in Chapter 4, Oka ardently supported, the other features, the "natural monuments" that were being set in place by reactionary statists during the late Meiji period were barriers to realizing his plans for a scientifically literate, technologically adept, superorganismic, developmental nation-state. Though Oka sidesteps the issue of a return to the agrarian world of villages and extended families, the emperor and, as Migita rightly suggests, the fundamentalist reading of the *kokutai* (national body) as an emperor-centered historical view presented formidable impediments to his evolutionism. Yet, as I have shown, Oka's initial strategy was simply to highlight the commonalities between his *shinkaron* and certain aspects of this orthodoxy in the faith that once scientific truth had a foothold it would gradually reform the whole. This metapolitical approach is best exemplified by the "human-way." Connecting with the deep meanings of community and moral customs, Oka hoped also to limn the constellation of ideological constructs that made up the middle strata, the commonsense meanings, with scientific truth. By presenting the corporatist biology derived from Haeckel's evolutionary morphology in popular form, he hoped to establish that community, civilization, and progress were all outgrowths of evolutionary processes. The Meiji era constructs—emperor and the emperor-centered historical view—would reform themselves, in an appropriate manner, once this truth was firmly entrenched.

What the reformist scientism and soft organicism of Oka's metapolitics initially failed to take into account were two interrelated matters: the aggressiveness of *kokutairon* (theory of the national body) and, more specifically, the tenacious resistance to programmatic transformation of the "deep social meanings" which *kokutairon* had co-opted. As we saw in Chapter 6, the efforts by the Home and Education Ministries after the Russo-Japanese War to promote reactionary Shintoism encroached on the very same nomic dimension that Oka was hoping to refurbish with the altruistic instincts of the "human-way." Despite the "Darwin boom" that his writings had helped inspire, the combination of shrine consolidation, emperor-centered school rituals, and the dissemination of Hozumi's orthodoxy began what seemed like a superstition-based correction of the incipient breakdown of norms and conventions in the final years of the Meiji period. Oka's failure to secure even honorable mention for evolutionary theory in the official 1911 elementary school textbooks must have looked like a total defeat for *shinkaron* and his superorganismic human-way.

The pervasiveness and value-positing power of the cosmological narrative enunciated by *kokutairon* inspired Oka to transcend mere reformism and tease out the temporal dimension of his scientism. For all its incongruence with the industrializing, urbanizing and increasingly pluralistic society of striving individuals that it was being foisted upon, the "emperor-centered historical view" of the family-state orthodoxy provided answers concerning ultimate values and national destiny. It was on this basis that it resonated with the communitarian proclivities of a nation whose members had overwhelmingly been raised in rural villages within extended family networks. *Kokutairon*, in other words, readily made available a temporal vision according to which these traditional arrangements could be preserved, even if its reactionary formula froze social relations in an unchanging past. Oka realized that he would need to match the orthodoxy in the business of cosmological construction—even if doing so would mean appealing to the nonrational and nonscientific predisposition that sacralized nomoi as manifestations of an overarching ontological order. Without saying so explicitly, his generative scientism and its temporal organicism would attempt to commandeer the deep communitarian meanings, the pretheoretical nomic disposition, by its own scientistic superstition: the grand palingenetic narrative of rise and fall, degeneration and regeneration, death and rebirth derived from evolutionary morphology.

The unexpected immovability of this deep nomic stratum where meanings reside explains why Oka was inspired to not just match superstition for superstition with his scientism, but envision a eugenic renewal of the *minzoku*. A thorough and comprehensive reconstitution of the nation-state in accordance with the historicist schema of corporatist biology: with this palingenetic move Oka's scientism takes on the features of what Griffin calls programmatic modernism. Remaking nomos as instinct, Oka came to see, would not occur solely on the basis of Lamarckian reform, which depended on an educated *minzoku* rationally comprehending the organicist structure of a hygienic nation and then acting in an altruistic manner that built up the human-way. The apparent success of state Shinto and *kokutairon* throughout society and, particularly, within the educational system in the late Meiji era illustrated that this rational appeal was insufficient. While he never abandoned Lamarckism, as we saw in Chapter 6, his theory of degeneration and his espousal of racial improvement show that Oka came to realize that remaking nomic instincts, preserving and regenerating the concrete body of the superorganism, would require a programmatic transformation of the very fiber of ethic nation. The palingenetic retrieval of a healthier, more cohesive past, the hygienic engineering of a future-ready, technologically adept body politic, and the affirmation of a developmental cosmology that evolved toward the reintegration of differentiated "individual" parts of this national body into a higher, organic unity—Oka's *shinkaron* sought to outmatch the Shintoist ontology and overcome nomic resistance to scientistic conversion via a closely-knit combination of these elements. Both anomic individualism and reactionary superstition would be superseded by an activist scientistic faith. As embodied in the national superorganism, Oka's generative scientism would posit the values and imagine the initiatives by which anomy would be overcome and concrete relations of a healthy *minzoku* would be regenerated.

While Oka explicitly rejects the revolutionary radicalism of the left, whether anarchist or socialist, this generative vision, despite its metapolitical origins, begins to contemplate a far more invasive and extreme reconstitution of the sociopolitical order. Regenerating the national body would mean understanding, utilizing, and adhering to the law-driven cosmic process of epigenetic development that decided the destiny of nation-states. Knowledge of this process would provide the "transparency of the real" required to eugenically engineer the nomic instincts needed to combat anomy. Simultaneously and more radically, evolutionary biology would supply the values that would guide and measure this regeneration. Despite Oka's abhorrence of state Shintoism in the schools, such generative scientism, like its more tepid reformist antecedent, did not seek to overthrow the political order. Instead it intended to resituate it within an historical-developmental schema that would act as the final arbitrator of meaning, value and purpose.

Yet for all its moderate intent this generative approach set a precedent that would have radicalizing ramifications. Though presented as straightforward science promotion, his immensely popular *shinkaron* was, with its theory of decadence, introducing a scientistic variety of programmatic modernism that would exert a subtle impact across the spectrum of Japanese life—and not least of all on the orthodoxy. Unlike Hozumi's family state, which hoped to reverse the decadence of the present by rejecting change and returning to the social past, Oka's return was, in the spirit of Haeckel's recapitulation-ism, a calculated palingenetic move of totalistic transformation: returning for him meant curing the fevers of modern life by beginning again from an earlier, healthier moment in the process of growth and replaying modern life without its maladies. As we have seen, chief among these maladies was in-dividualism which Oka, like many of his contemporaries, identified with an anomic egoism. Regrowing or regenerating the nation entailed, at its most basic level, eugenically refashioning differentiated and self-interested indi-viduals in a manner that reintegrated them back into the body politic and thereby reversed decline: social or, as we have dubbed them, nomic instincts would repair the consanguineous bonds that the conditions of degenerate modern existence had frayed. The nation-state would be technologically re-generated to a youthful, cohesive stage of the life cycle and grow into the fully differentiated state of modern existence in a healthy integrated manner. Through a program of racial improvement the palingenetic process of evolu-tion would overcome anomy and not only restore the organic nation but di-rect it toward a prosperous and hygienic future. An alternative modern mode of life, healthy and technologically proactive, would thereby be assured.

The absence of any such scientifically based, future orientation in Hozu-mi's orthodoxy left it open to challenge from programmatic visions such as Oka's. As Walter Skya argues, this orthodoxy, despite its success in the ed-ucation system and in reorganizing local shrines, faced a crisis in the 1910s and 1920s because its merely reactionary character rendered it incongru-ent with the experiences of the *kokumin*. In Chapter 5 we described how the mass mobilization of the Russo-Japanese War and the conditions of inten-sified urbanization and industrialization in its aftermath resulted in an ex-pectation of inclusion and participation on the part of imperial subjects. According to Skya and other scholars, the Hibiya Riot of 1905 signaled the emergence of "a nascent form of subjective freedom"[18] among the population that would doom Hozumi's family-state absolutism. The newly awakened masses would no longer submit to treatment as children of a coercively all-powerful paterfamilias, but require a political order that was relevant to their needs and solicitous of their support. In Skya's account, Hozumi's two most innovative and influential protégés at Tokyo University, Uesugi Shinkichi (1878–1929) and Kakehi Katsuhiko (1872–1961), worried that democracy and socialism were meeting this requirement and, in order that Hozumi's "Shinto ultranationalism" not be rendered obsolete, they set about transforming it into a program that aggressively co-opted the potentially subversive subjectivity of the masses. In Uesugi's case, "separation between the emperor and the individual" was "closed theoretically" so that "the emperor invaded the essence of one's very being, becoming the individual."[19] Having "totally internalized the emperor"[20] and established a "real relationship," subjects would work to "actively assist imperial rule" not out of self-interest or fear of retribution but as an apparently spontaneous enactment of "moral duty."[21] Similarly, in Kakehi's rendering "subjects cast aside their individual selves and 'enter into the emperor [*tennō no naka ni haite iru*].'"[22] With the widespread recognition that "one's life from the beginning was never one's own ... it came from the emperor," "a total identity between the individual and the collectively subsumed in the emperor"[23] is realized. As with Uesugi, the imperial subject becomes a willing extension of the imperial will: one assists the emperor and comes to "obey the will of the state voluntarily based on one's own sincere desires and one's own conscience."[24]

In neither of these versions of radical Shinto ultranationalism, however, does the account simply end with the total fusion of the emperor and imperial subjects. Instead both Uesugi and Kakehi extend this intimate, concrete relation to the nation-state as a whole and end up with political visions of a complete merging of society and state—visions that are both developmen-

---

18 Skya, *Japan's Holy War*, 156.
19 Ibid., 183–84.
20 Ibid., 183.
21 Ibid., 172.
22 Ibid., 195.
23 Ibid., 196.
24 Ibid., 195.

tal and organicist. What is particularly striking in light of this study is that these organicist visions not only arrived at renderings of a biologically homogeneous national body (*kokutai*) remarkably similar to Oka's superorganism, but they do so by emphatically rejecting "social Darwinism" on much the same terms as Oka did. Replacing politics with a correct nomic disposition, they hope to overcome internal division and struggle with a future rejuvenation of the organic unity that decadent individualism has interrupted.

This common logic is most stark in Uesugi who portrayed social Darwinism as the basis of a theory of "mechanistic organization" [*kikaiteki soshiki*] in which the individual is "a self-sufficient and complete entity in itself."[25] Evinced in the liberalism, laissez-faire capitalism and socialism of the contemporary West, this atomistic understanding of the individual assumed "conflict was at the basis of society" and was "the source of aggressive selfishness and vanity" epitomized by "personal advantage seeking at the expense of the state at large."[26] Believing that "social conflict was artificial, while social harmony was the natural condition of man,"[27] Uesugi imagined a political order in which "all people constituted one body" and "no one in society had any advantage over another."[28] This national body was an "ethnic nation-state [*minzoku kokka*]"[29] which, according to Skya, Uesugi envisioned as a "developing natural organism."[30] For Uesugi "man is a statist animal"[31] and "states were like organisms that developed and responded to laws of organic functional relationships between parts and wholes."[32] The fundamental law of development was that members of the *minzoku* were part of an organic "being as a totality" that provided a "spatial-temporal matrix" within which a mutually interdependent society would realize its "essential being [*honsei*]"[33]—the *völkisch* state.

For Kakehi, as well, the organicist collectivism of the *völkisch* state provided not only a response to laissez-faire social Darwinism, but a dynamic, future-oriented rendering of the *kokutai* more congruent with modern sen-

---

25 Ibid., 169.
26 Ibid.
27 Ibid., 170.
28 Ibid., 171.
29 Ibid., 173.
30 Ibid., 174.
31 Ibid., 167.
32 Ibid., 168.
33 Ibid., 166–67.

sibilities than Hozumi's reactionary Shinto ultranationalism. Proceeding from a Shinto fundamentalist perspective, Kakehi rejects Darwinism on what seem to be creationist grounds: "A dog is a dog; a monkey is a monkey; the descendent of the *kami* is a *kami*," he lectured before a provincial audience in 1915. "We here today are descendants of the *kami*. Our ancestors are not monkeys or pheasants. Our ancestors are humans—that is, gods—of the Age of the Gods."[34] Correspondingly, Kakehi attributed the problems of the modern world to rulers "who thought in Darwinist terms—that is, as struggle for existence."[35] Yet, somewhat paradoxically, Kakehi's own alternative to "Darwinism" was a conception of life as an existential struggle between organicist "universal selves" [*fuhenga*].[36] He regarded history as a contest between the most prominent of these universal selves, ethnic states which identified as examples of "great life" [*daiseimei*],[37] "a higher type among the categories of organic entities"[38]—"a kind of great ecological-biological system."[39] Kakehi argued that within the "universal great life"[40] of such corporate states individuals are physiologically joined to fellow imperial subjects, including their ancestors, as an extension of an organic-historical "life process"[41]: "[T]he self as a body is linked with other bodies within this environmental system, much like a large ecological system. It is in such a sense that the universal self may be considered the same body."[42] For Kakehi the Japanese state was founded on this organicist basis, a unique quality of the *kokutai* which he captured in the slogan "one heart, same body [*isshin dōtai*]."[43] Born from and residing within the emperor—whose body Kakehi regarded as equivalent to that of the state—the constituent cells of the historically developing "great life" of the state automatically followed the dictates of the imperial will without the need for coercion. Individuals were bereft of self-interest, identifying completely and instinctually with the higher individuality of the ethnic nation-state.

---

34 Ibid., 206.
35 Ibid.
36 Ibid., 198, 206.
37 Ibid., 198.
38 Ibid., 206.
39 Ibid., 200.
40 Ibid., 198.
41 Ibid., 199.
42 Ibid., 200.
43 Ibid., 192.

Skya argues that Uesugi and Kakehi's success in transforming Hozumi's absolutism to render it personally and politically relevant to the awakened modern masses can be seen in how their state theories proliferated after the First World War and lent ideological unity to politically fractured ultranationalist movement. In his account, it was their political religion of radical Shinto ultranationalism that animated both the Imperial Way and Control Factions in the 1930s and propelled Japan toward a "holy war" against decadent individualism in the 1940s. However, as we have just seen, the abundant use of concepts from corporatist evolutionism by both ideologues suggests that they were also keenly aware of the "incongruence" between Hozumi's backward-looking orthodoxy and what was more and more recognized as the ineluctable source of national power and historical change: modern science and technology. Threatened by the disembedding propensities of laissez-faire social Darwinism and the ideologies it apparently supported in the contemporary West, they seem to have relied on the organicist Darwinism—introduced to Japan by Katō and popularly disseminated by Oka—in order to reconcile their religious-political formulations with the inescapable progress of scientific knowledge. To become modern and relevant, Shinto ultranationalism had to describe a developmental trajectory wherein the nation-state recovered its original cohesion through a future natural process of growth. Whether conceived as Uesugi's spatial-temporal "being in totality" or Kakehi's "great universal life," the new orthodoxy would achieve an accommodation with science by intimating that the *kokutai* was akin to a superorganism.

As Skya himself shows in *Japan's Holy War*, such accommodation was the implicit aim of the *Kokutai no Hongi*, the "state religious document" that turned the radical Shinto ultranationalism of Uesugi and Kakehi into an official orthodoxy. According to Skya, this text points ahead to the "holy war" of the 1940s by making the eradication of anomic individualism into the sacred mission of the Japanese ethnic nation. Domestically, this eradication would entail imperial subjects "dying to the self and returning to the one [*botsuga kiitsu*]"—that is, "casting aside of our little selves"[44] and being absorbed completely into the harmonious "totalitarian structure"[45] of the

---

44   Ibid., 268.
45   Ibid., 278.

emperor-centered *kokutai*. Abroad the mission would require enforcing a "self-effacing totalitarian spirit"[46] by expunging Western individualism and the abstract political theories which based themselves upon it. Though Skya portrays this organicist hostility to individualism in the *Kokutai no Hongi* as the culmination of what he calls the "Japanese disenlightenment,"[47] it is evident from his own analysis that this sacred mission also entailed a reconciliation between orthodoxy and the modern science. The mission set before Japanese is, in other words, not just to expand the totalitarian spirit of primordial Japan over the planet but to "create a new Japanese culture by assimilating and sublimating foreign cultures which are the source of the various problems in keeping with the fundamental principles of our *kokutai*."[48] Such assimilation and sublimation constituted, according to the compilers of the *Kokutai no Hongi*, the signature historical achievement of the Japanese ethnic nation since its divine inception. Entire chapters of the *Kokutai no Hongi* were, in fact, dedicated to describing how foreign ideologies and intellectual systems such as Buddhism and Confucianism had been appropriated in a manner that successfully enhanced the imperial Way of Japan. "Sanitized and stripped of all concepts of universality,"[49] they had been used to bolster the unique *kokutai*. The problem with the contemporary West was that its contribution to the enhancement of imperial rule had not yet been adequately digested. In particular, the individualistic elements of the modern West still needed weeding out. Once this occurred, the text intimated, institutions and intellectual systems, such as modern science, could be assimilated and sublimated in harmony with the *kokutai*.

Perhaps the most telling indicator that such assimilation was being attempted is the six-volume, 3,127-page report, *An Investigation of Global Policy with the Yamato Race as Nucleus*, that John Dower discusses in his *War without Mercy*. Published in July 1943 by the biomedically trained bureaucrats of the Ministry of Health and Welfare, this "practical guide for policy makers and administrators"[50] in Japan's newly expanded empire sought not only to amalgamate, in the spirit of the *Kokutai no Hongi*, "Japanism" (*Nipponshugi*) by combining "purified Orientalism" and "the merits of Western

---

46 Ibid.
47 Ibid., 262.
48 Ibid., 275.
49 Ibid., 274.
50 Dower, *War without Mercy*, 263.

Civilization"[51] but ventured to do so, as the title of the report betrays, largely by finding organicist equivalents for the central features of family state orthodoxy. Dower especially emphasizes how the report, in applying the familialist notion of "proper place" to the empire, equated it to the division of labor—a term familiar to Ministry of Health and Welfare administrators from the disciplines of embryology and cell biology and that spoke to the epigenetic process whereby organic wholes differentiated and reintegrated as described in Chapters 2 and 3. Thus, the *minzoku kyōdōtai*—"the collectivity of peoples" or "racial cooperative body"[52]—that comprised the Greater East Asia Co-Prosperity Sphere cohered through an "organic" morality: the specialized "qualities" and "abilities," the national characteristics, of Asian nations were not to serve their own interests but instead were to fulfill "tasks, chores, and responsibilities"[53] that redounded to the well-being of the greater body of the entire empire. The family state of the Yamato *minzoku* that formed the "nucleus" of this quasi-biological entity was itself an emanation of genealogical-evolutionary processes: the "line of emperors unbroken for ages eternal" became a "main line" or "main race" that, through a "process of natural selection and assimilation" managed to absorb "the other racial states into a single 'enduring structure'" to produce a "uniform racial state."[54] Though the report admitted the resulting "organic community" encompassed "a fluid conjunction of blood, culture, history, and political form,"[55] it was, in the end, blood that mattered most—"blood told."[56] As "natural and spiritual communities which shared a common destiny" that was the extension of "a shared genetic and historical base," the Yamato *minzoku* depended on "a common genetic heritage" to forge the nomic "bonds of spiritual consciousness and cultural identity that were so crucial to the survival of the collectivity."[57] Only a national community founded on such blood unity could achieve enduring stability.

Like Oka, the Health and Welfare officials who wrote this report were worried that the conditions of modern life were threatening this natural or-

---

51 Ibid., 279.
52 Ibid.
53 Ibid.
54 Ibid., 269.
55 Ibid., 266.
56 Ibid., 268.
57 Ibid.

ganic collective of the nation with decline. While liberal individualism and urbanization were causing a downturn in the birth rate, the misguided focus of the medical profession on illness and infirmity was weakening the racial stock. As Dower points out, the Ministry of Health and Welfare had helped enact a National Eugenics Law[58] in 1940, and the report called for further "improvement in eugenic programs" that would promote "such methods as mental and physical training as well as selective marriage."[59] The ultimate means of attaining the "regeneration"[60] of the ethnic nation was the pursuit of imperium itself. Because "overseas expansion and colonization usually involves the most energetic and dynamic members of a population" the construction of the Greater East Asia Co-Prosperity Sphere would advance the "social evolution" and "racial development" of the Japanese *minzoku.*[61] And, as implied by Oka's evolutionary realpolitik, the failure to prepare for and pursue an outward trajectory would end growth, destroy cohesion and usher in decline.

While Dower continually links this report, with its frequent allusions to embryonic development, to contemporary national socialist ideas, a more direct and likely source is the corporate evolutionism that Oka and many of the officials in the Ministry of Health and Welfare had learned as part of their training. The failure to discern this connection is partly due to a lack of awareness of the rich and suggestive organicist *Weltanschauung* that informed Japanese *shinkaron*—a lack that this study is intended to begin addressing. However, an equally important factor has been the tendency to view *kokutairon* as constructed out of myths—deliberate fictions that were imposed on the population. Whether the feudal "emperor system" (*tennosei*) of highly influential Marxist scholars, the out-of-date yet often recycled modern myths that Gluck describes, or the totalitarian political religion of Skya's radical Shinto ultranationalists, devised to appeal to the awakened masses of the modern world, this treatment of ideology tends to block inroads from science. As a consequence, in a text such as *Tennosei to Shinkaron*, the author begins his discussion by underscoring that evolutionary science contains little ideological content and is inherently resistant to contributing to the for-

---

58 Ibid., 269.
59 Ibid., 270.
60 Ibid., 272.
61 Ibid.

mation of orthodoxy. To highlight the incompatibility of science and orthodoxy and the inevitable triumph of *shinkaron* over *kokutairon*, Migita's book
ends with a discussion of a 1947 *Life* magazine photograph of the now "human emperor" alongside busts of Abraham Lincoln and Charles Darwin.
Having renounced his divinity, the emperor, Migita suggests, was eager to
be seen embracing the inexorable body of scientific truth that the system of
orthodoxy concocted in his name had renounced and suppressed.

Migita's reluctance to recognize any sort of accommodation between
tennosei orthodoxy and biological science is especially curious: his own presentation not only provides ample evidence that such an accommodation
was attempted but points directly to a connection between Emperor Hirohito and the figure at the center of this study, Oka Asajirō. Migita, in fact
opens the final section of his *Tennosei to Shinkaron* with the quote from the
beginning of this epilogue which he attributes to Hirohito from around the
period of the Minobe Affair in 1935: "A time that tries to suppress and bypass science with ideological beliefs will be retarded in the progress of the
world. We have no choice but to be enveloped by things like the theory of
evolution."[62] Later, in the closing pages of his book, he cites Hirohito again,
this time from his diary: "there is from the beginning a need to believe in
an ideology. In the end I think that science and ideology must go together
in parallel fashion."[63] According to Migita, the Showa emperor's recognition of this imperative to align ideology with the ineluctable truths of evolution derives from the 1913 *Chūō Kōron* essay, that, as we saw in Chapter 6,
Oka published in the wake of the textbook committee's exclusion of evolutionary biology from its official readers. Entitled "Bite of the Sleeping Dog,"
this New Year's essay included, in the words of Fukuhara Rintarō, a "boldly
irreverent"[64] yet indirect attack on Shinto ultranationalism, warning that
a regime that enforces faith and squashes inquiry into natural phenomena
will miss out on the progress of ideas and find itself fatally handicapped in
competition with other nations. "In the end," Oka despairs, "going against
nations on all four sides that enthusiastically develop [scientifically], our nation alone has fallen behind to the extent that it cannot catch up."[65]

---

62 Migita, *Tennosei to Shinkaron*, 152.
63 Ibid., 213.
64 Ibid., 114.
65 Ibid., 112.

In Migita's account, Hirohito's enthusiasm for biology and the writings of its main popularizer, Oka, went together with widespread endorsement within the military, the ministries of state and society at large after the First World War of the reasoning lent expression in "Bite of the Sleeping Dog." New market opportunities, the growth of heavy and light industry, and, above all, the realities of total war convinced many in positions of authority of the need to nurture and passionately promote science. As a result, forty research institutes were created in Japan between 1919 and 1931, the number of science and technology courses offered in government sponsored higher education doubled from 1919 to 1925, and a marine biological investigation facility, the Straits Seaside Research Station, was established in 1922.[66] Though the editions of the nationally authorized school textbooks issued in 1918 and 1922 by the Ministry of Education still lacked any mention of evolution,[67] a "moment of conversion," according to Migita, occurred in 1923 when the official *Ordinary Elementary School National Language Reader* included a chapter celebrating Darwin.[68] Citing private magazines that advised teachers how to present this Darwin chapter to students, Migita says that it is obvious that school instructors used the occasion afforded by this chapter to elaborate fully on evolutionary theory in the classroom. Thus, despite his having quit the Ministry Education's textbook committee after the 1918 edition failed once again to mention evolution, "Oka's dream," as Migita calls it, of evolutionary science in schools was largely realized in the 1920s.

To reinforce its new found support for science, the government made use of Hirohito's interest in marine biology to vigorously promote an image of "the emperor as biologist"[69] to the general public. The young prince had been steered toward this avocation by Saionji Kinmochi, the last remaining *genrō*, and Admiral Tōgō Heihachirō, president of the Crown Prince's study center, who were worried that his earlier enthusiasm for historical studies "will become a seed for trouble" in the future.[70] By 1921 Hirohito was involved in research under his biology teacher Hattori Hirotarō and in 1925 he had a research lab constructed for himself at the Akasaka Detached Palace, a facility which was eventually relocated to the grounds of the Imperial

---

66 Ibid., 203–5.
67 Ibid., 118.
68 Ibid., 118–20.
69 Ibid., 152.
70 Ibid., 161–62.

Palace after he became emperor a year later. As early as 1921 government or-chestrated media reports began to appear concerning Hirohito's interest in marine biology.[71] In the coming years more and more magazine and news-paper articles were printed celebrating his "superiority as a biologist" and his "assiduous manner of doing research."[72] Claims were made that he had discovered new types of organisms, such as a novel variety of bacteria, and photos were displayed showing the emperor behind a microscope or posing before the Straits Biological Research Center.[73]

The culmination of these deliberate efforts to broadcast the image of the "biologist emperor" were a series of media events staged in conjunction with the emperor's research expeditions to various locales around the country. Spanning the decade roughly from Hirohito's enthronement to the Febru-ary 26 Incident (1936), these research excursions involved the close coor-dination of state ministers, local bureaucrats, and major metropolitan me-dia outlets. In some cases as many as fifty special correspondents covered these events and not only did headlines run as long as three weeks for a single expedition, but in certain instances the imperial research activities were filmed by newspaper companies and shown across the country in the-aters and at special outdoor screenings.[74] Because imperial expeditions of-ten doubled as military inspection tours, the military lent an enthusiastic hand, with the navy placing destroyers, battleships and torpedo boats, all equipped with research laboratory facilities, at the emperor's disposal, and even building and operating a special vessel for his collecting.[75] Not to be outdone, the army, at one point, helped to rig a mass search lamp to the sea bottom to facilitate these imperial investigations in marine biology.[76]

Though the emperor's collecting activities disappeared from the head-lines after the Marco Polo Bridge Incident in 1937, this was a response to critics, including both the May 15 and February 26 insurrectionists, who felt these expeditions were distracting and thwarting the imperial will in a time of war. It did not—Migita is emphatic—represent a turn against science.[77]

---

71   Ibid., 164–66.
72   Ibid., 173.
73   Ibid., 166–70.
74   Ibid., 178–92.
75   Ibid., 192–93.
76   Ibid., 194–96.
77   Ibid., 207–10.

The emperor, in fact, continued to pursue research into marine biology and go on investigative trips until the end of the war. He also publically granted awards to natural scientists and sponsored special New Year's lectures based on their works. Not only did the military-controlled press preserve the emperor's identity as a biologist, playing up his connection with scientists, but even Kihira Masami, a radical Shinto ultranationalist who attacked evolutionism from his high position at the "Spiritual Research Institute," praised the emperor for exercising his will based on his scientific research acumen.[78]

This persistence of the "emperor as biologist" image even after his research activities were concealed from the public was no doubt connected to what Migita calls "the sweeping over of eugenic thought and the theory of evolution"[79] in the Ministry of Education from the mid-1930s onward. As Fujino Yutaka has shown, the army, concerned about population decrease, the spread of diseases such as tuberculosis, and signs of a physical weakening of the *minzoku*, began to push for sterilization laws and other biomedical measures to counter these trends. Not only did these efforts culminate in the "People's Hereditary Law of 1940" but it led to attempts to spread eugenic thinking among the populace under the banner of "healthy people, healthy army."[80] Because eugenics was understood as a manifestation of evolutionary theory, the inspector general of education began to expand the teaching of evolution in the schools. This appears to have begun at the youth schools (*seinen gakkō*) that the Ministry of Education and the Army set up in the mid-1930s for laboring young men with an elementary school education in order to provide them with practical knowledge and introduce them to military training methods. Becoming compulsory in 1939 and enrolling three million students by 1943, such schools started to include lessons on evolution in 1938.[81] A similar trend was seen in middle schools and girl's high schools with syllabi during the Pacific War featuring lessons on the "Physique of the People" and "People's Eugenics."[82]

Migita is quick to underscore that this promotion of eugenics and evolutionary theory ran counter to efforts by fundamentalists within the Ministry of Education, such as Kihira, who laid plans to eradicate evolution from edu-

78 Ibid., 211–13.
79 Ibid., 136.
80 Ibid., 137.
81 Ibid., 136.
82 Ibid., 138.

cation. By 1938, even as eugenic thought was sweeping through other parts of the Ministry of Education, radical Shinto ultranationalists in Kihira's "People's Spiritual and Cultural Research Institute" had managed to get the Darwin chapter removed from elementary school readers and during the Pacific War inserted lessons into middle and high school textbooks that encouraged students to question whether evolution was something that really occurred in organisms.[83] According to Migita a state of confusion gripped the Ministry of Education and, by implication, Japanese society during the Second World War concerning evolutionary theory: while, especially in the wake of the Nomohan Incident that exposed Japan's technological inferiority,[84] rational planners from the army were pushing for eugenics education based on evolution, fundamentalists, possessed by the kind of "*kokutai* supremacism" that Skya dubs radical Shinto ultranationalism, schemed to eradicate evolutionism in the name of "clarifying the people's spiritual culture."[85]

This confusion stems, in Migita's view, from the basic irreconcilability of evolutionary science and Shintoist fundamentalism. Yet, as we have just seen, Kihira himself celebrated the emperor's research activities, and it is clear from Migita's own presentation that what concerned Kihira and the People's Spiritual and Cultural Research Institute was the "misuse of the natural science viewpoint."[86] Their fear was that according natural science the status of ultimate truth would open the floodgates of Marxism. Kihira's writings consistently attacked the scientific standing of evolutionary theory, calling it a fixation of intellectuals that was not verified by scientific observation.[87] While this sometimes goaded him to the point of seeming to reject evolution itself for its materialist and, therefore, universalist presumptions, the goal of Kihira and other radical Shinto ultranationalists was to subsume the contributions of the biological sciences to *kokutairon*. Kihira, after all, was one of the main compilers of the *Kokutai no Hongi*, the political catechism that, as we have just explained, sought to assimilate and sublimate the products of the Western enlightenment to Japan's unique national body (*kokutai*).[88]

---

83   Ibid., 133–35.
84   Ibid., 139.
85   Ibid., 125–26.
86   Ibid., 125.
87   Ibid., 129.
88   Skya, *Japan's Holy War*, 280.

Instead of the grudging "coexistence"[89] and self-contradictory "dualist thought" that Migita insists was adopted by not only the Ministry of Education but the entire "ruling class," the relationship between *shinkaron* and *kokutairon* can be better described as an unfinished synthesis. Migita's claim that there was "no overlap"[90] between *kokutai* orthodoxy and the "very dangerous knowledge"[91] made available by evolutionary theory has been completely undermined by our analysis of *Evolution and Human Life*, the seminal sociopolitical offering of early-twentieth-century Japan's premiere popularizer of evolutionary theory. As we have seen again and again, there was plenty in Oka's *shinkaron* that was ripe for assimilation, if not sublimation, to *kokutairon*, even despite its championing the common ancestry of human beings and the rest of living nature. From the very beginning Oka's metapolitics spoke in a modern idiom to the central concern of *kokutairon* orthodoxy: what Migita calls the "horizontal integration"[92] of the nation—or, in other words, the concern for social cohesion that Carol Gluck identifies as the impetus for ideological construction in the Meiji period. Oka's human-way matched the orthodoxy with regard to its main imperatives: it "denatured" politics by reducing conduct to altruistic nomic instincts; it rejected anomic laissez-faire social Darwinism in favor of a harmonious, organic community; it celebrated the concrete consanguineous bonds of the nation by likening the *minzoku* to superorganisms found in nature; and it emphasized totalistic national mobilization to meet outside threats by switching the level of evolutionary competition to the higher individuality of the nation-state and making the organic unity of such a supreme biological entity the prerequisite for national survival. On top of offering an evolutionary realpolitik that would have inherent appeal to military planners, it rendered the consanguineous nomos "natural" in the most literal and modern sense of the term. In short, Oka's organicist "consummate group" answered Hozumi's family-state on all its essentials.

Yet it is in how Oka's *shinkaron* moved beyond this common basis with Hozumi's original version of the orthodoxy that it, perhaps, wielded its greatest influence—for in doing so it anticipated the transformation that Shinto ultranationalism would have to undergo to remain congruent with

---

89 Migita, *Tennosei to Shinkaron*, 19.
90 Ibid., 14.
91 Ibid.
92 Ibid., 18.

modern experience and relevant to members of the ethnic nation. The temporal organicist logic of Oka's theory of decadence, as set down in "The Future of Humankind," not only prefigured but, in all likelihood, helped shape, as we have suggested above, the quasi-biological organicism of both Uesugi's "being as a totality" and Kakehi's "great life"—a universal self in which the nation as an individual beat with a single heart. As we have seen, these ideologists of radical Shinto ultranationalism were preoccupied with evolutionary theory at a time when Oka's writings were the main source of knowledge about biological science in Japanese society. Most crucially, by 1910 his *shinkaron* had come to constitute a form of programmatic modernism: it offered a vision of overcoming the anomic and degenerate individualism of the present by regenerating primordial cohesion to create a new national body whose constituent members were instinctively self-coordinating. Given the wide currency of Oka's vision and the programmatic modernist tendencies of radical Shinto ultranationalism the question arises: to what extent were ideological formulations such as "dying to the self and returning to the one" and "global policy with Yamato race as nucleus" the result of efforts to sublimate the contributions of Oka and other biologists who had been envisioning the future eugenic rejuvenation of an anomic nation?

A place where such an inquiry might begin is with the Showa emperor himself who, as we have seen, drew directly on Oka's most "boldly irreverent" essay in the midst of the 1935 crisis about his own station in the constitutional order and used it to argue for the need to coordinate ideology and evolutionary truth. As Migita explains, the relationship with Oka most likely extended far beyond the living god's close familiarity with the famous zoologist's popular writings. There existed profound ties between the two based on their common interest in marine biology. Oka, in fact, made a number of public statements at the monthly meetings of the Japan Academy thanking the emperor for having been providing him accesses to the imperial collection of marine specimens. Both Oka and the emperor did research into sea squirts and it was during the same year that we can confirm that the two of them were seen in public together—at the 1931 anniversary commemoration of the Tokyo Higher Normal School, from which Oka had retired two years earlier—that Oka helped organize and publish materials on the emperor's sea squirt investigations. The "Sagami Bay Sea Squirt Chart" that the emperor published in 1953 as part of the campaign to reassert his public identity as a biologist included an acknowledgement that Oka, who had passed away in 1944, participated in its creation. Migita strongly suggests that Oka and the emperor had been collaborating behind the scenes from the late 1920s onward, working on the same scientific questions and even sharing a similar worldview.

This intellectual intimacy between the Showa emperor and Japan's early-twentieth-century spokesman for evolutionary biology encapsulates what is perhaps the central dilemma of Japanese prewar and wartime ideology: how the "living god"—and, by extension, his divine nation—could also practice secular science? Oka's *shinkaron* attempted to put forth solutions to this dilemma not by compromising the "spirit of science" or endorsing "superstition," but by addressing the same concerns about national unity that had motivated the elaboration of Shinto ultranationalism into an orthodoxy. The organicism of evolutionary morphology enabled Oka, in his initial "metapolitical" stage, to depict the nation as a superorganism permanently mobilized by the nomic instincts of the human-way to survive the evolutionary realpolitik of the international arena. When the war hysteria that had motivated this vision of total war faded and a new seemingly anomic milieu of self-interested individuals manifested itself, Oka adjusted his *shinkaron* to answer ideologists who began to aggressively promote state Shintoism as a means to lend ontological permanence to the family-like national community for which they longed. By emphasizing the temporal aspects of organicism as a life-cycle process of differentiation and reintegration, Oka meant to provide an alternate escape from postwar anomy: the decadence of the individualistic socioeconomic order after the Russo-Japanese War could be overcome by regenerating the health and instinctual cohesion of the past.

Whether or not Shinto ultranationalists were provoked by Oka's "programmatic modernist" evolutionism, it is certainly this progressive vision that appealed to the "evolutionist"[93] living god who, perhaps more than anyone, wanted a way to synthesize the protocols of his station with the imperatives of a modern world that science so powerfully defined and described. That for Hirohito such a synthesis remained an unfinished project suggests that the complex interplay between science and ideology in early-twentieth-century Japan has not yet been adequately grasped.

93　Ibid., 152.

BIBLIOGRAPHY

Arendt, Hannah. *The Origins of Totalitarianism*. New York: Schocken, 2004.

Ariga, Nagao. *The Japanese Red Cross and the Russo-Japanese War*. London: Bradbury, Agnew, 1907.

Bartholomew, James. *The Formation of Science in Japan: Building a Research Tradition*. New Haven: Yale University Press, 1989.

Beiser, Frederick. *Hegel*. New York: Routledge, 2005.

Berger, Peter L. *The Sacred Canopy: Elements of a Sociological Theory of Religion*. New York: Anchor Books, 1990.

Bix, Herbert. *Hirohito and the Making of Modern Japan*. New York: Harper Perennial, 2001.

Bölsche, Wilhelm. *Haeckel: His Life and Work*. London: T. Fisher Unwin, 1906.

Bowler, Peter. *The Eclipse of Darwinism: Anti-Darwinian Theories in the Decades around 1900*. Baltimore: Johns Hopkins University Press, 1983.

———. *Evolution: The History of an Idea*. 3rd ed. Berkeley: University of California Press, 2003.

———. *The Non-Darwinian Revolution: Reinterpreting a Historical Myth*. Baltimore: Johns Hopkins University Press, 1988.

Boyle, John Hunter. *Modern Japan: The American Nexus*. New York: Harcourt Brace, 1993.

Braver, Lee. *Groundless Grounds: A Study of Wittgenstein and Heidegger*. Cambridge, MA: MIT Press, 2014.

Coker, Francis William. *Organismic Theories of the State: Nineteenth Century Interpretations of the State as Organism or Person*. Honolulu: University Press of the Pacific, 2002.

Coleman, William. *Biology in the Nineteenth Century: Problems of Form, Function and Transformation*. New York: Cambridge University Press, 1977.

Cumings, Bruce. "Webs with No Spiders: The Genealogy of the Developmental State." In *The Developmental State*, ed. Meredith Woo-Cumings, 61–92. Ithaca: Cornell University Press, 1999.

Davis, Winston. *The Moral and Political Naturalism of Baron Katō Hiroyuki*. Berkeley: Institute of East Asian Studies, 1996.

Dickenson, Frederick. *War and National Reinvention: Japan in the Great War, 1914–1919*. Cambridge, MA: Harvard University Press, 1999.

Di Gregori, Mario. *From Here to Eternity: Ernst Haeckel and Scientific Faith*. Gottingen: Vandenhoeck & Ruprecht, 2005.

Dorpalen, Andreas. *The World of General Haushofer: Geopolitics in Action*. New York: Ferris Printing Co., 1942.

Dower, John. *War without Mercy*. New York: Pantheon, 1986.

Driscoll, Mark. "Seeds and (Nest) Eggs of Empire: Sexology Manuals/Manual Sexology." In *Gendering Modern Japanese History*, ed. Barbara Molony, 191–224. Cambridge, MA: Harvard University Press, 2005.

Ferguson, Niall. *The War of the World: Twentieth-Century Conflict and the Descent of the West.* New York: Penguin, 2006.

Fridell, Wilbur M. "A Fresh Look at State Shinto," *Journal of the American Academy of Religion*, 44.3 (1976): 547–61.

———. "Government Ethics Textbooks in Late Meiji Japan." *Journal of Asian Studies* 29.4 (1970): 823–33.

———. "The Establishment of Shrine Shinto in Meiji Japan." *Japanese Journal of Religious Studies* 2.2–3 (1975): 137–68.

Gasman, Daniel. *The Scientific Origins of National Socialism: Social Darwinism in Ernst Haeckel and the Monist League.* London: Macdonald, 1971.

Gluck, Carol. *Japan's Modern Myths: Ideology in the Late Meiji Period.* Princeton: Princeton University Press, 1985.

Gordon, Andrew. *Labor and Imperial Democracy in Prewar Japan.* Berkeley: University of California Press, 1991.

———. *A Modern History of Japan: From Tokugawa Times to the Present.* New York: Oxford University Press, 2003.

Gould, Stephen Jay. *Ontogeny and Phylogeny.* Cambridge, MA: Harvard University Press, 1977.

Griffin, Roger. *Modernism and Fascism: The Sense of a Beginning under Mussolini and Hitler.* New York: Palgrave Macmillan, 2007.

Haeckel, Ernst. *The Evolution of Man: A Popular Exposition of the Principal Points of Human Ontogeny and Phylogeny.* New York: Appleton, 1879.

———. *The History of Creation: or the Development of the Earth and Its Inhabitants by the Action of Natural Causes. A Popular Exposition of the Doctrine of Evolution in General and That of Darwin, Goethe and Lamarck in Particular.* 2 vols. New York: D. Appleton and Co., 1876.

———. *Monism as Connecting Religion and Science: The Confession of Faith of a Man of Science.* Trans. J. Gilchrist. London: Adam and Charles Black, 1895.

———. *The Riddle of the Universe.* Buffalo: Prometheus Books, 1992.

———. *The Wonders of Life: A Popular Study of Biological Philosophy.* New York: Harper and Brothers, 1905.

Hardacre, Helen. *Shintō and the State, 1868–1988.* Princeton: Princeton University Press, 1989.

Hayashi, Makoto. "Cell Theory in Its Development and Inheritance in Meiji Japan." *Historia Scientiarum* 8.2 (1998): 115–32.

Hayek, Friedrich August. *The Counter-Revolution of Science: Studies on the Abuse of Reason.* Indianapolis: Liberty Press, 1979.

Hegel, George Wilhelm Friedrich. *Philosophy of Right.* Trans. T. M. Knox. New York: Oxford University Press, 1967.

Herman, Arthur. *The Idea of Decline in Western History.* New York: The Free Press, 1997.

Holtom, Daniel Clarence. *The Political Philosophy of Modern Shinto: A Study of the State Religion of Japan.* Chicago: University of Chicago Libraries, 1922.

Hozumi, Yatsuka. *Kokumin Kyouiku: Aikokushin* [National education: Patriotism]. Tokyo: Yuhikaku, 1897.

Ienaga, Saburo. *The Pacific War, 1931–1945.* New York: Pantheon Books, 1978.

Inoue, Tetsujirō. *Chokugo Engi* [Commentary on the rescript]. Tokyo: Keigyōsha, 1891.

———. *Kyoiku to Shūkyō no Shōtotsu* [The collision of education and religion]. Tokyo: Keigyōsha, 1893.

Irokawa, Daikichi. *The Culture of the Meiji Period*. Princeton: Princeton University Press, 1985.

Ishikawa, Chiyomatsu. "Jintai to demokurashii" [The human body and democracy]. In *Nihon kagaku gijutsushi taikei, Vol. 15*, ed. Nihon Kagakushi Gakkai. Tokyo: Daiichi Hōki Shuppan, 1967.

Johnston, William. *The Modern Epidemic: A History of Tuberculosis in Japan*. Cambridge, MA: Harvard University Asia Center, 1995.

Jordan, David K. "Filial Piety in Taiwanese Popular Thought." In *Confucianism and the Family*, ed. George A. De Vos, 267–284. Albany: State University of New York Press, 1998.

Josephson, Jason Ananda. *The Invention of Religion in Japan*. Chicago: University of Chicago Press, 2012.

Jünger, Ernst. *Copse 125: A Chronicle from Trench Warfare of 1918*. New York: Howard Fertig, 2003.

Jünger, Ernst. "Total Mobilization." in *The Heidegger Controversy: A Critical Reader*, ed. Richard Wolin, 119–139. Cambridge, MA: MIT Press, 1993.

Katō, Hiroyuki. *Katō Hiroyuki no bunsho* [Selected works of Katō Hiroyuki]. Vol. 3. Kyoto: Dōmeisha, 1990.

———. *Meisōteki Uchūkan "Waga Kokutai to Kirisuto-kyō" no Hihyō no Hihyō* [Critique of a critique: The fallacious outlook of the universe in "Our polity and Christianity"]. Tokyo: Hinoeuma Publishing, 1908.

Kim, Hoi-Eun. *Doctors of Empire: Medical and Cultural Encounters between Imperial Germany and Meiji Japan*. Toronto: University of Toronto Press, 2014.

Koestler, Arthur. *Darkness at Noon*. New York: Scribner, 2006.

Kowner, Rotem. "The War as a Turning Point in Modern Japanese History." In *The Impact of the Russo-Japanese War*, ed. Rotem Kowner, 29–46. New York: Routledge, 2007.

Kuga, Katsunan. *Katsunan Bushū*. Tokyo: 1910.

LaFeber, Walter. *The Clash: U.S.–Japan Relations throughout History*. New York: W. W. Norton & Co., 1998.

Lehmbruch, Gerhard. "The Institutional Embedding of Market Economies: The German 'Model' and Its Impact on Japan." In *The Origins of Nonliberal Capitalism: Germany and Japan in Comparison*, ed. Kozo Yamamura, 39–93. Ithaca: Cornell University Press, 2001.

Li, Dongmu. "Lu Xun and Oka Asajirō." *Journal of the Faculty of Letters Bukkyō University* 87 (2003): 63–80.

Lu, David. *Japan: A Documentary History, Vol. II*. New York: Routledge, 1997.

Maistre, Joseph de. *On God and Society: Essay on the Generative Principle of Political Constitutions and Other Human Institutions*. Ed. Elisha Greifer. Chicago: Regnery, 1959.

Martin, Bernd. *Japan and Germany in the Modern World*. Providence: Berghahn, 1995.

Maruyama, Masao. *Studies in the Intellectual History of Tokugawa Japan*. Princeton: Princeton University Press, 1974.

Matsunaga, Toshio. "Evolutionism in Early Twentieth Century Japan," *Historia Scientiarum* 11.3 (2002): 218–25.

McClain, James. *Japan: A Modern History*. New York: W. W. Norton and Co., 2002.

Migita, Hiroki. "Meijiki Chishikijin ni okeru seibutsu shinkaron no hayari saikou—jinjuu dosousetsu no inpakuto wo megutte." *Kagakusi Kenkyu* 42.225 (2003): 1-10".

———. *Tennosei to Shinkaron* [The emperor system and evolutionary theory]. Tokyo: Seikyusha, 2009.

Minear, Richard. *Japanese Tradition and Western Law: Emperor, State and Law in the Thought of Hozumi Yatsuka*. Cambridge, MA: Harvard University Press, 1970.

Nagai, Michio. "Herbert Spencer in Early Meiji Japan." *The Far Eastern Quarterly* 14 (Nov. 1954): 55–63.

Nakashima, Kosei. "Beyond the Shinto View." In *Report of the National Association of Shinto Priests* 103 (1907): 1-10.

———. "Shintoism," In *Report of the National Association of Shinto Priests* 108 (1908): 24-5.

Nishida, Kitarō. 1990. *An Inquiry into the Good.* New Haven: Yale University Press, 1990.

Nishiyama, Kaname. "Lorenz von Stein's Influence on Japan's Meiji Constitution of 1889." In *Lorenz von Steins "Bemerkungen über Verfassung und Verwaltung" von 1889 zu den Verfassungsarbeiten in Japan,* ed. Wilhelm Brauneder and Kaname Nishiyama, 39–59. Frankfurt am Main: Peter Lang, 1992.

Notehelfer, F. G. *Kōtoku Shusui: Portrait of a Japanese Radical.* Cambridge: Cambridge University Press, 1971.

Nyhart, Lynn. *Biology Takes Form: Animal Morphology and the German Universities, 1800–1900.* Chicago: University of Chicago Press, 1995.

Oda, Hidemi. "Oka Asajirō Sensei no Ōmokage." *Seibutsu Kagaku* 46.3 (1994): 113–28.

Oka, Asajirō. *Hanmon to Jiyu* [Anguish and freedom]. Tokyo: Yūseidō Shuppan, 1968.

———. "Jindō no Shōtai [The true character of humanity: the human-way]." In *Shinka to Jinsei* [Evolution and human life], 55-65. Tokyo: Yūseidō Shuppan, 1968.

———. *Jinrui no kako genzai oyobi mirai* [Past, present and future of mankind]. Tokyo: Yūseidō Shuppan, 1968.

———. "Jinrui no Seizon Kyōsō [Mankind's struggle for existence]." In *Shinka to Jinsei* [Evolution and human life], 76-84. Tokyo: Yūseidō Shuppan, 1968.

———. "Jinrui no shōrai [The future of humankind]." In *Shinka to Jinsei* [Evolution and human life], 204-232. Tokyo: Yūseidō Shuppan, 1968.

———. "Kyōiku to Meishin [Education and superstition]." In *Shinka to Jinsei* [Evolution and human life], 117-28. Tokyo: Yūseidō Shuppan, 1968.

———. "Minshu Kaizengaku no Jissai Kachi [The actual value of the study of racial improvement]." In *Shinka to Jinsei* [Evolution and human life], 196–203. Tokyo: Yūseidō Shuppan, 1968.

———. "Minzoku no Hatten to Rika [Science and the development of the race-nation]." In *Shinka to Jinsei* [Evolution and human life], 108–116. Tokyo: Yūseidō Shuppan, 1968.

———. *Oka Asajirō Shū.* Tokyo: Chikuma Shobō, 1974.

———. *Saru no Mura kara Kyowakoku made* [From monkey herd to the republic]. Tokyo: Yūseidō Shuppan, 1968.

———. "Risōteki Dantai Seikatsu [Ideal group life]." In *Shinka to Jinsei* [Evolution and human life], 66–75. Tokyo: Yūseidō Shuppan, 1968.

———. "Seibutsukai ni okeru Zen to Aku [Good and evil in the animal world]." In *Shinka to Jinsei* [Evolution and human life], 46–54. Tokyo: Yūseidō Shuppan, 1968.

———. "Sensō to Heiwa [War and peace]." In *Shinka to Jinsei* [Evolution and human life], 85–97. Tokyo: Yūseidō Shuppan, 1968.

———. "Shinkaron to Eisei [Evolutionary theory and hygiene]." In *Shinka to Jinsei* [Evolution and human life], 185–94. Tokyo: Yūseidō Shuppan, 1968.

———. *Shinkaron kōwa* [Lectures on evolutionary theory]. Tokyo: Tōkyō Kaiseikan, 1904.

Oka, Yoshitake. "Generational Conflict after the Russo-Japanese War," In *Conflict in Modern Japanese History: The Neglected Tradition,* ed. Tetsuo Najita, 197–225. Princeton: Princeton University Press, 1982.

Olsen, Richard. *Science and Scientism in Nineteenth-Century Europe.* Urbana: University of Illinois Press, 2008.

Otsubo, Sumiko. "Engendering Eugenics: Feminists and Marriage Restriction Legislation in the 1920s." In *Gendering Modern Japanese History,* ed. Barbara Molony, 225–256. Cambridge, MA: Harvard University Press, 2005.

Otsubo, Sumiko. "The Female Body and Eugenic Thought in Meiji Japan." In *Building a Modern Japan: Science, Technology, and Medicine in the Meiji Era and Beyond*, ed. Morris Low, 61-81. New York: Palgrave Macmillan, 2005.

Pittau, Joseph. *Political Thought in Early Meiji Japan, 1868-1889*. Cambridge, MA: Harvard University Press, 1967.

Popper, Karl. *The Open Society and Its Enemies, Volume 1: The Spell of Plato*. Princeton: Princeton University Press, 1971.

———. *The Open Society and Its Enemies, Volume 2: The High Tide of Prophecy: Hegel, Marx, and the Aftermath*. Princeton: Princeton University Press, 1971.

———. *The Poverty of Historicism*. New York: Routledge and Kegan Paul, 2002.

Pusey, James Reeve. *Lu Xun and Evolution*. Albany: State University of New York, 1998.

Pyle, Kenneth. "Advantages of Followership: German Economics and Japanese Bureaucrats, 1890–1925." *Journal of Japanese Studies* 1.1. (1974): 127–64.

———. *Japan Rising: The Resurgence of Japanese Power and Purpose*. New York: Public Affairs Books, 2007.

———. *The Making of Modern Japan*. 2nd ed. Lexington: D.C. Heath and Co., 1996.

———. "Meiji Conservatism." In *Modern Japanese Thought*, ed. Bob Wakabayashi, 98–146. Cambridge: Cambridge University Press, 1998.

———. *New Generation in Meiji Japan: Problems of Cultural Identity, 1885–1895*. Stanford: Stanford University Press, 1969.

———. "The Technology of Japanese Nationalism: The Local Improvement Movement, 1900–1918," *Journal of Asian Studies* 33.1 (1973): 51–65.

Richards, Robert. *The Meaning of Evolution: Morphological Construction and Ideological Reconstruction of Darwin's Theory*. Chicago: University of Chicago Press, 1992.

———. *The Romantic Conception of Life: Science and Philosophy in the Age of Goethe*. Chicago: University of Chicago Press, 2002.

———. *The Tragic Sense of Life: Ernst Haeckel and the Struggle over Evolutionary Thought*. Chicago: University of Chicago Press, 2008.

"Rinji Zōkan: Ōhaku jinshu shōtotsu." *Taiyō* 14:3 (15 February 1908).

Ryland, J. S. *Bryozoans*. London: Hutchinson, 1970.

Sanuki, Masakazu. "Kindai nihon ni okeru kyowashugi—1920 nendai no Oka Asajirō wo tsuujite." *Sokendai Bunaka Kagaku Kenkyu* 5 (March 2009): 29–68.

Sasaki, Takayuki. "Shinkaron yori mitaru Waga Teikoku" [Our empire seen by the theory of evolution], *Kokugakuin Zasshi* 7:23 (1907): 1-7.

Searle, John. *Intentionality*. Cambridge: Cambridge University Press, 1983.

Shimao, Eiko. "Darwinism in Japan, 1877–1927." *Annals of Science* 33 (1981): 93–102.

Shimazono, Susumu. "State Shinto in the Lives of the People: The Establishment of Emperor Worship, Modern Nationalism, and Shrine Shinto in Late Meiji." *Japanese Journal of Religious Studies* 36.1 (2009): 93–124.

Shimazu, Naoko. *Japanese Society at War: Death, Memory, and the Russo-Japanese War*. Cambridge: Cambridge University Press, 2009.

Silberman, Bernard S. *Cages of Reason: The Rise of the Rational State in France, Japan, the United States, and Great Britain*. Chicago: University of Chicago Press, 1993.

Skya, Walter. *Japan's Holy War: The Ideology of Radical Shintō Ultranationalism*. Durham: Duke University Press, 2009.

Takahashi, Aya. *The Development of the Japanese Nursing Profession: Adopting and Adapting Western Influences*. New York: RoutledgeCurzon, 2004.

Taylor, Charles. *Hegel*. New York: Cambridge University Press, 1975.

Todorov, Tzvetan. *Hope and Memory: Lessons from the Twentieth Century*. Princeton: Princeton University Press, 2003.

―――. *Imperfect Garden: The Legacy of Humanism*. Princeton: Princeton University Press, 2002.

Tolstoy, Leo. *"Bethink Yourselves!"* Boston: Ginn & Co., 1904.

Tsukuba, Hisaharu. *Oka Asajirō Shū*. Tokyo: Chikuma Shobo, 1974.

―――. "Kaisetsu" [Commentary], in Hisahiru Tsukuba, *Oka Asajirō Shū*. Tokyo: Chikuma Shobo, 1974, 430–63.

Turda, Marius. *Modernism and Eugenics*. New York: Palgrave Macmillan, 2010.

Von Stein, Lorenz. *The History of the Social Movement in France, 1789–1850*. Totowa: Bedminster Press, 1964.

Wakabayashi, Bob. *Anti-Foreignism and Western Learning in Early-Modern Japan: The New Theses of 1825*. Cambridge, MA: Harvard University Press, 1986.

Watanabe, Masao. *The Japanese and Western Science*. Philadelphia: University of Pennsylvania Press, 1976.

Weikart, Richard. *From Darwin to Hitler: Evolutionary Ethnics, Eugenics, and Racism in Germany*. New York: Palgrave Macmillan, 2004.

Weindling, Paul. *Health, Race and German Politics between National Unification and Nazism, 1870–1945*. New York: Cambridge, 1989.

Wells, David. "The Russo-Japanese War in Russian Literature." In *The Russo-Japanese War in Cultural Perspective, 1904–05*, ed. David Wells and Sandra Wilson, 108–133. New York: St. Martin's Press, 1999.

Wilson, Sandra. "The Russo-Japanese War and Japan." In *The Russo-Japanese War in Cultural Perspective, 1904–05*, ed. David Wells and Sandra Wilson, 160–193. New York: St. Martin's Press, 1999.

Wittgenstein, Ludwig. *On Certainty*. New York: Harper & Row, 1969.

Wray, Harold. "A Study in Contrasts: Japanese School Textbooks, 1903 and 1941–1945." *Monumenta Nipponica* 27.1 (1973): 69–85.

Yajima, Michiko. "Hilgendorf Predated Morse in Bringing Charles Darwin's Theory of Evolution to Japan." *Historia Scientiarum* 8.2 (1998): 133–40.

INDEX